Effects of Plant Extracts on Human Health

Effects of Plant Extracts on Human Health

Guest Editors

Fátima Regina Mena Barreto Silva
Diana Marcela Aragon Novoa

MDPI Basel • Beijing • Wuhan • Barcelona • Belgrade • Novi Sad • Cluj • Manchester

Guest Editors
Fátima Regina Mena Barreto Silva
Departament of Biochemistry
Federal University of Santa Catarina
Florianópolis
Brazil

Diana Marcela Aragon Novoa
Departamento de Farmácia
Universidad Nacional de Colombia
Bogotá
Colombia

Editorial Office
MDPI AG
Grosspeteranlage 5
4052 Basel, Switzerland

This is a reprint of the Special Issue, published open access by the journal *Nutrients* (ISSN 2072-6643), freely accessible at: https://www.mdpi.com/journal/nutrients/special_issues/90INO0372G.

For citation purposes, cite each article independently as indicated on the article page online and as indicated below:

Lastname, A.A.; Lastname, B.B. Article Title. *Journal Name* **Year**, *Volume Number*, Page Range.

ISBN 978-3-7258-6005-0 (Hbk)
ISBN 978-3-7258-6006-7 (PDF)
https://doi.org/10.3390/books978-3-7258-6006-7

Contents

About the Editors vii

Fátima Regina Mena Barreto Silva and Marcela Aragón Novoa
Effects of Plant Extracts on Human Health
Reprinted from: *Nutrients* **2025**, *17*, 1229, https://doi.org/10.3390/ nu17071229 1

Michał Wiciński, Anna Fajkiel-Madajczyk, Zuzanna Kurant, Sara Liss, Paweł Szyperski, Monika Szambelan, et al.
Ashwagandha's Multifaceted Effects on Human Health: Impact on Vascular Endothelium, Inflammation, Lipid Metabolism, and Cardiovascular Outcomes—A Review
Reprinted from: *Nutrients* **2024**, *16*, 2481, https://doi.org/10.3390/nu16152481 5

Dongsic Choi, Jun Gi Lee, Su-Hak Heo, Moon-Kyen Cho, Hae-Seon Nam, Sang-Han Lee and Yoon-Jin Lee
Curcumin and Its Potential to Target the Glycolytic Behavior of Lactate-Acclimated Prostate Carcinoma Cells with Docetaxel
Reprinted from: *Nutrients* **2024**, *16*, 4338, https://doi.org/10.3390/nu16244338 24

Na-Ra Han, Hi-Joon Park, Seong-Gyu Ko and Phil-Dong Moon
Tryptanthrin Down-Regulates Oncostatin M by Targeting GM-CSF-Mediated PI3K-AKT-NF-κB Axis
Reprinted from: *Nutrients* **2024**, *16*, 4109, https://doi.org/10.3390/nu16234109 42

Huda Abbasi, Maria Sharif, Peter John, Attya Bhatti, Muhammad Qasim Hayat and Qaisar Mansoor
Phytochemical, Cytoprotective Profiling, and Anti-Inflammatory Potential of *Colchicum luteum* in Rheumatoid Arthritis: An Experimental and Simulation Study
Reprinted from: *Nutrients* **2024**, *16*, 4020, https://doi.org/10.3390/nu16234020 51

Yoon-Young Sung, Seung-Hyung Kim, Won-Kyung Yang, Heung Joo Yuk, Mi-Sun Kim and Dong-Seon Kim
Lysimachia mauritiana Lam. Extract Alleviates Airway Inflammation Induced by Particulate Matter Plus Diesel Exhaust Particles in Mice
Reprinted from: *Nutrients* **2024**, *16*, 3732, https://doi.org/10.3390/nu16213732 73

Yiming Zhang, Shengying Zhu, Yueming Gu, Yanjing Feng and Bo Gao
Network Pharmacology Combined with Experimental Validation to Investigate the Mechanism of the Anti-Hyperuricemia Action of *Portulaca oleracea* Extract
Reprinted from: *Nutrients* **2024**, *16*, 3549, https://doi.org/10.3390/nu16203549 87

Maria Loreta Libero, Antonio J. Montero-Hidalgo, Lucia Recinella, Raúl M. Luque, Daniele Generali, Alessandra Acquaviva, et al.
The Protective Effects of an Aged Black Garlic Water Extract on the Prostate
Reprinted from: *Nutrients* **2024**, *16*, 3025, https://doi.org/10.3390/nu16173025 108

Isabel Rodriguez, Youn Hee Nam, Sung Woo Shin, Gyeong Jin Seo, Na Woo Kim, Wanlapa Nuankaew, et al.
Effects of *Castanopsis echinocarpa* on Sensorineural Hearing Loss via Neuronal Gene Regulation
Reprinted from: *Nutrients* **2024**, *16*, 2716, https://doi.org/10.3390/nu16162716 124

Won-Kyung Cho, Hee-Jeong Choi and Jin Yeul Ma
Selaginella tamariscina Ethanol Extract Attenuates Influenza A Virus Infection by Inhibiting Hemagglutinin and Neuraminidase
Reprinted from: *Nutrients* **2024**, *16*, 2377, https://doi.org/10.3390/nu16142377 . . . . **138**

Isabelly Teixeira Espinoça, Denise Caroline Luiz Soares Basilio, Anna Júlia Papa de Araujo, Rafael Seiji Nakano Ota, Kamylla Fernanda Souza de Souza, Nadla Soares Cassemiro, et al.
Antithrombotic Effect of Oil from the Pulp of Bocaiúva—*Acrocomia aculeata* (Jacq.) Lodd. ex Mart. (Arecaceae)
Reprinted from: *Nutrients* **2024**, *16*, 2024, https://doi.org/10.3390/nu16132024 . . . . **148**

Diana P. Rey, Sandra M. Echeverry, Ivonne H. Valderrama, Ingrid A. Rodriguez, Luis F. Ospina, Fatima Regina Mena Barreto Silva and Marcela Aragón
Antidiabetic Effect of *Passiflora ligularis* Leaves in High Fat-Diet/Streptozotocin-Induced Diabetic Mice
Reprinted from: *Nutrients* **2024**, *16*, 1669, https://doi.org/10.3390/nu16111669 . . . . **160**

About the Editors

Fátima Regina Mena Barreto Silva

Fátima Regina Mena Barreto Silva is full professor of Chemistry at the Universidade Federal de Santa Catarina in Florianópolis, Brazil and a coordinator of the "Instituto de Bioeletricidade Celular (IBIOCEL): Ciência & Saúde". She has participated in several projects related to diabetes, male fertility and cancer. Her research focus is on characterizing intracellular pathways mediated by hormones, toxicants, natural and synthetic compounds involving different programs and countries as follows: an international cooperation program with UNICAEN; an international project with the; projects for undergraduate and graduate (Master, PhD and Post-Doctoral) exchange students among UNICAEN and UFSC; and international projects in collaboration with the University of Guelph/Canada Sorbonne Universités, the University of California, Riverside; the Universidad Nacional de Colombia, Bogota; De Montfort University, Leicester, UK; the University of Coimbra; and the University of Porto. She has been a fellowship student of Japan International Cooperation Agency, Japan, a Visiting Scientist at UCR/USA and at UNICAEN, and an Invited Professor at UNICAEN/France in undergraduate and graduation Biology courses. As a researcher, she has developed studies in Pharmacy related to Pharmacognosy, Medicinal Chemistry and precision medicine. Key-words: Electrophysiology; Diagnostic strategies; Pathophysiology; Drugs development; Diabetes; Infertility; Cancer.

Diana Marcela Aragon Novoa

Diana Marcela Aragon Novoa is a pharmacist with a PhD in Pharmaceutical Science and a full professor at the National University of Colombia. She has experience in the research and development of new drug delivery systems, extract standardization, and the study of the pharmacokinetic and biopharmaceutical properties of different active pharmaceutical agents. She has supervised more than 25 Master's and PhD theses and has published more than 60 scientific papers, 10 scientific book chapters, and a book about the role of women in science. Her PhD thesis was awarded as a "Meritorious Thesis". She has been awarded for her performance as a researcher at the National University of Colombia, and has been named a senior researcher by the Ministry of Science of Colombia. She has led research projects funded by different organizations with Colombian and foreign participants and has been an invited researcher at different foreign universities. She is a member of the Ibero-American Pharmacometrics Network (RedIF) and the Organization for Women in Science for the Developing World (OWSD-Colombia).

nutrients

MDPI

Editorial

Effects of Plant Extracts on Human Health

Fátima Regina Mena Barreto Silva [1,*] and Marcela Aragón Novoa [1,2,*]

1 Instituto de Bioeletricidade Celular (IBIOCEL): Ciência & Saúde, Departamento de Bioquímica, Universidade Federal de Santa Catarina, Florianopólis 88049-900, SC, Brazil
2 Departamento de Farmacia, Universidad Nacional de Colombia, Av. Carrera 30 # 45-03 Edif 450, Bogota 111321, Colombia
* Correspondence: mena.barreto@ufsc.br (F.R.M.B.S.); dmaragonn@unal.edu.co (M.A.N.)

The extracts of plants exhibit a variety of bioactive compounds (polyphenols, carotenoids, fibers, essential oils, polysaccharides, alkaloids, and proteins), with the majority having biological effects, but their mechanisms of action are still unknown. Furthermore, in this kind of sample, the challenge is choosing between the variability of compounds in the crude extract, which exhibit activity in a selected cellular target for a specific disease of interest. This Special Issue is based on medicinal plants and explores the potential effect of their extracts and/or their compounds in specific experimental models of diseases. The effect of curcumin on hexokinase 2 was studied through cellular adaptation to lactic acidosis on intracellular energy metabolism and sensitivity to docetaxel in prostate carcinoma cells. From this set of data, it was observed that metabolic plasticity through enhanced glycolysis in lactate-acclimated prostatic cells may be one pathway for docetaxel resistance; therefore, targeting glycolysis using curcumin may provide potential for drug development and contribute to advancements in therapy for prostate cancer patients. Additionally, in an ex vivo model using C57BL/6 male mouse prostate and a prostate cancer cell line, the protective effects of aged black garlic water extract (ABGE) were evidenced; it exhibited anti-inflammatory and antioxidant effects in these preclinical models, partly attributed to catechin and garlic acid. In this ex vivo model, ABGE reduced the gene expression of COX-2, NF-κB, TNF-α, and IL-6. For in vitro studies, ABGE inhibited cell proliferation, colony and tumor sphere formation, and the cell migration of prostate cancer cells, emphasizing its potential therapeutic effects.

Different kinds of natural compounds act to inhibit inflammatory responses, such as, for example, the natural alkaloid, tryptanthrin. This compound significantly reduced the mRNA expression of oncostatin M (anti-inflammatory cytokin) in the granulocyte–macrophage, colony-stimulating factor (GM-CSF)-stimulated, neutrophil-like dHL-60 cells and inhibited the phosphorylation of phosphatidylinositol 3-kinase (PI3K), AKT, and nuclear factor (NF)-κB. In addition, tryptanthrin decreased the oncostatin M production in GM-CSF-stimulated neutrophils from mouse bone marrow. The potential anti-inflammatory effect of Colchicum luteum hydroethanolic extract (CLHE) compared with non-steroidal, anti-inflammatory drugs focused in on COX-2, and TNFα inhibition was studied in a collagen-induced arthritic mice model. Molecular docking identified that the two main non-toxic compounds possessed strong binding affinities to COX-2 and TNG-α. Therefore, as a whole, these data suggest that CLHE is a safer, anti-inflammatory, and multi-targeted alternative to NSAIDs for rheumatoid arthritis treatment. Another extract (*Lysimachia mauritiana* Lam. extract) alleviates the airway inflammation induced by particulate matter and diesel exhaust particles in mice. *Lysimachia mauritiana* alleviated the accumulation of neutrophils and the number of inflammatory cells in the lungs and the bronchoalveolar

https://doi.org/10.3390/nu17071229

lavage fluid of the mice exposed to particulate matter with a diameter of less than 10 μm, and also reduced the release of inflammatory mediators in the bronchoalveolar fluid and lungs. In addition, this extract inhibited MAPK and NF-κB signaling in the lungs. Altogether, this study indicates that this extract may be a promising therapeutic agent against inflammatory respiratory diseases.

For hyperuricemia, a metabolic disorder in the purine of the body discussed here, *Portulaca oleracea* (PO) inhibits xanthine oxidase activity through the effect of berberine and stachydrine isolated and purified from this plant and, therefore, reduces uric acid production. Furthermore, PO may reduce the body's reabsorption of urate and aid in its excretion out of the body by inhibiting the urate transporter proteins (GLUT9, URAT1) and promoting the high expression of urate excretory protein (ABCG2). The results of histology showed that, compared with the positive drug (allopurinol and benzbromarone) group, there was no obvious renal injury in the middle- and high-dose groups of PO extract. On the whole, PO represents a potential functional food for the treatment of hyperuricemia.

Another interesting point were the studies related to hearing loss. The variable etiology for sensorineural hearing loss includes noises above decibels considered bearable for the ear, ototoxic agents, and aging, which can damage the inner ear or the auditory nerve. Studies on *Castanopsis echinocarpa* explore this medicinal plant as a potential therapeutic agent for hearing loss via critical neuronal gene regulation. In addition, in vivo experiments using zebrafish and mouse revealed otic hair cell protection in zebrafish, improved auditory function, and the protection of cochlear sensory cells in a mouse model with induced hearing loss, ensuring neuron function and survival.

One of the studies published in this SI investigated whether *Selaginella tamariscina* has an antiviral effect against influenza A virus (IAV) infection. They used green fluorescent protein (GFP)-tagged influenza A virus (IAV) to examine the effect of Selaginella tamariscina ethanol extract (STE) on influenza viral infection. Fluorescence microscopy and flow cytometry showed that STE potently represses the GFP expression of the virus in a dose-dependent manner. STE significantly inhibited the expression of the IAV M2, NP, HA, NA, NS1, and PB2 proteins. Time-of-addition and hemagglutination inhibition assays showed that STE showed an inhibitory effect on hemagglutinin and viral binding on the cells at an early infection stage. In addition, STE exerted a suppressive effect on the neuraminidase activity of the H1N1 and H3N2 IAVs. Furthermore, in a dose-dependent way, STE inhibited the cytopathic effect induced by H3N2, as well as by H1N1 IAV. Especially in the presence of STE, the cytopathic effect was completely blocked. Overall, these data suggest that STE has antiviral efficacy against IAV infection; thus, it could be developed as a natural IAV inhibitor.

The study that evaluated the antithrombotic action of *Acrocomia aculeata* pulp oil (AAPO) in natura in an in vitro experimental model reported that ADP/epinephrine induced platelet aggregation after treatment with AAPO, as evaluated using turbidimetry, and that coagulation was determined by the prothrombin activity time and activated partial thromboplastin time. Promising results showed that AAPO has major components such as oleic acid, palmitic acid, lauric acid, caprylic acid, and squalene. AAPO showed no toxicity in vitro or in vivo. Platelet aggregation decreased against agonists when using treatments with different concentrations of AAPO. The oil did not interfere with the prothrombin time or the activated partial thromboplastin time. Moreover, it expressly decreased ROS-induced platelet activation and P-selectin expression. Therefore, AAPO showed antiplatelet action, given that it decreased the platelet activation verified by the decrease in P-selectin expression as well as in ROS production.

The extract from the leaves of *Passiflora ligularis* (*P. ligularis*) showed significant effects on lowering serum glucose levels; it reduced insulin resistance, preserved pancreatic tissue, contributed antioxidant effects, and ameliorated the serum lipid profile in studies carried out in adult mice. Based on this experimental approach, the extract of *P. ligularis* exhibits a potential role in the treatment of type 2 diabetes. Finally, this SI discussed the multifaceted effects of extracts from plants on human health based on *Withania somnifera*, popularly known as Ashwagandha. The wide spectrum of action of this plant stems from its observed anti-inflammatory, neuroprotective, immunomodulatory, hepatoprotective, cardioprotective, anti-diabetic, adaptogenic, anti-arthritic, anti-stress, and antimicrobial effects.

The description above summarizes the updated data related to the extracts of plants and, in some cases, highlights specific extracts/plants characterized by major compounds in different disease models, such as in the prostate cancer cell line and C57BL/6 mouse prostate, rheumatoid arthritis, respiratory diseases, hyperuricemia, hearing loss, influenza A, thrombose, and diabetes, as well as reports on the multifaceted effects of extracts on inflammation, neuroprotection, immunomodulation, hepatoprotection, cardio protection, diabetes, arthritis, stress, and microbial factors. Therefore, we invite our readers who are passionate about this area to enjoy a pleasant read.

Author Contributions: Writing—original draft, F.R.M.B.S.; revision and editing, F.R.M.B.S. and M.A.N. All authors have read and agreed to the published version of the manuscript.

Conflicts of Interest: The authors declare no conflicts of interest.

List of Contributions:

1. Choi, D.; Lee, J.G.; Heo, S.-H.; Cho, M.-K.; Nam, H.-S.; Lee, S.-H.; Lee, Y.-J. Curcumin and Its Potential to Target the Glycolytic Behavior of Lactate-Acclimated Prostate Carcinoma Cells with Docetaxel. *Nutrients* **2024**, *16*, 4338. https://doi.org/10.3390/nu16244338.
2. Han, N.-R.; Park, H.-J.; Ko, S.-G.; Moon, P.-D. Tryptanthrin Down-Regulates Oncostatin M by Targeting GM-CSF-Mediated PI3K-AKT-NF-κB Axis. *Nutrients* **2024**, *16*, 4109. https://doi.org/10.3390/nu16234109.
3. Abbasi, H.; Sharif, M.; John, P.; Bhatti, A.; Hayat, M.Q.; Mansoor, Q. Phytochemical, Cytoprotective Profiling, and Anti-Inflammatory Potential of *Colchicum luteum* in Rheumatoid Arthritis: An Experimental and Simulation Study. *Nutrients* **2024**, *16*, 4020. https://doi.org/10.3390/nu16234020.
4. Sung, Y.-Y.; Kim, S.-H.; Yang, W.-K.; Yuk, H.J.; Kim, M.-S.; Kim, D.-S. *Lysimachia mauritiana* Lam. Extract Alleviates Airway Inflammation Induced by Particulate Matter Plus Diesel Exhaust Particles in Mice. *Nutrients* **2024**, *16*, 3732. https://doi.org/10.3390/nu16213732.
5. Zhang, Y.; Zhu, S.; Gu, Y.; Feng, Y.; Gao, B. Network Pharmacology Combined with Experimental Validation to Investigate the Mechanism of the Anti-Hyperuricemia Action of *Portulaca oleracea* Extract. *Nutrients* **2024**, *16*, 3549. https://doi.org/10.3390/nu16203549.
6. Libero, M.L.; Montero-Hidalgo, A.J.; Recinella, L.; Luque, R.M.; Generali, D.; Acquaviva, A.; Orlando, G.; Ferrante, C.; Menghini, L.; Di Simone, S.C.; et al. The Protective Effects of an Aged Black Garlic Water Extract on the Prostate. *Nutrients* **2024**, *16*, 3025. https://doi.org/10.3390/nu16173025.
7. Rodriguez, I.; Nam, Y.H.; Shin, S.W.; Seo, G.J.; Kim, N.W.; Nuankaew, W.; Kim, D.H.; Park, Y.H.; Lee, H.Y.; Peng, X.H.; et al. Effects of *Castanopsis echinocarpa* on Sensorineural Hearing Loss via Neuronal Gene Regulation. *Nutrients* **2024**, *16*, 2716. https://doi.org/10.3390/nu16162716.
8. Cho, W.-K.; Choi, H.-J.; Ma, J.Y. *Selaginella tamariscina* Ethanol Extract Attenuates Influenza A Virus Infection by Inhibiting Hemagglutinin and Neuraminidase. *Nutrients* **2024**, *16*, 2377. https://doi.org/10.3390/nu16142377
9. Espinoça, I.T.; Basilio, D.C.L.S.; de Araujo, A.J.P.; Ota, R.S.N.; de Souza, K.F.S.; Cassemiro, N.S.; Lagatta, D.C.; Paredes-Gamero, E.J.; Macedo, M.L.R.; Silva, D.B.; et al. Antithrombotic Effect of Oil from the Pulp of Bocaiúva—*Acrocomia aculeata* (Jacq.) Lodd. ex Mart. (Arecaceae). *Nutrients* **2024**, *16*, 2024. https://doi.org/10.3390/nu16132024.
10. Rey, D.P.; Echeverry, S.M.; Valderrama, I.H.; Rodriguez, I.A.; Ospina, L.F.; Mena Barreto Silva, F.R.; Aragón, M. Antidiabetic Effect of *Passiflora ligularis* Leaves in High Fat-Diet/Streptozotocin-Induced Diabetic Mice. *Nutrients* **2024**, *16*, 1669. https://doi.org/10.3390/nu16111669

11. Wiciński, M.; Fajkiel-Madajczyk, A.; Kurant, Z.; Liss, S.; Szyperski, P.; Szambelan, M.; Gromadzki, B.; Rupniak, I.; Słupski, M.; Sadowska-Krawczenko, I. Ashwagandha's Multifaceted Effects on Human Health: Impact on Vascular Endothelium, Inflammation, Lipid Metabolism, and Cardiovascular Outcomes—A Review. *Nutrients* **2024**, *16*, 2481. https://doi.org/10.3390/nu16152481.

nutrients

MDPI

Review

Ashwagandha's Multifaceted Effects on Human Health: Impact on Vascular Endothelium, Inflammation, Lipid Metabolism, and Cardiovascular Outcomes—A Review

Michał Wiciński [1], Anna Fajkiel-Madajczyk [1,*], Zuzanna Kurant [1], Sara Liss [1], Paweł Szyperski [1], Monika Szambelan [1], Bartłomiej Gromadzki [1], Iga Rupniak [2], Maciej Słupski [3] and Iwona Sadowska-Krawczenko [2]

[1] Department of Pharmacology and Therapeutics, Faculty of Medicine, Collegium Medicum in Bydgoszcz, Nicolaus Copernicus University, M. Curie Skłodowskiej 9, 85-094 Bydgoszcz, Poland; michal.wicinski@cm.umk.pl (M.W.); zuzanna.kurant@cm.umk.pl (Z.K.); sara.liss@cm.umk.pl (S.L.); pawel.szyperski@cm.umk.pl (P.S.); monika.szambelan@cm.umk.pl (M.S.); bartlomiej.gromadzki@cm.umk.pl (B.G.)

[2] Department of Neonatology, Ludwik Rydygier Collegium Medicum in Bydgoszcz, Nicolaus Copernicus University in Torun, ul. Ujejskiego 75, 85-168 Bydgoszcz, Poland; iga.rupniak@cm.umk.pl (I.R.); iwonasadowska@cm.umk.pl (I.S.-K.)

[3] Department of Hepatobiliary and General Surgery, Faculty of Medicine, Collegium Medicum in Bydgoszcz, Nicolaus Copernicus University, M. Curie Skłodowskiej 9, 85-094 Bydgoszcz, Poland; maciej.slupski@cm.umk.pl

* Correspondence: anna.fajkiel@cm.umk.pl

Abstract: *Withania somnifera*, commonly known as Ashwagandha, has been popular for many years. Numerous studies have shown that the extract of this plant, due to its wealth of active substances, can induce anti-inflammatory, neuroprotective, immunomodulatory, hepatoprotective, cardioprotective, anti-diabetic, adaptogenic, anti-arthritic, anti-stress, and antimicrobial effects. This review examines the impact of Ashwagandha extract on the vascular endothelium, inflammation, lipid metabolism, and cardiovascular outcomes. Studies have shown that Ashwagandha extracts exhibit an anti-angiogenic effect by inhibiting vascular endothelial growth factor (VEGF)-induced capillary sprouting and formation by lowering the mean density of microvessels. Furthermore, the results of numerous studies highlight the anti-inflammatory role of Ashwagandha extract, as the action of this plant causes a decrease in the expression of pro-inflammatory cytokines. Interestingly, withanolides, present in Ashwagandha root, have shown the ability to inhibit the differentiation of preadipocytes into adipocytes. Research results have also proved that *W. somnifera* demonstrates cardioprotective effects due to its antioxidant properties and reduces ischemia/reperfusion-induced apoptosis. It seems that this plant can be successfully used as a potential treatment for several conditions, mainly those with increased inflammation. More research is needed to elucidate the exact mechanisms by which the substances contained in *W. somnifera* extracts can act in the human body.

Keywords: ashwagandha; lipid metabolism; inflammation; vascular endothelium; cardiovascular outcomes

1. Introduction

The increased risk of developing lifestyle diseases in the global population has led scientists to search for natural products that may have a beneficial effect in treating these conditions. Preparations of plant origin often seem to be safer than synthetic drugs, which can cause dangerous side effects and do not change the progression of some diseases in the long run [1]. Medicinal plant extracts are of great interest as potential drugs and elements of complementary therapies that can reduce the amount of drugs taken by the patient. Moreover, substances of plant origin have multidirectional effects, thanks to which they can be used in preventive treatments, which allows for maintaining appropriate homeostasis in the body. Finally, they can be used as a part of conventional treatment, which requires adequate evidence of their effectiveness [2].

Ashwagandha is the name of *Withania somnifera* in Sanskrit. Other terms for this therapeutic plant are Indian ginseng or winter cherry. *W. somnifera* has been known in traditional medicine (Ayurveda and Unani Systems of Medicine) for over 5000 years. The Latin word "somnifera" means "sleep-inducer", but the therapeutic effects of this plant have been reported in many different fields of medicine [3,4]. A wide range of treatment indications is found due to the anti-inflammatory, antihypoxic, antiischemic, neuroprotective, immunomodulatory, hepatoprotective, cardioprotective, anti-diabetic, adaptogenic, anti-arthritic, anti-stress, and antimicrobial effects [5–7]. Nowadays, Ashwagandha supplementation is popular mainly as an anti-stress solution and is believed to improve overall health and longevity.

All parts of the plant (leaves, flowers, seeds, root) have health potential, but the root is the part that is mostly used medicinally [7]. The major phytochemical components contained in roots are alkaloids (convolamine, convoline, convolidine, convolvine), withanolides (withanolide A, withasomnine, withanosides), sitoindosides (β-sitosterol and d-glycoside), and steroids [8,9]. Withanolides are responsible for the best-documented pharmacological activity [9,10]. Withaferin A, one of the most representative withanolides found in *W. somnifera*, is well known for its anti-inflammatory, antioxidant, immunomodulatory, pro-apoptotic, anti-angiogenesis, and anti-adipogenesis effects [11,12].

This review examines the impact of Ashwagandha extract on the vascular endothelium, inflammation, lipid metabolism, and cardiovascular outcomes. The PubMed and Google Scholar databases were searched using combinations of the following keywords: Ashwagandha, *Withania somnifera*, withanolides, inflammation, lipid metabolism, vascular endothelium, blood pressure, and cardiovascular outcomes. The search mainly included research published in the years 2003–2023.

2. Vascular Endothelium

The vascular endothelium, the inner lining of the vascular wall, comprises a single layer of endothelial cells (ECs), providing a barrier between blood and tissues [13]. ECs are physiologically active, participating in various critical processes. These include the regulation of vascular tone, coagulation, platelet adhesion and aggregation, inflammation, immune responses, cell proliferation, and angiogenesis [13,14]. As a result, ECs play a significant role in the pathogenesis of conditions such as cardiovascular diseases [15], diabetes mellitus [14], and cancers [14]. Therefore, this has led to a growing field of research focused on substances that could potentially target ECs for therapeutic purposes. *W. somnifera*, for its wealth of active substances, influences the vascular endothelium through multiple mechanisms.

It is recognized that angiogenesis, the process of forming new capillaries, plays a crucial role in many diseases [16,17]. This process is facilitated by the angiogenic vascular endothelial growth factor (VEGF). VEGF interacts with specific receptors—VEGF-1 and VEGF-2—located on the surface of endothelial cells, leading to the formation of new vessels [18]. Mathur et al. conducted a study investigating the anticancer effects of *W. somnifera*, with a particular focus on its impact on angiogenesis [19]. In the chick-chorioallantoic membrane (CAM) assay, the test group was exposed to 10 ng of VEGF along with extracts or fractions of *W. somnifera* at concentrations of 2.5 ng, 5 ng, and 10 ng. Additionally, subcutaneous gel foam sponges were implanted in mice using higher concentrations (100 ng of VEGF in combination with 100 ng of the plant extract) to measure the density and number of vessels formed. After 12 days of in vitro incubation and 14 days of follow-up in mice, the results indicated that *W. somnifera*, particularly at higher concentrations (10 ng in vitro and 100 ng in vivo), inhibited VEGF-induced capillary sprouting and formation by lowering the mean microvessel density (number of blood vessels per unit area), thereby reinforcing Ashwagandha's role as an anti-angiogenic agent [19].

The ubiquitin–proteasome pathway (UPP) is one of the main pathways that selectively degrades cellular proteins and regulates most processes essential for maintaining cellular function balance [20]. This process involves the covalent attachment of ubiquitin to a substrate protein, forming a polyubiquitin chain (ubiquitylation), which signals the proteolysis of this protein with the involvement of proteasomes [21]. One of the proteins degraded by the UPP is the hypoxia-inducible factor (HIF), which partially promotes new blood vessel formation through the transcription of factors such as VEGF [22]. Another example is the degradation and phosphorylation of nuclear factor kappa B (IκBα), leading to the activation of nuclear factor κB (NF-κB) and its subsequent role in angiogenesis, the cell cycle, apoptosis, carcinogenesis, and immune responses [23,24]. NF-κB activation occurs in response to various factors, including pro-inflammatory cytokines, with tumor necrosis factor-alpha (TNF-α) being the most extensively studied [25]. Mohan et al. carried out a study investigating the effect of *W. somnifera* on these pathways [26]. In their research, human umbilical vein endothelial cells (HUVECs) were induced by growth factors (FGF-2 at 30 ng/mL) and then treated with various concentrations of Ashwagandha fractions (5, 10, and 50 μg/mL). After 24 h of coincubation, the length and quantity of vessels were reduced. This study also found out that *W. somnifera*, at various concentrations (0.2, 1, 5 μM), inhibited NF-κB activation in TNF-α (10 ng/mL)-stimulated HUVECs, as measured by the electrophoretic mobility shift assay (EMSA). Additionally, there was an increase in the level of polyubiquitinated proteins, suggesting the involvement of the UPP in the process of NF-κB inhibition [26].

Further research on Ashwagandha's role in endothelial-cell-mediated angiogenesis was conducted by Bargagna-Mohan et al. [27]. They pre-treated human choroidal endothelial cells (HCECs) and HUVECs with different concentrations of Ashwagandha extract (0.25, 0.5, 1 μM) for 30 min and then stimulated with TNF-α (10 ng/mL) for 20 min. The study discovered that *W. somnifera* in a dose-dependent manner inhibited the induction of inflammatory IκBα degradation and increased the levels of ubiquitinated species, targeting the UPP and suppressing angiogenic sprouting in an in vitro tube formation assay. Moreover, the use of *W. somnifera* resulted in the induction of the expression of the antioxidant enzyme heme oxygenase-1 (HO-1) in ECs, providing cytoprotective effects and contributing to maintaining vascular homeostasis [27].

Nitric oxide (NO) is an important compound produced in ECs by the constitutive calcium-dependent enzyme nitric oxide synthase (NOS) [28]. There are three NOS isoforms—endothelial NOS (eNOS), neuronal NOS (nNOS), and inducible NOS (iNOS) [29]. NO exerts a potent vasodilating and anti-inflammatory effect, contributing to the maintenance of vascular homeostasis [30]. In a study using rat aortic rings and a human endothelial cell line, Pathak et al. presented a significant increase in NO production mediated by *W. somnifera* (more specifically two extracts from Ashwagandha—standardized root extract of the plant NMITLI-118R (NM) and withanolide A) with the highest NO generation at a concentration of 50 μg/mL for the NM extract and 5 μg/mL for the withanolide A extract [29]. Research has shown that the increase in NO production is mediated through upregulating the expression of eNOS genes and proteins, as measured by Real-Time PCR. NO-induced vasorelaxation is achieved by activating guanylyl cyclase, an enzyme in vascular smooth muscle cells that converts guanosine-5′-triphosphate (GTP) into cyclic guanosine monophosphate (cGMP). This research underscores Ashwagandha's vasoprotective potential [29].

Furthermore, Iuvone et al. explored the plant's immunostimulating properties [31]. They examined the impact of *W. somnifera* on NO synthesis in mouse macrophages by stimulating them with various concentrations (1–256 μg/mL) of the Ashwagandha extract. After 24 h, they measured the nitrite levels in the culture and found a significant, concentration-dependent increase in NO production starting from 4 μg/mL of the extract. They also observed the upregulation of iNOS, one of the NOS isoforms, typically synthesized by cells in response to inflammation, possibly mediated through NF-κB transactivation [31].

Endothelial cell dysfunction is triggered by an imbalance between antioxidants and reactive oxygen species (ROS) [32]. This endothelial activation eventually results in a decreased bioavailability of NO, impaired vascular tone [32], initiation of EC apoptosis, and alteration in their angiogenic potential [33]. Khalil et al. carried out a study on rats where induced myocardial infarction caused oxidative stress by generating free radicals [34]. This led to a reduction in the levels of antioxidant enzymes—specifically superoxide dismutase (SOD) and glutathione peroxidase (GPx)—which are responsible for scavenging free radicals. The study showed that treating the animals with 100 mg/kg of *W. somnifera* for 4 weeks enhanced the activity of these enzymes, thereby bolstering the endogenous antioxidant system [34]. A similar study was previously conducted by Kaur et al. on rats with induced pulmonary hypertension and right ventricular hypertrophy [35]. They demonstrated that *W. somnifera*, administered for 5 weeks in doses of 50 and 100 mg/kg, alleviates oxidative stress (more effectively at higher concentrations) by reducing ROS levels. This is achieved through an enhancement in endogenous antioxidant enzymes such as SOD, thereby improving the function of the pulmonary vascular endothelium [35]. Moreover, the effects of Ashwagandha have been associated with an increase in eNOS expression in the lungs of rats, which elevates NO levels and exhibits vasodilatory, antiproliferative, and apoptosis-inducing effects [35]. The results of this study also outlined the anti-inflammatory role of Ashwagandha extract, as the plant's action resulted in a decrease in the level of expression of pro-inflammatory cytokines TNF-α and NF-κB and an increase in the level of the anti-inflammatory cytokine interleukin-10 (IL-10) [35].

However, not all research findings are consistent with the aforementioned data. For instance, in the study by Kim et al., AGS human gastric epithelial cell lines infected with *Helicobacter pylori* were examined for, among others, VEGF production and HIF-1α levels in the absence or presence of one of the compounds of *W. somnifera*—withaferin A (10–500 nM). The results showed that pre-treatment, as well as co-treatment with withaferin A, did not inhibit the basal or *H. pylori*-induced VEGF production and did not affect HIF-1α stabilization in gastric epithelial cells [36].

Additionally, not every component of *W. somnifera* exhibits the same effect on the vascular endothelium. An example is the study by Chaudhary et al., which compared the properties of withaferin A with its natural and structurally similar analog—2,3-dihydro-3β-methoxy-withaferin A (3βmWi-A). This study demonstrated that in cancer cells, withaferin A reduced the level of VEGF, whereas 3βmWi-A did not have this property. Thereby, the authors of the study suggested that 3βmWi-A does not exhibit anti-metastatic potential [37].

In the studies discussed in this chapter, *W. somnifera* was mainly used as a standalone therapeutic agent, so it can be ruled out that the results were due to a more complex treatment regimen. Despite the promising research results, the referenced studies show that to assess the role and effects of *W. somnifera*, it is essential to conduct more studies that would provide a definitive position on the impact of Ashwagandha on the vascular endothelium. Most of the conducted studies are in vitro or in vivo in rats. There is a lack of typical clinical trials that would allow for the prediction of clinical applications in specific human diseases associated with vascular endothelial dysfunction.

In summary, *W. somnifera* exerts multiple effects on the vascular endothelium. By inhibiting VEGF, preventing NF-κB activation, modulating NO production, inducing antioxidant enzymes like HO-1, SOD, and GPx, and reducing ROS levels, it demonstrates anti-angiogenic, vasodilatory, and anti-inflammatory properties. These findings suggest that Ashwagandha may enhance vascular endothelial function, potentially expanding its medical applications by leveraging its mentioned properties. Table 1 shows a summary of the research discussed in this chapter.

Table 1. Summary of reviewed research.

Authors	Subject of Study	Dose	Results
Kaur et al. (2015) [35]	MCT-challenged rats with PH (pulmonary hypertension)	*W. somnifera* root powder (50 and 100 mg/kg/d, p.o.)	↓ RVP, ↓ RVH; ↑ TUNEL-positive cells, ↓ procaspase-3; ↑ IL-10, ↓ TNF-α, ↓ NF-κB; ↑ eNOS, ↓ HIF-1α
Khalil et al. (2015) [34]	Wistar albino rats (n = 40)	WSLEt (100 mg/kg) for 4 weeks	↓ heart weight, ↓ cTnI; ↓ TC, ↓ TGs, ↓ VLDL-C, ↑ HDL-C; ↑ SOD, ↑ GRx, ↑ GPx, ↑ GST, ↓ LPO; ↓ inflammatory cells
Iuvone et al. (2003) [31]	The monocyte/macrophage cell line J774	WS (1–256 μg/mL)	↑ NO; ↓ NO synthase inhibitor L-NAME; ↓ TLCK—an inhibitor of NF-κB activation
Mathur et al. (2006) [19]	Chick-chorioallantoic membrane (CAM) with VEGF	2.5, 5, and 10 ng of WS root extract and fractions	↓ mean microvessel density; ↓ MVD
	Subcutaneous implantation of gel foam sponges with VEGF in male Swiss albino mice (25–35 g)	100 ng of WS root extract and fractions	
Mohan et al. (2004) [26]	Human umbilical vein endothelial cells induced by FGF-2	5, 10, and 50 μg/mL of WS fractions; 24 h of coincubation	↓ sprouting index
	Human umbilical vein endothelial cells stimulated with TNF-α	0.2, 1, and 5 μM of withaferin A; 30 min of treatment + 20 min of TNF-α coincubation	↓ TNF-α-induced NF-κB activation; ↑ polyubiquitinated proteins
Bargagna-Mohan et al. (2006) [27]	Human choroidal endothelial cells and human umbilical vein endothelial cells, both stimulated with TNF-α	0.25, 0.5, and 1 μM of withanolide D; 30 min of treatment + 20 min of TNF-α coincubation	↑ IκBα; ↑ ubiquitinated species
	Human choroidal endothelial cells and human umbilical vein endothelial cells, both stimulated with VEGF	0.5, 1, and 2 μM of withaferin A; 12 h	↑ HO-1
Pathak et al. (2017) [29]	Transverse aortic rings (4 mm) of 10-week-old male Wistar rats (250 g)	0.1–100 μg/mL of standardized WS root extract (NM) and 0.1–100 μg/mL of marker compound withanolide A	↑ vasorelaxation
	Human endothelial cell line EA.hy926	3 h of treatment with 0.5–100 μg/mL of NM and 0.5–50 μg/mL of withanolide A	↑ NO; ↑ eNOS
Kim et al. (2015) [36]	AGS cells infected with *H. pylori* in the absence or presence of withaferin A (pre-treated and co-treated)	10–500 nM of withaferin A; 24 h of experiment	↔ VEGF
Chaudhary et al. (2019) [37]	AGS cells pre-treated with withaferin A and infected with *H. pylori* Osteosarcoma cell lines treated with WA and 3βmWi-A	500 nM of withaferin A; 6 h of experiment; 0.3 and 0.6 μM of withaferin A and 3βmWi-A for 48 h	↔ HIF-1α; ↓ VEGF (for withaferin A); ↑ VEGF (for 3βmWi-A)

Note: ↓ reduction, ↑ increase, and ↔ irrelevant; abbreviations: RVP—right ventricle pressure; RVH—right ventricle hypertrophy; cTnI—cardiac troponin I; TC—total cholesterol; TGs—triglycerides; HDL-C—high-density lipoprotein cholesterol; VLDL-C—very-low-density lipoprotein cholesterol; TLCK—trypsin-like serine protease inhibitor; MVD—mitral valve disease; WS—*W. somnifera*.

3. Inflammation

Chronic inflammation underlies various diseases, including cardiovascular disorders, neurodegenerative conditions, and immune dysfunctions. Also aging, despite the lack of coexistence of diseases, is now considered to be the result of low-grade inflammation. The term "inflammaging" was created, describing the deteriorating organ dysfunction with age [38]. Key pro-inflammatory cytokines like TNF-α and interleukin-1 (IL-1) exacerbate these conditions, while anti-inflammatory cytokines such as IL-10 and transforming growth factor beta (TGF-β) provide a counterbalance [39].

The influence of the external environment, as well as internal processes such as telomere attrition and genome alterations, are factors that modulate inflammation and aging [40]. A wide range of studies have shown that extracts of *W. somnifera* have many properties which modulate multiple pathways of the immune system in rats [41], cats [42], and humans [43].

Immunoglobulin E (IgE) recognizes the foreign antigen and informs mast cells and basophils about it. Subsequent exposure to the same antigen induces a type 2 allergic reaction aimed at activating T helper 2 (Th2) and B lymphocytes and consecutively producing IgE, group 2 innate lymphoid cells (ILC2), eosinophils, and elevated Th2 cytokines—interleukins (IL-4, IL-5, IL-13) [44]. Clinical symptoms of an excessively activated immune system in this pathway include asthma, skin rash, excessive mucus production, and pollen or food allergies. *W. somnifera* has properties that attenuate type 2 allergic reactions by a reduction in cytokines IL-4, IL-13, TNF-α, and IgE [45,46].

Many of the substances contained in Ashwagandha extract have immunomodulatory effects [47]. Withanolides, which are steroid derivatives, influence the hypothalamic–pituitary–adrenal (HPA) axis. Lopresti et al. carried out a double-blind randomized controlled trial (RCT) in which patients took a 240 mg extract of *W. somnifera* with 84 mg of withanolide glycosides. They showed a reduction in morning cortisol and dehydroepiandrosterone (DHEA) after 15 days of use. Clinically, this was reflected in improved mood and reduced anxiety, which was measured using the HAM-A (Hamilton Anxiety Rating Scale) and DASS-21 (Depression Anxiety Stress Scale-21) compared to the placebo group [48]. A reduction in cortisol levels, as well as stress as measured using the Perceived Stress Scale (PSS) and HAM-A depending on the dose of *W. somnifera* extract, was shown in an 8-week study by Salve J. et al. The researchers divided the participants into groups: the first group was given a placebo, the second 250 mg, and the third a 600 mg extract of Ashwagandha. An improvement in emotional state and a reduction in cortisol levels were seen in both groups receiving the root extract, but the higher dose had a better effect [49].

On the one hand, withanolides diminish the level of cortisol, which has an anti-inflammatory effect, and on the other hand, selectively block cyclooxygenase-2 (COX2) and inhibit lipopolysaccharide (LPS)-induced inflammation [50]. Withaferin A inhibits NF-κB, activator protein 1 (AP1), and alpha-2 macroglobulin [51]. Withaferin A in combination with withanolide E can silence the proliferation of B and T lymphocytes and affect the recognition of antigens [26]. The modulation of T lymphocyte activity is based on the effect of withaferin on blocking the activity of Zap70 kinase. The potential advantage could be the prevention of autoimmune-mediated pathologies [52].

Singh et al. showed that the extract from *W. somnifera* root in add-on therapy influences the improvement in forced expiratory volume in one second—FEV1% (increased by 14.36% after 12 weeks of therapy); quality of life; and exercise tolerance in GOLD 2 and 3 categories of chronic obstructive pulmonary disease (COPD) patients. It was proved that withanolides are the most potent in inhibiting the activity of angiotensin-converting enzyme 2 (ACE2), myeloperoxidase (MPO), and interleukin-6 (IL-6), which significantly enhances lung function. Simultaneous anti-inflammatory and free radical lowering effects alleviate obstructive symptoms [53].

The adaptogenic function of *W. somnifera* was proved in influencing transcription RNA, resulting in the regulation of cellular metabolism and the maintenance of homeostasis. Advanced glycation end products (AGEs) are secreted by microglia, and they are a marker of aging and degenerative processes in the brain. They induce iNOS expression and bind to RAGE in neurons, which leads to cells damage and apoptosis. AGEs cause the augmentation of the formation of the amyloid-beta precursor protein (APP) and its derivative amyloid-beta Aβ and tau protein. They create toxins for neuron oligomers. Aβ similarly to AGEs binds to RAGE and activates the extracellular-signal-regulated kinase (ERK) 1/2 pathway and further NF-κB. The effect of this is an increase in the expression of COX2, interleukin-1β (IL-1β), or iNOS. All these factors intensify neuroinflammation [54]. The ability of Ashwagandha to inhibit at a transcriptional level the biosynthesis of Aβ and IL-1β leads to the suppression of neurodegeneration [55].

Panossian et al. proved the ability of *W. somnifera* to downregulate the expression of arachidonate 12-lipoxygenase (ALOX12), leukotriene C4 synthase, and dipeptidase 2 (DPEP2) genes in human neuroglia cells. This leads to the inhibition of neuroinflammation and neurodegeneration [56].

Extended inflammation contributes to chronic organ dysfunction. Cytokines circulating in the blood and those synthesized by the epithelium of the renal tubes make the kidneys extremely sensitive to inflammation. In the kidneys, angiotensin II and TNFα stimulate the signaling pathway of NF-κB [57,58]. The result is the increased expression of genes C-C Motif Chemokine Ligand 2 (CCL2) and C-C Motif Chemokine Ligand 5 (CCL5) and further renal fibrosis. The progressive remodeling of kidneys by increasing fibrosis leads to their loss of function. *W. somnifera* by the downregulation of TNF-α, CCL2, and CCL5 protects the kidneys. A study of the effects of various herbal extracts on rat kidney NRK-52E cells showed that a formulation containing 250 mg of Ashwagandha (including 2.5% withanolides) at a dilution of 1:100 after 24 h of incubation prevents TNF-α- and LPS-induced CCL5 gene expression [59].

The anti-inflammatory and antioxidant properties of Ashwagandha were proven in the liver. *W. somnifera* extract rich in the withanolide fraction reduces the expression of COX-2, iNOS, IL-1β, and TNFα. This was proved by Devkar et al. in a study with acetaminophen-treated rats. The hepatoprotective effect of the withanolide-rich extract was significant and dose-dependent. The doses used in the study were 50 mg/kg, 100 mg/kg, and 200 mg/kg. The downregulation of TNF-α and IL-1β mRNA expression in a dose-dependent manner was observed. iNOS and COX-2 mRNA expressions were reduced only when a 200 mg/kg dose was used [60].

Kaileh et al. in their study focused on the discovery of the mechanisms of action of Ashwagandha and showed using cell cultures (murine fibrosarcoma cells, human kidney cells, IKK-α- and IKK-β-deficient mouse embryonic fibroblasts, cervix cancer cells, human breast cancer cells) that the pre-treatment of the leaf extract of *W. somnifera* blocks the TNF effect by the inhibition of the IκB kinase (IKK) complex. The task of IKK is to phosphorylate IκB inhibitor proteins, under the influence of pro-inflammatory factors, and then release NF-κB. The blockade of this reaction by Ashwagandha prevents NF-κB from entering the cell nucleus and attaching to DNA [61].

An indispensable element of the human organism's homeostasis is coping with harmful external factors, inflammation, destructive processes, or aging. *W. somnifera* is an adaptogen that helps to adjust and survive the negative effects of damage at the gene expression level. Improving the functioning of the cells, and secondarily of organs, inhibits the effects of aging and extends life. Table 2 shows a summary of the research discussed in this chapter.

Table 2. Summary of reviewed research.

Authors	Subject of Study	Dose	Results
Lopresti et al. (2019) [48]	Stressed, healthy adults	240 mg of a standardized Ashwagandha extract (Shoden)	↓ morning serum cortisol and ↓ DHEA
Salve et al. (2019) [49]	Stressed healthy adults	250 mg and 600 mg of Ashwagandha extract	↓ morning serum cortisol; 600 mg better effect
Fazil et al. (2021) [52]	T cells	0.3–1.25 μM withaferin A	Inhibition of the ZAP70 kinase and retardation of T-cell motility
Singh et al. 2022 [53]	COPD patients qualified as GOLD 2 and 3	250 mg of WS root capsules	↓ ACE-2, ↓ MPO, and ↓ IL-6
Atluri et al. (2020) [55]	SH-APP cells	50 nM–1 μM of withaferin A	↓ Aβ, ↓ IL-1β, and ↓ NF-κB
Panossian et al. (2018) [56]	Cultivated neuroglial cells	WS (5.0 μg/mL) corresponding dose in humans 300 mg; WSL (1.5 μg/mL) corresponding dose in humans 90 mg	↓ ALOX12, ↓ DPEP2, and ↓ leukotriene C4 synthetase
Grunz-Borgmann et al. (2015) [59]	Rat kidney NRK-52E cell line	450 mg of a standardized extract containing a minimum of 2.5% total withanolides	Inhibition of TNFα on CCL2 and CCL5 gene expression
Devkar et al. (2016) [60]	Male Swiss albino mice	50 mg/kg, 100 mg/kg, and 200 mg/kg of the withanolide-rich extract	Every dose: ↓ TNFα and ↓ IL-1β mRNA expression; 200 mg/kg: ↓ iNOS and ↓ COX-2 mRNA expression
Kaileh et al. (2007) [61]	Murine fibrosarcoma L929sA cells and human embryonic kidney 293T cells, IKK-α- and IKK-β-deficient mouse embryonic fibroblasts and cervix cancer cells (HeLa), and MDA-MB-231 human breast cancer cells	Withaferin A, withanolide A, and 12-deoxywithastramonolide (1 mg/mL)	↓ IL-6; ↓ NFκB B-driven gene expression; ↑ AP1-driven gene expression; ↓ NFκB/DNA binding; ↓ NFκB translocation; ↓ TNF-induced phosphorylation and degradation of IκBα; ↓ TNF-induced IKKβ activity; ↑ induces the phosphorylation of IKKβ through the MEK/ERK Pathway

Note: ↓ reduction, ↑ increase; abbreviations: MEK/ERK—mitogen-activated protein kinase/extracellular-signal-regulated kinase; WS—*W. somnifera*.

4. Lipid Metabolism Disorders

Lipid metabolism disorders encompass a range of conditions characterized by abnormalities in the body's synthesis, breakdown, and transport of lipids. These disorders can lead to elevated levels of cholesterol and triglycerides in the blood, contributing to serious health issues such as cardiovascular disease, diabetes, and metabolic syndrome. Common lipid metabolism disorders include hyperlipidemia, atherosclerosis, and obesity [62,63]. Hyperlipidemia refers to elevated levels of lipids in the blood, which can predispose individuals to atherosclerosis. In this condition, plaque builds up in the arterial walls, leading to reduced blood flow and an increased risk of heart attacks and strokes [64]. Obesity, defined by excessive fat accumulation, further exacerbates these risks and is often associated with insulin resistance and type 2 diabetes [65].

The management of lipid metabolism disorders traditionally involves lifestyle modifications such as diet and exercise and, in many cases, pharmacological treatment. Examples of substances used in treatment are statins or fibrates [64,66]. However, these treatments may not be effective for all patients and sometimes can come with significant side effects. This has spurred interest in complementary therapies, including the use of medicinal plants. Among these, *W. somnifera* has emerged as a promising candidate due to its multiple therapeutic properties.

A pivotal study identified anti-adipogenic withanolides from the root of *W. somnifera*, demonstrating their ability to inhibit the differentiation of preadipocytes into adipocytes [10]. This anti-adipogenic effect is significant as it prevents the formation of new fat cells, playing a crucial role in preventing and managing obesity—a major risk factor for lipid metabolism disorders. In the study, they used 25 μM of withanolides [10]. Further research has shown that *W. somnifera* extract can enhance energy expenditure by improving mitochondrial function in adipose tissue and skeletal muscle [67]. Enhanced mitochondrial activity leads to a higher metabolic rate and increased energy expenditure, which helps reduce body fat and improve lipid profiles. These findings underscore the herb's potential in addressing metabolic syndrome, often associated with lipid metabolism disorders.

Another study on Nile tilapia found that dietary supplementation with *W. somnifera* improved the fish's lipid profile and intestinal histomorphology [68]. Additionally, the study observed a modulation of cytokine responses to *Streptococcus iniae* infection, suggesting an overall enhancement in health and immune response. It is important to point out that this research was performed on fish. However, the implications for human health are still noteworthy, indicating that *W. somnifera* could also enhance human lipid metabolism and immune function.

Withaferin A, a bioactive compound in Ashwagandha, modulated oxidative damage by regulating inflammatory mediators and apoptosis through the phosphatidylinositol 3-kinase/protein kinase B (PI3K/AKT) signaling pathway in high-cholesterol-induced atherosclerosis in experimental rats [69]. By reducing oxidative stress and inflammation, withaferin A helps to mitigate the progression of atherosclerosis and other lipid-related disorders. This modulation of oxidative damage is crucial for the management of lipid metabolism disorders, as oxidative stress and inflammation are key contributors to their pathogenesis. In another significant study, withaferin A demonstrated protective effects against high-fat-diet-induced obesity by attenuating oxidative stress, inflammation, and insulin resistance [70]. This protective action is vital for preventing obesity and associated lipid metabolism disorders. The attenuation of oxidative stress and inflammation, coupled with improved insulin sensitivity, highlights the comprehensive benefits of *W. somnifera* in managing high-fat-diet-related health issues.

Research on withanolide A, another compound from *W. somnifera*, showed cytoprotective effects against 7-ketocholesterol-induced cytotoxicity in human brain endothelial cells [71]. This protection is essential for maintaining brain health, especially in conditions where lipid metabolism disorders might lead to neurological complications. By safeguarding brain endothelial cells from lipid-induced damage, withanolide A supports overall metabolic health and highlights the broad therapeutic potential of Ashwagandha.

A review of traditional knowledge and recent research findings has consolidated evidence supporting the role of Ashwagandha in managing metabolic syndrome [72]. This review emphasizes the herb's efficacy in improving various metabolic parameters, including lipid metabolism, offering a holistic approach to treating metabolic disorders. The integration of traditional knowledge with contemporary scientific research can pave the way for novel therapeutic strategies. Additionally, new anti-adipogenic withanolides, such as withasomniferol D, have been identified from the root of Ashwagandha [73]. These newly discovered compounds expand the potential therapeutic applications of *W. somnifera* in lipid metabolism disorders, presenting new opportunities for research and development. The study investigated withanolides at a concentration of 25 μM.

Lastly, an in vitro study demonstrated the hypolipidemic effects of Ashwagandha and Arjuna, showing a significant reduction in lipid levels [74]. This supports the traditional use of these herbs in managing hyperlipidemia and underscores the importance of integrating traditional practices with modern scientific validation.

The accumulating evidence highlights *W. somnifera*'s multifaceted role in managing lipid metabolism disorders. Its anti-adipogenic properties, enhancement in energy expenditure, improvement in lipid profiles, and protective effects against oxidative stress and inflammation make it a promising candidate for further research and clinical application. Integrating traditional knowledge with modern scientific insights can foster the development of innovative therapeutic strategies for lipid metabolism disorders, offering hope for improved management and better health outcomes. Unfortunately, there is a lack of data on clinical trials testing the potential use of *W. somnifera* in diseases related to lipid metabolism, which should be taken into consideration when using extracts of this plant to improve the organism's lipid metabolism.

5. Cardiovascular Outcomes

According to the WHO (World Health Organization), cardiovascular diseases are the leading cause of death worldwide—they cause about 17.9 deaths each year [75]. The challenge this poses to the world keeps us looking for ways to reduce this statistic.

It is already a well-known fact that blood pressure (BP) is closely related to cardiovascular risk and also to renal function, organs of vision, or endothelial epithelium damage, as we mentioned before in this article [76–78]. Therefore, the limit of normal values of BP was determined to be able to start the treatment of hypertension early enough to prevent the consequences caused by its too-high values and to reduce the cardiovascular risk. We decided to review the articles to find out whether *W. somnifera* becoming more and more popular and its active compounds could be used in hypertension treatment and how its properties relate to cardiovascular risk. Does it have any potential?

First, it is important to raise the issue that several studies confirm the anti-anxiety and anti-stress effects of Ashwagandha [79–83]. It is known that prolonged stress is related to hypertension development and thus bears the risk of cardiovascular events [84,85]. The question is as follows: could we draw such a far-reaching conclusion that Ashwagandha, by reducing stress, has a long-term protective effect on vessels and blood pressure and can reduce cardiovascular risk?

In a randomized, double-blind, placebo-controlled trial scientists investigated the efficacy and safety of Ashwagandha root extract in adults experiencing high stress and fatigue. The authors divided 120 overweight or mildly obese women and men feeling stressed and fatigued into two groups—60 of them received the placebo, and the remaining 60 received 200 mg of *W. somnifera* root extract standardized to 1.5% total withanolides, twice daily, for 12 weeks [79]. It turned out that despite a reduction in perceived stress over time, Ashwagandha did not significantly affect the blood pressure among responders.

Our question is, since the effects of hypertension occur in the long term, should the trial and observation not take longer? In fact, should we not address how long-term stress reduction from *W. somnifera* extract supplementation affects the overall cardiovascular risk?

The results of this study seem to be similar to those of another, in which 40 males and 40 females took 300 mg of Ashwagandha or placebo, for 8 weeks, twice daily, orally. According to the scientists, there were no significant changes between these two groups when it comes to body weight, body temperature, pulse rate, respiratory rate, and most interesting to us—systolic (SBP) and diastolic (DBP) BP. The measurements were collected at the baseline and after 8 weeks of supplementation. So, another study does not confirm the effect of Ashwagandha on BP nor on factors related to cardiovascular risk, such as weight [86].

However, existing research suggests that Ashwagandha may influence BP. In a further study, researchers investigated the effect of *W. somnifera* on a group of 51 people with hypertension. The first group received 2 g of Ashwagandha root powder with milk, and the second group received the same substance but with water. Before supplementation, in both groups, the mean SBP was, respectively, 164 mmHg and 157 mmHg, and after supplementation, this decreased to 158 mmHg in the first group and 154 mmHg in the second group. The difference was not significant. Surprisingly, the mean DBP after supplementation with Ashwagandha root extract decreased in the first group from 100.5 mmHg to 85 mmHg and in the second from 101.2 mmHg to 92 mmHg [87]. It seems that the hypotensive effect after *W. somnifera* supplementation is significant and more visible when it comes to DBP than SBP. Moreover, Ashwagandha root extract supplemented with milk is more effective in decreasing BP in comparison to its supplementation with water. To explain the effect of *W. somnifera* action, the authors refer to other studies. They propose that this contributes to reducing stress by *W. somnifera*, which in turn decreases activating HPA and oxidative stress, having a cardioprotective function in this way [87]. Regarding this, we maintain our earlier consideration that there may be a correlation between the stress-reducing effects of Ashwagandha and a potential reduced risk of developing cardiovascular disease, but this requires further research.

The above-mentioned results are quite different to the conclusions from another randomized, controlled, parallel-group, single-blinded study, where a group of healthy college-going young adults between 18 and 25 years old were supplemented with 500 mg capsules of *W. somnifera* extract, once daily, for 8 weeks [88]. According to the authors, in the present study, after the administration of Ashwagandha, the maximum oxygen consumption capacity increased by 6.8% at a moderate intensity, but no significant change was observed in the balance and resting BP. What is interesting in the same study was another study group in which participants were supplemented with *Terminalia arjuna*—it seems that this plant is effective in resting SBP reduction, but what is more, the biggest resting SBP reduction was observed in a group supplemented simultaneously with *W. somnifera* and *Terminalia arjuna* extract [88]. Unfortunately, a few limitations can be noted—the authors did not describe the used dosage of extracts, and more research is needed to investigate which active substances cause these effects. Are these substances contained in *Terminalia arjuna*, or in *W. somnifera*? Maybe the active substances from both of these plants interact and thus lower BP?

The studies discussed above show that Ashwagandha's effect on BP is questionable, and more research should be conducted to find out how it actually works in this area. Based on the current state of knowledge, we must conclude that *W. somnifera*'s effect on BP is doubtful. More research is needed.

Undeterred by these findings, we went a step further to find out if *W. somnifera* could be used in patients with the lethal manifestation of cardiovascular disease which myocardial infarction potentially is. It turns out that in isoprenaline (synthetic, cardiotoxic catecholamine)-induced myocardial infarction (MI) in rats, Ashwagandha gives cardioprotective effects. The authors investigated how the markers of myocardial damage were changing under the influence of Ashwagandha administration [89]. For a better assessment, they take into account the correlation between biochemical parameters (such as lipid peroxidation product malondialdehyde, endogenous antioxidants such as glutathione, antioxidant enzymes superoxide dismutase, catalase, and glutathione peroxidase, and myocardial enzymes creatinine phosphokinase and lactate dehydrogenase), functional parameters (such as mean arterial pressure, heart rate, left ventricular peak positive pressure change, left ventricular rate of peak negative pressure change, and elevated left ventricular end-diastolic pressure), and histopathological parameters in the examined hearts. It turns out that isoprenaline-induced MI caused a significant decrease in antioxidant enzymes. Interestingly, in the group treated with *W. somnifera*, the level of some antioxidant enzymes increased [89]. These data indicate that Ashwagandha has a protective effect on the myocardium by counteracting the destructive oxidative stress induced by ischemia. However, when it comes to hemodynamic parameters, as in previous studies, Ashwagandha did not improve blood pressure recordings significantly as compared to the isoprenaline control group. It also had no influence on the heart rate, but it has to be mentioned that it reduced the left ventricular end-diastolic pressure, and the myocardial relaxation (left ventricular pressure decline) was notably restored as compared to the isoprenaline control. It also improved contractility. The effects were dose-dependent.

Finishing, the authors referred to histopathological parameters and remarked that Ashwagandha did not significantly prevent myofiber loss but significantly prevented myonecrosis, as indicated by a significant reduction in the infiltration of inflammatory cells and vascular changes as well as edema as compared to the isoprenaline control group [89].

To consolidate the above knowledge, we will refer to the next study, which confirms the cardioprotective effect of *W. somnifera*. The authors divided rats into three groups—a saline control group (sham group) and an ischemia and reperfusion group (control group) where on the 31st day rats were given 45 min of left anterior descending (LAD) coronary artery ligation and 60 min of reperfusion-induced myocardial injury [90]. In the last group, the rats were administered Ashwagandha extract in a dose of 50 mg/kg, for 30 days, as an independent treatment of ischemia. On the 31st day, these rats were also given 45 min of LAD coronary artery ligation and 60 min of reperfusion-induced myocardial injury. The conclusion was drawn that *W. somnifera* significantly reduced lipid peroxidation expressed by a significant reduction in thiobarbituric acid reactive substance (TBARS) levels and restored the creatinine phosphokinase (CPK) in comparison to the control group. When it comes to the histological results, in a sham group, the myocardium had an organized pattern as a normal architecture. In rat hearts subjected to ischemia and reperfusion, the authors observed edema, myonecrosis, inflammation, and myofiber loss. In contrast to this, in a group of pre-treated Ashwagandha rats subjected to ischemia and reperfusion, the occasional focal myofiber loss, necrosis, edema, and inflammation were significantly less as compared to the control group. To summarize the immunohistochemical results, it has to be distinguished that in the Ashwagandha-treated group, the Bax (proapoptotic protein) expression was attenuated in comparison to in the control group (the results of which, in turn, showed an increase in Bax expression compared to the sham group), which suggests that *W. somnifera* may inhibit the apoptosis in injured myocardium. Pre-treatment with Ashwagandha was also associated with greater Bcl-2 expression, which is in turn an anti-apoptotic protein, in comparison to the control group [90].

The results from extensive studies present that *W. somnifera* shows cardioprotective effects due to its antioxidant properties and reduced ischemic/reperfusion-provoked apoptosis, which was confirmed biochemically, histologically, and immunohistochemically.

Another study examined the effect of Ashwagandha on ischemic/reperfused myocytes (MI/R). The subject of the research was primary neonatal cardiomyocytes (NRVMs) isolated from 1- to 2-day-old Sprague Dawley rats administered withaferin A. The apoptotic death was induced by simulated ischemia/reperfusion (SI/R) and hydrogen peroxide (H_2O_2) exposure (as a model of oxidative stress). The administration of withaferin A in cells under stress conditions—both SI/R and H_2O_2 exposure—caused increased lactate dehydrogenase (LDH) release (as an intracellular enzyme and marker of cell breakdown and apoptosis). When it comes to the molecular mechanism, the authors propose that withaferin A modulates oxidative stress/apoptosis by inducing Akt expression, which is a kinase upregulating peroxiredoxins (Prdx-1), and SOD2 and SOD3 enzymes involved in antioxidant signaling pathways. This study allows major conclusions to be drawn—oxidative stress is the cause of cell death as a result of ischemia and reperfusion, which can be prevented by administering withaferin A which modulates antioxidant processes [91].

It is also worth mentioning a study examining the influence of withaferin A on MI/R injury in wild-type and AMP-activated protein kinase domain-negative (AMPK-DN) gene transgenic mice with reduced infarct size and improved cardiac function. The authors believe that the mechanism behind this effect is the decreased activation of caspase 9 (involved in an intrinsic apoptotic way), upregulating AMP-activated protein kinase (AMPK) phosphorylation and increasing the MI/R-inhibited ratio of Bcl2/Bax. It turned out that in AMPK-DN gene transgenic mice, withaferin A administration did not reduce cardiac dysfunction and infarct size nor did it restore the Bcl2/Bax ratio, which only proves that the cardioprotective mechanism of this substance's action in the ischemic myocardium is based on the upregulation of the anti-apoptotic mitochondrial pathway in an AMPK-dependent manner [12].

These studies proved that Ashwagandha and its active compounds via its upregulation of the anti-apoptotic mitochondrial pathway and antioxidative action play a cardioprotective role. It cannot be ignored that withaferin A is more effective in the case of smaller doses in both of the research works.

In the studies discussed above, the perceived limitations include the lack of descriptions of the active substances responsible for specific effects, the lack of standardization of doses, and the limited number of clinical trials conducted on the protective effects of Ashwagandha on the cardiovascular system. It seems that *W. somnifera* may have potential cardioprotective properties, but more research is needed to clarify the mechanisms of its action and the reasons for the discrepancies in the above-described studies. Table 3 shows a summary of the research discussed in this chapter.

Table 3. Summary of reviewed research.

Authors	Subject of Study	Dose	Results
Smith et al. (2023) [79]	120 overweight or mildly obese women and men	200 mg of WS root extract standardized to 1.5% total withanolides, twice daily, for 12 weeks	↓ stress; No significant change in BP
Verma et al. (2021) [86]	Randomized, double-blind, placebo-controlled, and parallel-group study; 80 healthy participants	Ashwagandha root extract 300 mg for 8 weeks	No AE reported; ↔ BW, BP; ↔ ALT, AST, ALP; ↔ TSH, fT3, fT4
Kushwaha et al. (2012) [87]	51 stress-oriented hypertensive subjects in the age group of 40 to 70 years old	2 g Ashwagandha root powder, orally, for 91 days (with milk or with water)	↔ BMI; ↔ SBP; ↓ DBP
Sandhu et al. (2010) [88]	Healthy college-going young adults between 18 and 25 years old	500 mg capsules of WS extract (no information about used dosage in capsules) once daily, for 8 weeks	↑ maximum oxygen consumption capacity at moderate intensity; No significant change was observed in balance and resting BP; ↓ resting SBP when supplemented simultaneously with WS and *Terminalia arjuna* extract
Mohanty et al. (2004) [89]	Wistar albino male rats	25, 50, and 100 mg/kg orally for 4 weeks	↑ glutathione (50 and 100 mg/kg); ↑ antioxidant enzyme glutathione peroxidase; ↑ superoxide dismutase; ↑ lactate dehydrogenase; ↑ creatinine phosphokinase; ↔ blood pressure; ↓ left ventricular end-diastolic pressure; ↑ myocardial relaxation (left ventricular pressure decline); ↑ contractility (50 mg/kg); ↓ myonecrosis and ↓ edema
Mohanty et al. (2008) [90]	Adult male Wistar rats	Hydro-alcoholic extract of WS (50 mg/kg) orally, for 30 days	↑ GSH, ↓ TBARS, ↑ CPK; ↓ Bax protein, ↑ Bcl-2; ↓ TUNEL-positive cells
Langade et al. (2019) [83]	Randomized, double-blind, placebo-controlled study of 60 patients with insomnia	Ashwagandha root extract, 300 mg	↓ SOL, ↓ WASO; ↑ TST, ↑ TIB, ↑ SE; ↓ PSQI; ↓ HAM-A
Yan et al. (2018) [91]	Primary neonatal cardiomyocytes (NRVMs) were isolated from 1- to 2-day-old Sprague Dawley rats; 8–10-week-old wild-type mice	fWFA (0 nM, 100 nM, 1000 nM)	↓ apoptotic cell death; ↑ HO-1, ↑ Prdx-1, ↑ SOD-2 (via activation of Akt pathway); ↓ ROS
Guo et al. (2019) [12]	Adult male wild-type (WT) mice and adult male AMPK-DN mice [dominant negative α2-subunit (D157A) of AMPK]	Low-dose (1 mg/kg) or high-dose (5 mg/kg) WFA	(1 mg/kg) ↑ LVEF, ↑ dP/dtmax and dP/dtmin, ↓ infarct size; (5 mg/kg) ↓ dP/dtmax and dP/dtmin (both) ↓ TUNEL staining, ↓ caspase-3 activity; ↑ Bcl2, ↓ Bcl2/ Bax; ↑ AMPK

Note: ↓ reduction, ↑ increase, and ↔ irrelevant; abbreviations: BW—body weight; ALT—alanine transaminase; AST—aspartate transaminase; ALP—alkaline phosphatase; TSH—thyroid-stimulating hormone; fT3—free tri-iodothyronine; fT4—free thyroxine; SOL—sleep onset latency; WASO—wage after sleep onset; TST—total sleep time; TIB—total time in bed; SE—sleep efficiency; PSQI—Pittsburgh Sleep Quality Index; LVEF—left ventricular ejection fraction; GSH—glutathione; WS—*W. somnifera*.

6. Limitations

Despite the promising results of the studies discussed in the chapters above, there are several limitations worth considering. Data from large clinical trials examining Ashwagandha as a medicine are still lacking. It seems reasonable to ask whether Ashwagandha extracts can be used as a standalone treatment for a specific condition or rather as a complementary therapy—an adjuvant to conventional treatment. It is also worth mentioning that most preparations with this plant extract are dietary supplements, which is associated with an easier registration procedure for such products [92].

Ashwagandha root extract is widely regarded as safe and well tolerated [48,86]. On the other hand, it is important to note that plant extracts can have many side effects and contraindications [93]. Recent studies have shown that Ashwagandha is a factor in herbal-induced liver injury (HILI). Ashwagandha-induced HILI manifests as cholestatic hepatitis. In addition, it can lead to acute and chronic liver failure syndrome, which is associated with a high mortality rate. There is an increased risk in people with pre-existing liver disease [94]. In patients with hyperthyroidism, *W. somnifera* extracts can cause symptoms such as irritability, restlessness, nervousness, hand tremors, palpitations, psychomotor agitation, muscle fatigue, and reduced libido [3]. Due to the enhancement in testosterone production by Ashwagandha, men with hormone-sensitive prostate cancer should avoid its use, as it intensifies the progression of the disease [7]. Furthermore, for women planning pregnancies, the use of higher doses of *W. somnifera* root extract can cause miscarriages [7]. Moreover, Ashwagandha has additive effects with anticonvulsants, anti-anxiety medications, and antidepressants, which may lead to a dangerous increase in their side effects [95]. Therefore, despite the relative safety of this plant preparation, it is important to educate patients and medical staff whenever such products are recommended. Importantly, patients' self-administration of Ashwagandha runs the risk of not controlling other therapies they receive [3].

Another important issue regarding *W. somnifera* is the standardization of the raw material and the assessment of the bioavailability of the active substances from these preparations [3]. The studies discussed above often lacked the standardization of the extracts to a specific content of active substances; hence, the interpretation of the results and comparison between studies are challenging. Some studies have shown that the active compounds contained in Ashwagandha extracts, e.g., withaferin A, have low bioavailability. This fact results in a lower therapeutic effect caused by these substances. Therefore, an important issue seems to be the development of an appropriate formulation of potential drugs, which poses a major challenge for subsequent researchers [3,96]. An additional challenge is that *W. somnifera* is a plant consisting of various components with differing properties. This creates a broad scope for further research in this area to enable the use of *W. somnifera* for disease prevention or treatment.

7. Conclusions

This review of the research presented above shows the wide range of effects of Ashwagandha extract on metabolism. Several substances in it (alkaloids, steroids, and probably the most important withanolides) influence various metabolic pathways, thus causing various effects and possibly modifying the course of diseases.

Ashwagandha has a broad effect on the endothelium. It shows an anti-angiogenic impact by inhibiting VEGF-induced capillary sprouting and formation by lowering the mean microvessel density. Also, it causes a significant increase in NO production and alleviates oxidative stress by reducing reactive oxygen species levels.

The text above discusses research on the multidirectional impact of *W. somnifera* on the immune system, producing an anti-inflammatory effect. Ashwagandha has properties that attenuate type 2 allergic reactions by a reduction in cytokines IL-4, IL-13, TNF-α, and IgE, reduction in cortisol levels, as well as stress, the selective blocking of COX2 and inhibition of LPS-induced inflammation, and the inhibition of the activity of ACE2, MPO, and IL-6. Anti-inflammatory and antioxidant properties were proven in the liver and kidney. Additionally, the adaptogenic function of *W. somnifera* was proved to influence transcription RNA, resulting in the regulation of cellular metabolism and maintenance of homeostasis.

Ashwagandha extract also affects lipid metabolism. It inhibits the differentiation of preadipocytes into adipocytes, can enhance energy expenditure by improving mitochondrial function in adipose tissue and skeletal muscle, and shows a significant reduction in lipid levels.

These results suggest that Ashwagandha has many benefits. By exhibiting the above-mentioned effects, this plant can be expected to have a major impact on cardiovascular disease and thus improve cardiovascular outcomes. However, the implications for human health are still noteworthy. There are discrepancies in the scientific research performed.

On the one hand, Ashwagandha did not affect significantly blood pressure. The effect on BP is questionable, and more research should be conducted. There is no significant effect on body weight, body temperature, pulse rate, or respiratory rate. On the other hand, Ashwagandha has a protective effect on the myocardium by counteracting the destructive oxidative stress induced by ischemia. Cardioprotective effects (due to its antioxidant properties and reduced ischemic/reperfusion-provoked apoptosis) have been biochemically, histologically, and immunohistochemically proven.

It seems that *W. somnifera* may have potential mainly anti-inflammatory effects and hence cardioprotective, immunomodulatory, neuroprotective, hepatoprotective, anti-diabetic, adaptogenic, anti-arthritic, and anti-stress effects, but it is still unknown to what extent it has a real impact on the course of diseases. More research is needed to explain the mechanism of action of the substances contained in Ashwagandha to clarify the reasons for the discrepancies in the above-described studies and, most importantly, what real impact they have on patients' health.

Author Contributions: Conceptualization, M.W.; methodology, M.W. and A.F.-M.; writing—original draft preparation, Z.K., S.L., P.S., M.S. (Monika Szambelan), B.G. and I.R.; writing—review and editing, A.F.-M., Z.K., S.L., P.S., M.S. (Monika Szambelan), B.G. and I.R.; visualization, A.F.-M.; supervision, M.W., M.S. (Maciej Słupski) and I.S.-K.; project administration, M.W.; funding acquisition, M.W. All authors have read and agreed to the published version of the manuscript.

Funding: This research received no external funding.

Conflicts of Interest: The authors declare no conflicts of interest.

References

1. Gregory, J.; Vengalasetti, Y.V.; Bredesen, D.E.; Rao, R.V. Neuroprotective Herbs for the Management of Alzheimer's Disease. *Biomolecules* **2021**, *11*, 543. [CrossRef]
2. Luthra, R.; Roy, A. Role of Medicinal Plants against Neurodegenerative Diseases. *Curr. Pharm. Biotechnol.* **2022**, *23*, 123–139. [CrossRef]
3. Wiciński, M.; Fajkiel-Madajczyk, A.; Kurant, Z.; Kurant, D.; Gryczka, K.; Falkowski, M.; Wiśniewska, M.; Słupski, M.; Ohla, J.; Zabrzyński, J. Can Ashwagandha Benefit the Endocrine System?—A Review. *Int. J. Mol. Sci.* **2023**, *24*, 16513. [CrossRef]
4. Kashyap, V.K.; Peasah-Darkwah, G.; Dhasmana, A.; Jaggi, M.; Yallapu, M.M.; Chauhan, S.C. *Withania somnifera*: Progress towards a Pharmaceutical Agent for Immunomodulation and Cancer Therapeutics. *Pharmaceutics* **2022**, *14*, 611. [CrossRef]
5. Della Porta, M.; Maier, J.A.; Cazzola, R. Effects of *Withania somnifera* on Cortisol Levels in Stressed Human Subjects: A Systematic Review. *Nutrients* **2023**, *15*, 5015. [CrossRef]
6. Leonard, M.; Dickerson, B.; Estes, L.; Gonzalez, D.E.; Jenkins, V.; Johnson, S.; Xing, D.; Yoo, C.; Ko, J.; Purpura, M.; et al. Acute and Repeated Ashwagandha Supplementation Improves Markers of Cognitive Function and Mood. *Nutrients* **2024**, *16*, 1813. [CrossRef]
7. Mikulska, P.; Malinowska, M.; Ignacyk, M.; Szustowski, P.; Nowak, J.; Pesta, K.; Szeląg, M.; Szklanny, D.; Judasz, E.; Kaczmarek, G.; et al. Ashwagandha (*Withania somnifera*)—Current Research on the Health-Promoting Activities: A Narrative Review. *Pharmaceutics* **2023**, *15*, 1057. [CrossRef]
8. Mandlik Ingawale, D.S.; Namdeo, A.G. Pharmacological evaluation of Ashwagandha highlighting its healthcare claims, safety, and toxicity aspects. *J. Diet. Suppl.* **2021**, *18*, 183–226. [CrossRef]
9. Afewerky, H.K.; Ayodeji, A.E.; Tiamiyu, B.B.; Orege, J.I.; Okeke, E.S.; Oyejobi, A.O.; Bate, P.N.N.; Adeyemi, S.B. Critical review of the *Withania somnifera* (L.) Dunal: Ethnobotany, pharmacological efficacy, and commercialization significance in Africa. *Bull. Natl. Res. Cent.* **2021**, *45*, 176. [CrossRef]
10. Lee, S.R.; Lee, B.S.; Yu, J.S.; Kang, H.; Yoo, M.J.; Yi, S.A.; Han, J.W.; Kim, S.; Kim, J.K.; Kim, J.C.; et al. Identification of anti-adipogenic withanolides from the roots of Indian ginseng (*Withania somnifera*). *J. Ginseng Res.* **2022**, *46*, 357–366. [CrossRef]

11. Cavaleri, F.; Chattopadhyay, S.; Palsule, V.; Kar, P.K.; Chatterjee, R. Study of Drug Target Identification and Associated Molecular Mechanisms for the Therapeutic Activity and Hair Follicle Induction of Two Ashwagandha Extracts Having Differential Withanolide Constitutions. *J. Nutr. Metab.* **2023**, *2023*, 9599744. [CrossRef]
12. Guo, R.; Gan, L.; Lau, W.B.; Yan, Z.; Xie, D.; Gao, E.; Christopher, T.A.; Lopez, B.L.; Ma, X.; Wang, Y. Withaferin A Prevents Myocardial Ischemia/Reperfusion Injury by Upregulating AMP-Activated Protein Kinase-Dependent B-Cell Lymphoma2 Signaling. *Circ. J.* **2019**, *83*, 1726–1736. [CrossRef]
13. Krüger-Genge, A.; Blocki, A.; Franke, R.-P.; Jung, F. Vascular Endothelial Cell Biology: An Update. *Int. J. Mol. Sci.* **2019**, *20*, 4411. [CrossRef]
14. Rajendran, P.; Rengarajan, T.; Thangavel, J.; Nishigaki, Y.; Sakthisekaran, D.; Sethi, G.; Nishigaki, I. The vascular endothelium and human diseases. *Int. J. Biol. Sci.* **2013**, *9*, 1057–1069. [CrossRef]
15. Cahill, P.A.; Redmond, E.M. Vascular endothelium—Gatekeeper of vessel health. *Atherosclerosis* **2016**, *248*, 97–109. [CrossRef]
16. La Mendola, D.; Trincavelli, M.L.; Martini, C. Angiogenesis in Disease. *Int. J. Mol. Sci.* **2022**, *23*, 10962. [CrossRef]
17. Griffioen, A.W.; Dudley, A.C. The rising impact of angiogenesis research. *Angiogenesis* **2022**, *25*, 435–437. [CrossRef]
18. Carmeliet, P. VEGF as a key mediator of angiogenesis in cancer. *Oncology* **2005**, *69*, 4–10. [CrossRef]
19. Mathur, R.; Gupta, S.K.; Singh, N.; Mathur, S.; Kochupillai, V.; Velpandian, T. Evaluation of the effect of *Withania somnifera* root extracts on cell cycle and angiogenesis. *J. Ethnopharmacol.* **2006**, *105*, 336–341. [CrossRef]
20. Wang, Y.; Le, W.D. Autophagy and Ubiquitin-Proteasome System. *Adv. Exp. Med. Biol.* **2019**, *1206*, 527–550. [CrossRef]
21. Staszczak, M. Szlak ubikwityna-proteasom jako cel strategii terapeutycznych [Ubiquitin-proteasome pathway as a target for therapeutic strategies]. *Postepy Biochem.* **2017**, *63*, 287–303. [PubMed]
22. Shang, F.; Taylor, A. Roles for the ubiquitin-proteasome pathway in protein quality control and signaling in the retina: Implications in the pathogenesis of age-related macular degeneration. *Mol. Aspects Med.* **2012**, *33*, 446–466. [CrossRef] [PubMed]
23. Bakshi, H.A.; Quinn, G.A.; Nasef, M.M.; Mishra, V.; Aljabali, A.A.A.; El-Tanani, M.; Serrano-Aroca, Á.; Webba Da Silva, M.; McCarron, P.A.; Tambuwala, M.M. Crocin Inhibits Angiogenesis and Metastasis in Colon Cancer via TNF-α/NF-kB/VEGF Pathways. *Cells* **2022**, *11*, 1502. [CrossRef] [PubMed]
24. Bąska, P.; Norbury, L.J. The Role of Nuclear Factor Kappa B (NF-κB) in the Immune Response against Parasites. *Pathogens* **2022**, *11*, 310. [CrossRef] [PubMed]
25. Thoma, A.; Lightfoot, A.P. NF-kB and Inflammatory Cytokine Signalling: Role in Skeletal Muscle Atrophy. *Adv. Exp. Med. Biol.* **2018**, *1088*, 267–279. [CrossRef] [PubMed]
26. Mohan, R.; Hammers, H.J.; Bargagna-Mohan, P.; Zhan, X.H.; Herbstritt, C.J.; Ruiz, A.; Zhang, L.; Hanson, A.D.; Conner, B.P.; Rougas, J.; et al. Withaferin A is a potent inhibitor of angiogenesis. *Angiogenesis* **2004**, *7*, 115–122. [CrossRef] [PubMed]
27. Bargagna-Mohan, P.; Ravindranath, P.P.; Mohan, R. Small molecule anti-angiogenic probes of the ubiquitin proteasome pathway: Potential application to choroidal neovascularization. *Investig. Ophthalmol. Vis. Sci.* **2006**, *47*, 4138–4145. [CrossRef] [PubMed]
28. Tousoulis, D.; Kampoli, A.M.; Tentolouris, C.; Papageorgiou, N.; Stefanadis, C. The role of nitric oxide on endothelial function. *Curr. Vasc. Pharmacol.* **2012**, *10*, 4–18. [CrossRef]
29. Pathak, P.; Shukla, P.; Kanshana, J.S.; Jagavelu, K.; Sangwan, N.S.; Dwivedi, A.K.; Dikshit, M. Standardized root extract of *Withania somnifera* and Withanolide A exert moderate vasorelaxant effect in the rat aortic rings by enhancing nitric oxide generation. *J. Ethnopharmacol.* **2021**, *278*, 114296. [CrossRef]
30. Cyr, A.R.; Huckaby, L.V.; Shiva, S.S.; Zuckerbraun, B.S. Nitric Oxide and Endothelial Dysfunction. *Crit. Care Clin.* **2020**, *36*, 307–321. [CrossRef]
31. Iuvone, T.; Esposito, G.; Capasso, F.; Izzo, A.A. Induction of nitric oxide synthase expression by *Withania somnifera* in macrophages. *Life Sci.* **2003**, *72*, 1617–1625. [CrossRef]
32. Incalza, M.A.; D'Oria, R.; Natalicchio, A.; Perrini, S.; Laviola, L.; Giorgino, F. Oxidative stress and reactive oxygen species in endothelial dysfunction associated with cardiovascular and metabolic diseases. *Vascul Pharmacol.* **2018**, *100*, 1–19. [CrossRef]
33. Shaito, A.; Aramouni, K.; Assaf, R.; Parenti, A.; Orekhov, A.; Yazbi, A.E.; Pintus, G.; Eid, A.H. Oxidative Stress-Induced Endothelial Dysfunction in Cardiovascular Diseases. *Front. Biosci.* **2022**, *27*, 105. [CrossRef] [PubMed]
34. Khalil, M.I.; Ahmmed, I.; Ahmed, R.; Tanvir, E.M.; Afroz, R.; Paul, S.; Gan, S.H.; Alam, N. Amelioration of Isoproterenol-Induced Oxidative Damage in Rat Myocardium by *Withania somnifera* Leaf Extract. *Biomed. Res. Int.* **2015**, *2015*, 624159. [CrossRef]
35. Kaur, G.; Singh, N.; Samuel, S.S.; Bora, H.K.; Sharma, S.; Pachauri, S.D.; Dwivedi, A.K.; Siddiqui, H.H.; Hanif, K. *Withania somnifera* shows a protective effect in monocrotaline-induced pulmonary hypertension. *Pharm. Biol.* **2015**, *53*, 147–157. [CrossRef] [PubMed]
36. Kim, G.; Kim, T.H.; Kang, M.J.; Choi, J.A.; Pack, D.Y.; Lee, I.R.; Kim, M.G.; Han, S.S.; Kim, B.Y.; Oh, S.M.; et al. Inhibitory effect of withaferin A on Helicobacter pylori-induced IL-8 production and NF-κB activation in gastric epithelial cells. *Mol. Med. Rep.* **2016**, *13*, 967–972. [CrossRef]
37. Chaudhary, A.; Kalra, R.S.; Malik, V.; Katiyar, S.P.; Sundar, D.; Kaul, S.C.; Wadhwa, R. 2,3-Dihydro-3β-methoxy Withaferin-A Lacks Anti-Metastasis Potency: Bioinformatics and Experimental Evidences. *Sci. Rep.* **2019**, *9*, 17344. [CrossRef]
38. Sanada, F.; Taniyama, Y.; Muratsu, J.; Otsu, R.; Shimizu, H.; Rakugi, H.; Morishita, R. Source of chronic inflammation in aging. *Front. Cardiovasc. Med.* **2018**, *5*, 12. [CrossRef] [PubMed]
39. Kany, S.; Vollrath, J.; Relja, B. Cytokines in Inflammatory Disease. *Int. J. Mol. Sci.* **2019**, *20*, 6008. [CrossRef]

40. Jiapaer, Z.; Su, D.; Hua, L.; Lehmann, H.I.; Gokulnath, P.; Vulugundam, G.; Li, G. Regulation and roles of RNA modifications in aging-related diseases. *Aging Cell* **2022**, *21*, e13657. [CrossRef]
41. Kiran, R.G. Comparative study of anti-inflammatory activity of *Withania somnifera* (Ashwagandha) with hydrocortisone in experimental animals (Albino rats). *J. Med. Plants Stud.* **2016**, *4*, 78–83.
42. Devarasetti, A.K.; Bharani, K.K.; Anand, A.K.S.; Kollipaka, R.; Saranu, V.D.T. Adaptogenic Ashwagandha root extract modulates inflammatory markers in feline stress management: A double-blind placebo-controlled clinical trial. *J. Appl. Anim. Res.* **2023**, *52*, 2335921. [CrossRef]
43. Kanjilal, S.; Gupta, A.K.; Patnaik, R.S.; Dey, A. Analysis of Clinical Trial Registry of India for Evidence of Anti-Arthritic Properties of *Withania somnifera* (Ashwagandha). *Altern. Ther. Health Med.* **2021**, *27*, 58–66. [PubMed]
44. Galli, S.J.; Tsai, M.; Piliponsky, A.M. The development of allergic inflammation. *Nature* **2008**, *454*, 445–454. [CrossRef] [PubMed]
45. Saggam, A.; Limgaokar, K.; Borse, S.; Chavan-Gautam, P.; Dixit, S.; Tillu, G.; Patwardhan, B. *Withania somnifera* (L.) dunal: Opportunity for clinical repurposing in COVID-19 management. *Front. Pharmacol.* **2021**, *12*, 623795. [CrossRef] [PubMed]
46. Zhao, H.M.; Gao, Z.W.; Xie, S.X.; Han, X.; Sun, Q.S. Withaferin A attenuates ovalbumin induced airway inflammation. *Front. Biosci.* **2019**, *24*, 576–596. [CrossRef] [PubMed]
47. Paul, S.; Chakraborty, S.; Anand, U.; Dey, S.; Nandy, S.; Ghorai, M.; Saha, S.C.; Patil, M.T.; Kandimalla, R.; Proćków, J.; et al. *Withania somnifera* (L.) Dunal (Ashwagandha): A comprehensive review on ethnopharmacology, pharmacotherapeutics, biomedicinal and toxicological aspects. *Biomed. Pharmacother* **2021**, *143*, 112175. [CrossRef] [PubMed]
48. Lopresti, A.L.; Smith, S.J.; Malvi, H.; Kodgule, R. An investigation into the stress-relieving and pharmacological actions of an ashwagandha (*Withania somnifera*) extract: A randomized, double-blind, placebo-controlled study. *Medicine* **2019**, *98*, e17186. [CrossRef]
49. Salve, J.; Pate, S.; Debnath, K.; Langade, D. Adaptogenic and Anxiolytic Effects of Ashwagandha Root Extract in Healthy Adults: A Double-blind, Randomized, Placebo-controlled Clinical Study. *Cureus* **2019**, *11*, e6466. [CrossRef]
50. Orrù, A.; Marchese, G.; Ruiu, S. Alkaloids in *Withania somnifera* (L.) Dunal root extract contribute to its anti-inflammatory activity. *Pharmacology* **2023**, *108*, 301–307. [CrossRef]
51. Saleem, S.; Muhammad, G.; Hussain, M.A.; Altaf, M.; Bukhari, S.N.A. *Withania somnifera* L.: Insights into the phytochemical profile, therapeutic potential, clinical trials, and future prospective. Iran. *J. Basic. Med. Sci.* **2020**, *23*, 1501–1526. [CrossRef]
52. Fazil, M.H.U.T.; Chirumamilla, C.S.; Perez-Novo, C.; Wong, B.H.S.; Kumar, S.; Sze, S.K.; Berghe, W.V.; Verma, N.K. The steroidal lactone withaferin A impedes T-cell motility by inhibiting the kinase ZAP70 and subsequent kinome signaling. *J. Biol. Chem.* **2021**, *297*, 101377. [CrossRef]
53. Singh, P.; Salman, K.A.; Shameem, M.; Warsi, M.S. *Withania somnifera* (L.) Dunal as Add-On Therapy for COPD Patients: A Randomized, Placebo-Controlled, Double-Blind Study. *Front. Pharmacol.* **2022**, *13*, 901710. [CrossRef] [PubMed]
54. Rungratanawanich, W.; Qu, Y.; Wang, X.; Essa, M.M.; Song, B.J. Advanced glycation end products (AGEs) and other adducts in aging-related diseases and alcoholmediated tissue injury. *Exp. Mol. Med.* **2021**, *53*, 168–188. [CrossRef] [PubMed]
55. Atluri, V.S.R.; Tiwari, S.; Rodriguez, M.; Kaushik, A.; Yndart, A.; Kolishetti, N.; Nair, M. Inhibition of amyloid-Beta production, associated Neuroinflammation, and histone deacetylase 2-mediated epigenetic modifications prevent neuropathology in Alzheimer's disease in vitro model. *Front. Aging Neurosci.* **2020**, *11*, 342. [CrossRef] [PubMed]
56. Panossian, A.; Seo, E.J.; Efferth, T. Novel molecular mechanisms for the adaptogenic effects of herbal extracts on isolated brain cells using systems biology. *Phytomedicine* **2018**, *50*, 257–284. [CrossRef] [PubMed]
57. Lin, H.; Hou, C.C.; Cheng, C.F.; Chiu, T.H.; Hsu, Y.H.; Sue, Y.M.; Chen, C.H. Peroxisomal proliferator-activated receptor-alpha protects renal tubular cells from doxorubicin-induced apoptosis. *Mol. Pharmacol.* **2007**, *72*, 1238–1245. [CrossRef] [PubMed]
58. Esteban, V.; Lorenzo, O.; Suzuki, Y.; Mezzano, S.; Blanco, J.; Kretzler, M.; Ruiz-Ortega, M. Angiotensin II, via AT1 and AT2 receptors and NF-kappaB pathway, regulates the inflammatory response in unilateral ureteral obstruction. *J. Am. Soc. Nephrol.* **2004**, *15*, 1514–1529. [CrossRef] [PubMed]
59. Grunz-Borgmann, E.; Mossine, V.; Fritsche, K.; Parrish, A.R. Ashwagandha attenuates TNF-α- and LPS-induced NF-κB activation and CCL2 and CCL5 gene expression in NRK-52E cells. *BMC Complement. Altern. Med.* **2015**, *15*, 434. [CrossRef]
60. Devkar, S.T.; Kandhare, A.D.; Zanwar, A.A.; Jagtap, S.D.; Katyare, S.S.; Bodhankar, S.L.; Hegde, M.V. Hepatoprotective effect of withanolide-rich fraction in acetaminophen-intoxicated rat: Decisive role of TNF-α, IL-1β, COX-II and iNOS. *Pharm. Biol.* **2016**, *54*, 2394–2403. [CrossRef]
61. Kaileh, M.; Vanden Berghe, W.; Heyerick, A.; Horion, J.; Piette, J.; Libert, C.; De Keukeleire, D.; Essawi, T.; Haegeman, G. Withaferin a strongly elicits IkappaB kinase beta hyperphosphorylation concomitant with potent inhibition of its kinase activity. *J. Biol. Chem.* **2007**, *282*, 4253–4264. [CrossRef] [PubMed]
62. Zheng, W.; Zhang, J.; Jiang, Y.; Wang, S.; Yang, Z. Overlapping Pattern of the Four Individual Components of Dyslipidemia in Adults: Analysis of Nationally Representative Data. *J. Clin. Med.* **2024**, *13*, 3624. [CrossRef] [PubMed]
63. Sharebiani, H.; Mokaram, M.; Mirghani, M.; Fazeli, B.; Stanek, A. The Effects of Antioxidant Supplementation on the Pathologic Mechanisms of Metabolic Syndrome and Cardiovascular Disease Development. *Nutrients* **2024**, *16*, 1641. [CrossRef] [PubMed]
64. Stewart, J.; McCallin, T.; Martinez, J.; Chacko, S.; Yusuf, S. Hyperlipidemia. *Pediatr. Rev.* **2020**, *41*, 393–402. [CrossRef]
65. Ruze, R.; Liu, T.; Zou, X.; Song, J.; Chen, Y.; Xu, R.; Yin, X.; Xu, Q. Obesity and type 2 diabetes mellitus: Connections in epidemiology, pathogenesis, and treatments. *Front. Endocrinol* **2023**, *14*, 1161521. [CrossRef] [PubMed]
66. Karr, S. Epidemiology and management of hyperlipidemia. *Am. J. Manag. Care.* **2017**, *23*, S139–S148.

67. Lee, D.-H.; Ahn, J.; Jang, Y.-J.; Seo, H.-D.; Ha, T.-Y.; Kim, M.J.; Huh, Y.H.; Jung, C.H. *Withania somnifera* Extract Enhances Energy Expenditure via Improving Mitochondrial Function in Adipose Tissue and Skeletal Muscle. *Nutrients* **2020**, *12*, 431. [CrossRef]
68. Zahran, E.; El Sebaei, M.G.; Awadin, W.; Elbahnaswy, S.; Risha, E.; Elseady, Y. *Withania somnifera* dietary supplementation improves lipid profile, intestinal histomorphology in healthy Nile tilapia (*Oreochromis niloticus*), and modulates cytokines response to *Streptococcus* infection. *Fish. Shellfish. Immunol.* **2020**, *106*, 133–141. [CrossRef] [PubMed]
69. Zhang, L.; Shi, Y.; Yan, M.; Zhang, G. Modulatory action of withaferin-A on oxidative damage through regulation of inflammatory mediators and apoptosis via PI3K/AKT signaling pathway in high cholesterol-induced atherosclerosis in experimental rats. *J. Biochem. Mol. Toxicol.* **2022**, *36*, e23154. [CrossRef]
70. Abu Bakar, M.H.; Azmi, M.N.; Shariff, K.A.; Tan, J.S. Withaferin A Protects Against High-Fat Diet-Induced Obesity Via Attenuation of Oxidative Stress, Inflammation, and Insulin Resistance. *Appl. Biochem. Biotechnol.* **2019**, *188*, 241–259. [CrossRef]
71. Soh, S.; Ong, W.-Y. Effect of Withanolide A on 7-Ketocholesterol Induced Cytotoxicity in hCMEC/D3 Brain Endothelial Cells. *Cells* **2022**, *11*, 457. [CrossRef]
72. Rakha, A.; Ramzan, Z.; Umar, N.; Rasheed, H.; Fatima, A.; Ahmed, Z.; Kieliszek, M.; Aadil, R.M. The Role of Ashwagandha in Metabolic Syndrome: A Review of Traditional Knowledge and Recent Research Findings. *J. Biol. Regul. Homeost. Agents* **2023**, *37*, 5091–5103. [CrossRef]
73. Lee, B.S.; Yoo, M.J.; Kang, H.; Lee, S.R.; Kim, S.; Yu, J.S.; Kim, J.C.; Jang, T.S.; Pang, C.; Kim, K.H. Withasomniferol D, a New Anti-Adipogenic Withanolide from the Roots of Ashwagandha (*Withania somnifera*). *Pharmaceuticals* **2021**, *14*, 1017. [CrossRef] [PubMed]
74. Akhani, S.; Gotmare, S.R. Hypolipidemic effect of Ashwagandha (*Withania somnifera*) and Arjuna (Terminalia arjuna): An in vitro study. *Natl. J. Physiol. Pharm. Pharmacol.* **2023**, *13*, 1084–1087. [CrossRef]
75. Cardiovascular Diseases. Available online: https://www.who.int/health-topics/cardiovascular-diseases#tab=tab_1 (accessed on 11 June 2024).
76. Wiciński, M.; Górski, K.; Wódkiewicz, E.; Walczak, M.; Nowaczewska, M.; Malinowski, B. Vasculoprotective Effects of Vildagliptin. Focus on Atherogenesis. *Int. J. Mol. Sci.* **2020**, *21*, 2275. [CrossRef] [PubMed]
77. Bidani, A.K.; Griffin, K.A. Long-term renal consequences of hypertension for normal and diseased kidneys. *Curr. Opin. Nephrol. Hypertens.* **2002**, *11*, 73–80. [CrossRef]
78. Dziedziak, J.; Zaleska-Zmijewska, A.; Szaflik, J.P.; Cudnoch-Jędrzejewska, A. Impact of Arterial Hypertension on the Eye: A Review of the Pathogenesis, Diagnostic Methods, and Treatment of Hypertensive Retinopathy. *Med. Sci. Monit.* **2022**, *28*, e935135. [CrossRef] [PubMed]
79. Smith, S.J.; Lopresti, A.L.; Fairchild, T.J. Exploring the efficacy and safety of a novel standardized ashwagandha (*Withania somnifera*) root extract (Witholytin®) in adults experiencing high stress and fatigue in a randomized, double-blind, placebo-controlled trial. *J. Psychopharmacol.* **2023**, *37*, 1091. [CrossRef] [PubMed]
80. Gopukumar, K.; Thanawala, S.; Somepalli, V.; Rao, T.S.S.; Thamatam, V.B.; Chauhan, S. Efficacy and Safety of Ashwagandha Root Extract on Cognitive Functions in Healthy, Stressed Adults: A Randomized, Double-Blind, Placebo-Controlled Study. *Evid. Based Complement. Alternat. Med.* **2021**, *2021*, 8254344. [CrossRef]
81. Esmaealzadeh, N.; Iranpanah, A.; Sarris, J.; Rahimi, R. A literature review of the studies concerning selected plant-derived adaptogens and their general function in body with a focus on animal studies. *Phytomedicine* **2022**, *105*, 154354. [CrossRef]
82. Speers, A.B.; Cabey, K.A.; Soumyanath, A.; Wright, K.M. Effects of *Withania somnifera* (Ashwagandha) on Stress and the Stress-Related Neuropsychiatric Disorders Anxiety, Depression, and Insomnia. *Curr. Neuropharmacol.* **2021**, *19*, 1468–1495. [CrossRef] [PubMed]
83. Langade, D.; Kanchi, S.; Salve, J.; Debnath, K.; Ambegaokar, D. Efficacy and Safety of Ashwagandha (*Withania somnifera*) Root Extract in Insomnia and Anxiety: A Double-blind, Randomized, Placebo-controlled Study. *Cureus* **2019**, *11*, e5797. [CrossRef] [PubMed]
84. Osborne, M.T.; Shin, L.M.; Mehta, N.N.; Pitman, R.K.; Fayad, Z.A.; Tawakol, A. Disentangling the Links Between Psychosocial Stress and Cardiovascular Disease. *Circ. Cardiovasc. Imaging* **2020**, *13*, e010931. [CrossRef] [PubMed]
85. Matthews, K.A.; Katholi, C.R.; McCreath, H.; Whooley, M.A.; Williams, D.R.; Zhu, S.; Markovitz, J.H. Blood pressure reactivity to psychological stress predicts hypertension in the CARDIA study. *Circulation* **2004**, *110*, 74–78. [CrossRef] [PubMed]
86. Verma, N.; Gupta, S.K.; Tiwari, S.; Mishra, A.K. Safety of Ashwagandha Root Extract: A Randomized, Placebo-Controlled, study in Healthy Volunteers. *Complement. Ther. Med.* **2021**, *57*, 102642. [CrossRef]
87. Kushwaha, S.; Betsy, A.; Chawla, P. Effect of Ashwagandha (*Withania somnifera*) root powder supplementation in treatment of hypertension. *Stud. Ethno-Med.* **2012**, *6*, 111–115. [CrossRef]
88. Sandhu, J.S.; Shah, B.; Shenoy, S.; Chauhan, S.; Lavekar, G.S.; Padhi, M.M. Effects of *Withania somnifera* (Ashwagandha) and Terminalia arjuna (Arjuna) on physical performance and cardiorespiratory endurance in healthy young adults. *Int. J. Ayurveda Res.* **2010**, *1*, 144. [CrossRef] [PubMed]
89. Mohanty, I.; Arya, D.S.; Dinda, A.; Talwar, K.K.; Joshi, S.; Gupta, S.K. Mechanisms of cardioprotective effect of *Withania somnifera* in experimentally induced myocardial infarction. *Basic. Clin. Pharmacol. Toxicol.* **2004**, *94*, 184–190. [CrossRef]
90. Mohanty, I.R.; Arya, D.S.; Gupta, S.K. *Withania somnifera* provides cardioprotection and attenuates ischemia-reperfusion-induced apoptosis. *Clin. Nutr.* **2008**, *27*, 635–642. [CrossRef]

91. Yan, Z.; Guo, R.; Gan, L.; Lau, W.B.; Cao, X.; Zhao, J.; Ma, X.; Christopher, T.A.; Lopez, B.L.; Wang, Y. Withaferin A inhibits apoptosis via activated Akt-mediated inhibition of oxidative stress. *Life Sci.* **2018**, *211*, 91–101. [CrossRef]
92. Thakkar, S.; Anklam, E.; Xu, A.; Ulberth, F.; Li, J.; Li, B.; Hugas, M.; Sarma, N.; Crerar, S.; Swift, S.; et al. Regulatory landscape of dietary supplements and herbal medicines from a global perspective. *Regul. Toxicol. Pharmacol.* **2020**, *114*, 104647. [CrossRef] [PubMed]
93. Vazirani, S.; Kothari, A.; Fujimoto, J.; Gomez, M. Supplements Are Not a Synonym for Safe: Suspected Liver Injury from Ashwagandha. *Fed. Pract.* **2023**, *40*, 315–319. [CrossRef] [PubMed]
94. Philips, C.A.; Valsan, A.; Theruvath, A.H.; Ravindran, R.; Oommen, T.T.; Rajesh, S.; Augustine, P.; Liver Research Club India. Ashwagandha-induced liver injury-A case series from India and literature review. *Hepatol. Commun.* **2023**, *7*, e0270. [CrossRef] [PubMed]
95. Akhgarjand, C.; Asoudeh, F.; Bagheri, A.; Kalantar, Z.; Vahabi, Z.; Shab-bidar, S.; Rezvani, H.; Djafarian, K. Does Ashwagandha supplementation have a beneficial effect on the management of anxiety and stress? A systematic review and meta-analysis of randomized controlled trials. *Phyther. Res.* **2022**, *36*, 4115–4124. [CrossRef]
96. Pires, N.; Gota, V.; Gulia, A.; Hingorani, L.; Agarwal, M.; Puri, A. Safety and pharmacokinetics of Withaferin-A in advanced stage high grade osteosarcoma: A phase I trial. *J. Ayurveda Integr. Med.* **2020**, *11*, 68–72. [CrossRef]

nutrients

MDPI

Article

Curcumin and Its Potential to Target the Glycolytic Behavior of Lactate-Acclimated Prostate Carcinoma Cells with Docetaxel

Dongsic Choi [1], Jun Gi Lee [2], Su-Hak Heo [3], Moon-Kyen Cho [4], Hae-Seon Nam [4], Sang-Han Lee [1] and Yoon-Jin Lee [1,*]

1 Department of Biochemistry, College of Medicine, Soonchunhyang University, Cheonan 31511, Republic of Korea; dongsic@sch.ac.kr (D.C.); m1037624@sch.ac.kr (S.-H.L.)
2 Biochemistry and Molecular Biology, Marquette University, Milwaukee, WI 53233, USA; jungi0714@gmail.com
3 Department of Medicinal Bioscience, College of Biomedical and Health Science, Konkuk University Glocal Campus, Chungju 27478, Republic of Korea; cableshh@gmail.com
4 Division of Molecular Cancer Research, Soonchunhyang Medical Research Institute, Soonchunhyang University, Cheonan 31151, Republic of Korea; mkcho@schmc.ac.kr (M.-K.C.); namhs@sch.ac.kr (H.-S.N.)
* Correspondence: leeyj@sch.ac.kr; Tel.: +82-41-570-2443

Abstract: Background: Dysregulated cellular metabolism is known to be associated with drug resistance in cancer treatment. **Methods:** In this study, we investigated the impact of cellular adaptation to lactic acidosis on intracellular energy metabolism and sensitivity to docetaxel in prostate carcinoma (PC) cells. The effects of curcumin and the role of hexokinase 2 (HK2) in this process were also examined. **Results:** PC-3AcT and DU145AcT cells that preadapted to lactic acid displayed increased growth behavior, increased dependence on glycolysis, and reduced sensitivity to docetaxel compared to parental PC-3 and DU145 cells. Molecular analyses revealed activation of the c-Raf/MEK/ERK pathway, upregulation of cyclin D1, cyclin B1, and p-cdc2Thr161, and increased levels and activities of key regulatory enzymes in glycolysis, including HK2, in lactate-acclimated cells. HK2 knockdown resulted in decreased cell growth and glycolytic activity, decreased levels of complexes I–V in the mitochondrial electron transport chain, loss of mitochondrial membrane potential, and depletion of intracellular ATP, ultimately leading to cell death. In a xenograft animal model, curcumin combined with docetaxel reduced tumor size and weight, induced downregulation of glycolytic enzymes, and stimulated the upregulation of apoptotic and necroptotic proteins. This was consistent with the in vitro results from 2D monolayer and 3D spheroid cultures, suggesting that the efficacy of curcumin is not affected by docetaxel. **Conclusions:** Overall, our findings suggest that metabolic plasticity through enhanced glycolysis observed in lactate-acclimated PC cells may be one of the underlying causes of docetaxel resistance, and targeting glycolysis by curcumin may provide potential for drug development that could improve treatment outcomes in PC patients.

Keywords: curcumin; glycolysis; lactic acid; prostate cancer cells; chemoresistance; apoptosis; necroptosis

1. Introduction

Unlike normal cells, cancer cells tend to rely on the low energy yield of glycolysis to make ATP, even when sufficient levels of oxygen are present [1]. Glycolysis produces 18 times less ATP than mitochondrial oxidation, but is 100 times faster than oxidative phosphorylation, which may benefit cancer cells by providing them with greater energy [2]. Additionally, the provision of metabolic intermediates or precursors and NADPH generated from glycolysis and hexose monophosphate shunts can promote rapid cell proliferation of cancer cells and help maintain intracellular redox status, respectively [3].

High dependence on glycolysis can promote drug resistance, angiogenesis, and metastatic behavior of cancer cells by releasing excess generated protons into the extracellular space and maintaining an alkaline intracellular pH and acidic extracellular pH [4]. Lactic acid is produced intracellularly as a result of high glycolysis. It is one of the major metabolites that accumulates in the tumor microenvironment and causes acidification. Although excess lactic acid can also be utilized for energy provision, increased lactate production and subsequent acidification of the tumor microenvironment (TME) appear to promote several important malignant progressions, including angiogenesis, tissue invasion/metastasis, and drug resistance [4]. Previous studies have demonstrated that lactic acid levels in prostate cancer (PC) are closely related to cancer progression [5]. While healthy prostate cells produce ATP primarily through glucose oxidation even under aerobic conditions, prostate cells undergoing neoplastic transformation or early-stage PC use citric acid from the tricarboxylic acid cycle (TCA) cycle for oxidative phosphorylation. At advanced stages, PC cells exhibit the glycolysis-dependent Warburg phenotype, thereby increasing lactate production [6,7]. A systemic increase in lactate is associated with disease recurrence and is known to have a poor prognosis for survival [8,9]. Therefore, targeting the glycolytic pathway as a therapeutic strategy to combat cancer may provide an effective approach for the development of new targeted anticancer drugs in cancers that exhibit a prevalence of the glycolytic phenotype.

Docetaxel, a semisynthetic analog of the natural product paclitaxel, is the most widely used chemotherapeutic drug for the treatment of metastatic castrate-resistant PC (mCRPC). It preferentially binds to β-tubulin, altering cellular microtubule dynamics, thus leading to cell cycle arrest and apoptosis [10]. Although it has transient efficacy, patients receiving long-term treatment with docetaxel are known to exhibit drug resistance and systemic cytotoxicity, limiting the clinical use of taxane-based chemotherapy in CRPC [11]. PC cells are known to acquire resistance to docetaxel through tubulin alterations, enhanced survival signaling pathways, decreased drug influx and increased drug efflux, altered androgen receptor signaling, centrosome clustering, and cancer stem cells [11]. Recently, there has been increasing evidence that metabolic reprogramming is involved in docetaxel resistance in PC cells [12,13]. The Warburg effect is a type of metabolic reprogramming characterized by increased glycolysis and consequently high lactate production. This change not only allows cancer cells to adapt to various conditions of the TME by providing them with sufficient energy and metabolic intermediates essential for rapid proliferation and malignant progression, but also induces immunosuppression and immune evasion of cancer cells, making them more prone to developing resistance to chemotherapy [14,15]. Moreover, TME components plays a central role in shaping and maintaining these metabolic changes in cancer cells [16]. However, although direct evidence for metabolic reorganization and anticancer drug resistance through crosstalk between the TME and cancer cells is limited and further studies are needed, targeting altered metabolism in conjunction with chemotherapy might be a rational therapeutic strategy to improve therapeutic response and overcome drug resistance. Therefore, recent studies have attempted to develop natural-based agents that can enhance the therapeutic efficacy of conventional chemotherapies to improve the current cure rates for PCs while minimizing adverse effects on healthy cells [17].

Curcumin, a flavonoid found in the roots of turmeric or *Curcuma longa*, has been shown to have antioxidant, anti-inflammatory, and anti-proliferative properties [18]. Anti-carcinogenic effects of curcumin have been demonstrated in several cancers, including PC, by modulating various signaling pathways, including p53, mitogen-activated protein (MAP) kinase, phosphoinositol-3 kinases/protein kinase B (P13K/Akt), Janus kinase/signal transducer and activator of transcription (JAK/STAT), sonic hedgehog, and nuclear factor kappa-light-chain-enhancer of activated B cells (NF-κB) pathways [19]. Curcumin is a natural product that is less toxic and has fewer side effects than existing chemotherapy drugs and can be used safely. It is also known to be advantageous in sensitizing cancer cells when used in combination with chemotherapeutic drugs [20]. In previous studies, we first reported that the preferential cytotoxic effect of curcumin on PC-3AcT cells pre-adapted to a lactate-containing medium with increased tolerance to docetaxel was associated with its anti-glycolytic role through inhibition of MEK/ERK signaling, suggesting that there is a relationship between the dependence of PC cells on glycolysis and the effect of protecting them from chemotherapeutic drugs [21,22].

In this study, we performed the following experiments to further confirm the anti-cancer properties of curcumin, which showed a better killing effect on lactate-acclimated cells with an increased glycolytic and docetaxel-resistant phenotype. First, we investigated whether there were differences in cell growth, glycolysis, and bioenergetics at the basal level between lactate-acclimated PC-3AcT or DU145AcT cells and their parental PC-3 or DU145 cells. Next, by examining the knockdown effect of hexokinase 2 (HK2), a key target of curcumin's anti-glycolytic role, we sought to elucidate the importance of this enzyme as an attractive target for the development of PC therapeutics. Finally, we evaluated whether the antiglycolytic effects of curcumin demonstrated in 2D monolayer cultures were not affected by co-treatment with docetaxel in 3D spheroid cultures and a nude mouse xenograft model.

2. Materials and Methods

2.1. Cell Culture and Assays

Human prostate epithelial cell lines HPrEC and RWPE-1 and human PC cell lines PC-3 and DU145 were purchased from the American Type Culture Collection (ATCC; Manassas, VA, USA). Acidic pre-adapted cells designated as PC-3AcT and DU145AcT were established by continuously exposing PC-3 and DU145 cells, respectively, to lactic acid (final concentration: 3.8 μM) over four passages for 15 days. Cells were seeded at a density of 10^4 cells/well in 96-well cell culture plates and cultured in in Dulbecco's Modified Eagles Medium (DMEM, Welgene Inc., Gyeongsan, Republic of Korea) containing lactic acid (final concentration: 3.8 μM) and 5% fetal bovine serum and cultured at 37 °C in a 5% CO_2 incubator. They were then treated with fixed (40 μM) or increasing concentrations (0, 5, 10, 20, 40, 80, and 100 μM) of curcumin with or without docetaxel (40 nM) for the cell viability assay. Negative control cells were treated with 0.1% dimethyl sulfoxide. Cell viability was determined by MTT assay, as previously described [23]. The effect of combined treatment of the two compounds was assessed using the combination index (CI), as previously described [23]. To measure the activities of HK and pyruvate dehydrogenase (PDH), an HK Colorimetric Assay Kit (cat. no. K789-100) and PDH Activity Colorimetric Assay Kit (cat. no. K679-100) were used, respectively, according to the manufacturer's instructions (BioVision, Inc., Milpotas, CA, USA). Glucose consumption was determined by assessing glucose contents in the culture media using a Glucose Colorimetric Assay Kit (cat. no. K606-100; Biovision, Inc., Milpotas, CA, USA) according to the manufacturer's instructions. Intracellular ATP content was determined by measuring luminescence using a CellTiter-Glo Luminescent Cell Viability Assay Kit (Promega Corporation, Madison, WI, USA) according to the protocols provided by the manufacturer. Absorbance and luminescence values were measured with a GloMax-Multi microplate multimode reader (Promega Corporation, Madison, WI, USA).

2.2. Western Blotting

Cells were seeded at a density of 10^5 cells/well in 6-well cell culture plates, and cultured in DMEM containing lactic acid (final concentration: 3.8 μM) and 5% fetal bovine serum at 37 °C in a 5% CO_2 incubator. After combined treatment with curcumin (40 μM) and docetaxel (40 nM) for 48 h, whole cell lysates were extracted from samples obtained from cell culture and animal experiments using 1× RIPA buffer (1× PBS, 0.5% sodium deoxycholate, 1% NP-40, 0.1% sodium dodecyl sulfate, 10 mg/mL phenylmethylsulfonyl fluoride). Mitochondrial and cytosolic extracts were prepared with a Mitochondria Isolation Kit for Mammalian Cells according to the instruction provided (cat no. 89874; Thermo Scientific, Rockford, IL, USA). Protein concentration was determined with a BCA Protein Assay (cat no. 23225; Thermo Scientific). Forty micrograms of proteins were loaded onto 4–12% NuPAGE gels (Invitrogen, Carlsbad, CA, USA), separated, and transferred to a polyvinylidenefluoride membrane (Cytiva Life Sciences, Marlborough, MA, USA). Blots were blocked with 1× casein solution (cat. no; 37528; Thermo Fisher Scientific, Inc.,

Waltham, MA, USA) for 2 h at room temperature and then incubated with the primary antibody overnight at 4 °C. After washing three times with 1x PBS-Tween 20, horseradish peroxidase (HRP)-conjugated secondary antibodies was applied for 2 h at room temperature. The signal was visualized using an Enhanced Chemiluminescence (ECL) Detection Kit (cat. no. W1001; Promega). Densitometry was performed on blots using TINA 2.09 software (Raytest Isotopen Messgeraete GmbH, Straubenhardt, Germany) and normalized to β-actin. Oxphos human WB antibody cocktail (cat. no. 45-8199) and antibodies to cyclin B1 (cat. no. 4138), phosphorylated (p)-cyclin dependent kinase (CDK) 2, p-Cdc2^{Thr161} (cat. no. 9114) and p-cdc2^{Tyr15} (cat. no. 4539), p-mitogen-activated protein kinase 1/2 (p-MEK1/2; cat. no. 9154), p-extracellular-signal-regulated kinase 1/2 (p-ERK1/2; cat. no. 4370), ERK (cat. no. 9102), HK2 (cat. no. 2867), phosphofructokinase platelet (PFKP; cat. no. 93654), PDH (cat. no. 3205), voltage-dependent anion channel (VDAC; cat. no. 4661), α-tubulin (cat. no. 2144), p-mixed lineage kinase domain-like (p-MLKL; cat. no. 91689), MLKL (cat. no. 14993), p-receptor-interacting protein 3 (p-RIP3; cat. no. 93654), RIP3 (cat. no. 13526), B-cell lymphoma 2 (Bcl-2; cat. no. 2870), Bcl-2 associated X (Bax; cat. no. 5023), poly (ADP-ribose) polymerase (PARP; cat. no. 9542), cleaved PARP (cat. no. 9541), caspase-3 (cat. no. 14220), and cleaved caspase-3 (cat. no. 9664) were purchased from Cell Signaling Technology, Inc. (Danvers, CO, USA) and diluted 1:500. HRP-coupled goat anti-rabbit IgG (1:5000; cat. no. sc-2004), goat anti-mouse IgG (1:5000; cat. no. sc-2005), and antibodies to cyclin D1 (1:500; cat. no. SC-718), p53 (1:500; cat. no. sc-126), and MEK (1:500; cat. no. SC-436) were purchased from Santa-Cruz Biotechnology, Inc. (Dallas, TX, USA). Membranes were re-probed with antibodies to β-actin (1000; cat. no. A2228; Sigma-Aldrich, St. Louis, MO, USA), MEK1/2, ERK1/2, VDAC, α-tubulin, MLKL, and RIP3 as loading controls.

2.3. Mitochondrial Fractionation

Mitochondrial-enriched fractions were prepared according to the instruction of the Mitochondria Isolation Kit for Cultured Cells (cat no. 89874; Thermo Scientific). Briefly, cells (2×10^7) were incubated in 800 μL of Mitochondria Isolation Reagent A on ice for 2 min, 10 μL of Mitochondria Isolation Reagent B on ice for 5 min, and 800 μL of Mitochondria Isolation Reagent C at 4 °C for 10 min. After centrifugation at 700× *g* for 10 min at 4 °C, the supernatant was transferred to a new 2.0 mL tube and centrifuged at 12,000× *g* for 15 min at 4 °C. The supernatant was stored as the cytosolic fraction. The pellet was resuspended in 500 μL Mitochondria Isolation Reagent C, and the mitochondrial pellet was obtained by centrifugation at 12,000× *g* for 5 min. This was defined as the mitochondrial fraction and stored at −80 °C for Western blot analysis.

2.4. Mitochondrial Membrane Potential (ΔΨ)

In each well of a 6-well culture plate, cells (1×10^5) were seeded and incubated overnight in lactic acid-containing DMEM. Cells were then treated with or without 40 nM docetaxel for 48 h. After trypsinization, cells were harvested by centrifugation at 500× *g* for 7 min, adjusted to 10^6 cells/mL, and incubated in serum-free DMEM containing 30 nM rhodamine 123 (Sigma-Aldrich) at 37 °C for 30 min in the dark. Then, the cells were centrifuged at 500× *g* for 5 min to discard the supernatant, and washed twice in pre-warmed medium. The fluorescence intensity of the cells was measured using a MACSQuant analyzer and MACSQuantify software version 2.5 (Miltenyi Biotec GmbH, Bergisch Gladbach, Germany).

2.5. Reactive Oxygen Species

Cells (1×10^5) were seeded per well of a 6-well culture plate and incubated overnight in lactic acid-containing DMEM. Cells were then treated with or without 40 nM docetaxel for 48 h. Trypsinized cells were collected by centrifugation at 500× *g* for 7 min, adjusted to 10^6 cells/mL, and incubated in serum-free DMEM containing 10 μM 2′,7′-dichlorodihydrofluorescein diacetate (Sigma-Aldrich) at 37 °C for 30 min in the dark, and then the reactive oxygen species (ROS) were measured. The fluorescence intensity of the cells was measured using a MACSQuant analyzer and MACSQuantify software version 2.5 (Miltenyi Biotec GmbH, Bergisch Gladbach, Germany).

2.6. Annexin V-PE/7-AAD Double Staining

To analyze the distribution of apoptotic and necrotic cells, the Muse Annexin V & Dead Cell Assay Kit (cat. no. MCH100105; Merck KGaA, Darmstadt, Germany) was used according to the manufacturer's instructions. Cells were treated with or without 40 nM docetaxel for 48 h. Cells were then harvested by trypsinization and resuspended in 200 μL of Muse Annexin V & Dead Cell reagent for 30 min at room temperature in the dark. These cells were analyzed with a Muse cell analyzer (Merck KGaA). Annexin V-phycoerythrin (PE)-positive apoptotic and 7-amino-actinomycin D (AAD)-positive necrotic cells were detected by double staining using Annexin V-PE and 7-AAD.

2.7. Cell Cycle Analysis

The cell cycle distribution at each phase was measured by staining with propidium iodide (PI). Trypsinized cells were harvested by centrifugation at 500× *g* for 7 min at 4 °C, and then fixed overnight at −20 °C with ice-cold 70% ethanol. Cells (1×10^6) were washed with 1× phosphate-buffered saline (PBS) and incubated with 200 μL of Muse Cell Cycle Reagent (cat. no. MCH100106; Merck KGaA) containing PI and RNase for 30 min at room temperature in the dark. Data from 10,000 cells were analyzed using MACSQuant analyzer and MACSQuantify software version 2.5 (Miltenyi Biotec GmbH).

2.8. HK2-Targeting siRNA Transfection

RNA interference of HK2 was performed using a HK2-targeting small interfering RNA (siHK2) duplex from Invitrogen (Oligo ID, HSS179239). Cells (1×10^5) were seeded into 6-well plates and transfected at 40% confluency with siHK2 using Lipofectamine™ RNAiMAX Transfecton Reagent (Invitrogen) according to the manufacturer's recommendations. Stealth RNAi negative control duplex (siC, Oligo ID, 452001) was used as a negative control. 250 μL. Two hundred and fifty μL of Opti-MEM medium containing siRNAse (25 pmol) and 7.5 μL of Lipofectamine™ RNAiMAX Transfecton Reagent was added to each well. At 24 h after transfection, cells were treated with or without curcumin for another 48 h and then harvested with trypsin for ΔΨ measurement, Annexin V-PE binding assay, cell cycle analysis, and Western blot analysis.

2.9. Spheroid Culture and Viability Assay

Spheroid culture was performed in ultra-low attachment 96-well plates, as previously described [24]. Plates seeded with 1×10^4 cells/well were centrifuged at 500× *g* for 10 min to allow cells to cluster in the wells, and then maintained in complete DMEM containing lactic acid for 5 days. Spheroids were treated with curcumin (40 μM) and docetaxel (40 nM) for 48 h. To detect live and dead cells, the green fluorescence of fluorescein diacetate (FDA; Sigma-Aldrich, 5 μg/mL) and red fluorescence for PI (Sigma-Aldrich, 10 μg/mL) were used, respectively. After staining for 5 min, the spheroids were washed with 1× PBS and observed using a Leica EL6000 fluorescence microscope (Leica Microsystems GmbH, Wetzlar, Germany). Spheroid viability was determined with an Enhanced Cell Viability Assay Kit (Young In Frontier Co., Ltd., Geumcheon, Republic of Korea) according to the manufacturer's instructions. Briefly, 10 μL of Cellvia solution was added to each well, left at room temperature for 1 h, and then mixed for 1 min until the formed formazan crystal dissolved. The amount of formazan formed by living cells was measured spectrophotometrically at 450 nm using a GloMax-Multi microplate multimode reader (Promega Corporation).

2.10. Xenograft Assay Using Nude Mice

Five-week-old male mice (*n* = 9, starting size 22–24 g), BklNbt:BALB/c/nu/nu, were acclimated to specific pathogen-free conditions for 1 week, and fed pellets and water ad libitum. They were then randomly divided into two groups (control, 4 mice; treatment,

5 mice) and injected subcutaneously with PC-3AcT cells (2×10^6) suspended in 0.2 mL 1× PBS. Among these, mice in which xenografts were not formed or were too small were excluded, and as a result, 4 mice and 3 mice were used as the control group and the group administered curcumin and docetaxel together, respectively. Curcumin (15 mg/kg) and docetaxel (0.5 mg/kg) were administered intratumorally at three-day intervals. Body weight and tumor growth were observed every 3 days until the 24th day of the experiment. During the experimental period, the mice were observed for clinical signs of distress, including posture, movement, ease of handling, fur condition, arousal, and diarrhea. There were no restrictions on food, water, or exercise during the experimental period, and no animals were subject to humane endpoints or euthanasia due to extreme pain or clinical symptoms. Mice were euthanized by cervical dislocation. The excised tumors were measured for their volume using a Vernier caliper and stored at −80 °C for Western blot analysis. Tumor volume was calculated with the following formula: volume (mm^3) = length (mm) × width (mm) × width (mm)/2. The animal study was approved by the Institutional Animal Care and Use Committee of Soonchunhyang University on 8 March 2021 (Approval No. SCH20-0060). Animal welfare and experimental procedures were strictly conducted in accordance with the Experimental Animal Welfare Guidelines of the Animal Experiment Center at Soonchunhyang Institute of Medi-Bio Science (Cheonan, Republic of Korea).

2.11. Statistical Analysis

All experimental data were analyzed with SPSS version 17.0 (SPSS, Inc., Chicago, IL, USA) and expressed as the mean ± standard deviation of three independent experiments. Comparison between two groups was performed by one-way analysis of variance and Tukey's post hoc correction. Statistical significance was considered when the *p*-value was less than 0.05.

3. Results

3.1. Preadaptation of PC Cells to Lactic Acid Makes Them Tolerate Docetaxel Better with an Increase of Glycolytic Flux

To evaluate the effect of pre-adaptation to lactic acid-containing medium for 15 days, we first measured the growth status and expression of CDKs (p-cdc2Thr161 and p-cdc2Tyr15) and its regulatory subunits (cyclins D1 and B1) of PC-3AcT and DU145AcT cells while culturing them in medium containing 3.8 μM lactic acid. On the first day of culture, some floating cells were observed in the acidic medium, but there was no noticeable difference in the confluency of adherent cells. Compared with their parental PC-3 and DU145 cells, PC-3AcT and DU145AcT cells showed significantly faster growth, with an approximate 1.8-fold and 1.4-fold increase at 48 h and 72 h, respectively ($p < 0.05$, Figure 1A). This was probably as a result of pre-adaptation to acidic medium containing lactic acid, accompanied by upregulation of cyclin D1, cyclin B1, and p-cdc2Thr161, and downregulation of p-cdc2Tyr15 based on Western blot analysis (Figure 1B). The c-Raf/MEK/ERK pathway was also activated in PC-3AcT and DU145AcT cells, as shown by increased levels of p-MEK1/2 and p-ERK1/2 (Figure 1C).

Next, we analyzed proteins or enzymes that are known to play critical roles in aerobic glycolysis and oxidative phosphorylation to investigate the effect of lactic acid on bioenergetics. As shown in Figure 1D, higher levels of HK2, PFKP, and PDH were observed in PC-3AcT and DU145AcT cells than in their parental PC-3 and DU145 cells. After 48 h of culture, the activities of HK and PDH increased (Figure 1E), consistent with results of Western blotting, and the glucose concentration in the culture medium decreased by approximately 74.1% and 69.8% in PC-3AcT and DU145AcT cells compared to PC-3 and DU145 cells, respectively (Figure 1F).

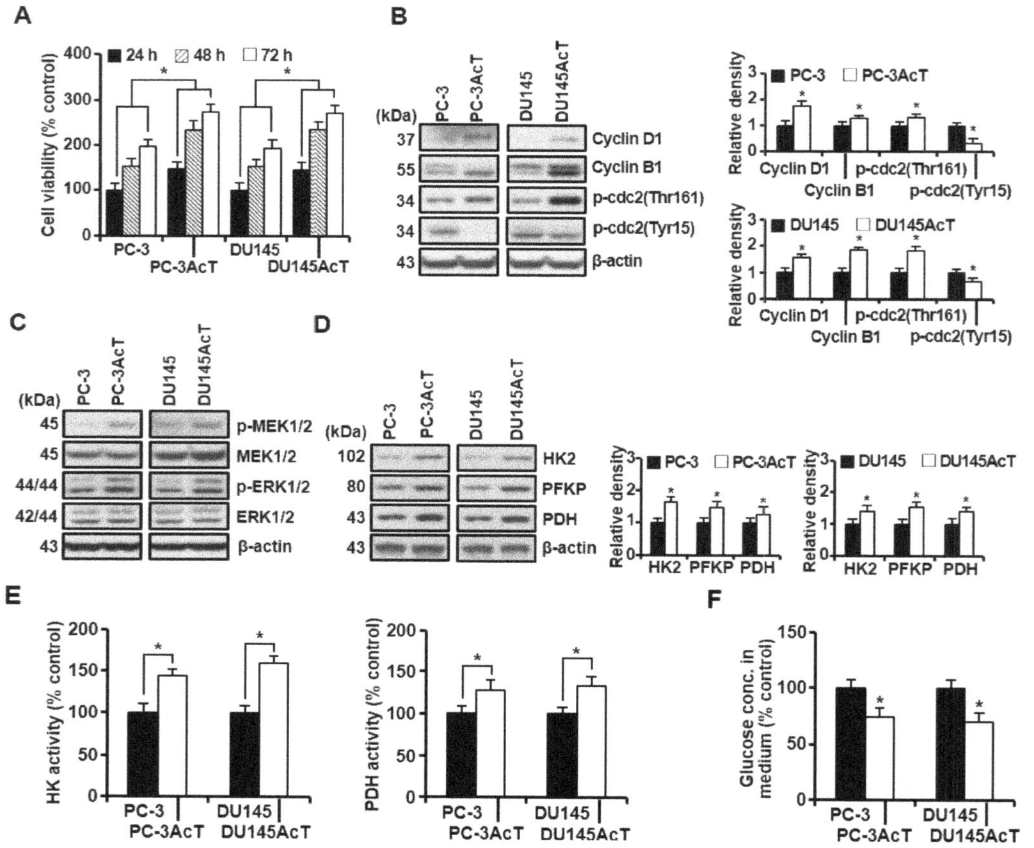

Figure 1. Increased glycolytic flux in PC-3AcT and DU145AcT cells pre-adapted to lactic acid. Cellular responses were examined after culturing cells in DMEM containing 3.8 μM lactic acid for the indicated time (or 48 h, otherwise). (**A**) Percent cell viability. (**B–D**) Western blot analysis of cell cycle-regulatory (**B**), MEK/ERK signaling (**C**), and key regulatory enzymes in glycolysis (**D**). (**E**) Activities of hexokinase and pyruvate dehydrogenase. (**F**) Changes in glucose concentration in culture medium. Data are expressed as the mean ± standard deviation of three independent experiments. Statistical significance comparing respective PC-3 or DU145 cells was considered at * $p < 0.05$ using one-way ANOVA and Tukey's post hoc correction. HK, hexokinase; PFKP, phosphofructokinase platelet; PDH, pyruvate dehydrogenase.

The proportion of HK2 was increased in the mitochondrial fractions of PC-3AcT and DU145AcT cells compared to PC-3 and DU145 cells (Figure 2A). Base-level analysis of the five complexes in the mitochondrial respiratory chain showed no significant changes except for a slight increase in complex II (SDHB, succinate dehydrogenase subunit B) (Figure 2B). The fractions of cells showing ΔΨ loss, indicative of mitochondrial dysfunction, were slightly reduced in PC-3AcT and DU145AcT cells (Figure 2C). During this process, the ATP contents of these cells were increased significantly, with an approximate 1.2-fold and 1.3-fold increase in PC-3AcT and DU145AcT, respectively ($p < 0.05$, Figure 2D). In the viability assay of PC-3AcT and Du145AcT cells treated with 40 nM docetaxel, both cell lines (approximately 39% and 34% growth inhibition in PC-3AcT and DU145AcT, respectively) showed more resistance to docetaxel than their parental cells (approximately 49% and 47% growth inhibition in PC-3 and DU145, respectively) ($p < 0.05$, Figure 2E). In line with this, the percentage of Annexin V-PE positive cells, indicating an apoptotic fraction, and the percentage of cells with ΔΨ loss, indicating mitochondrial dysfunction, were low in PC-3AcT and DU145AcT cells in response to docetaxel treatment (Figure 2F,G).

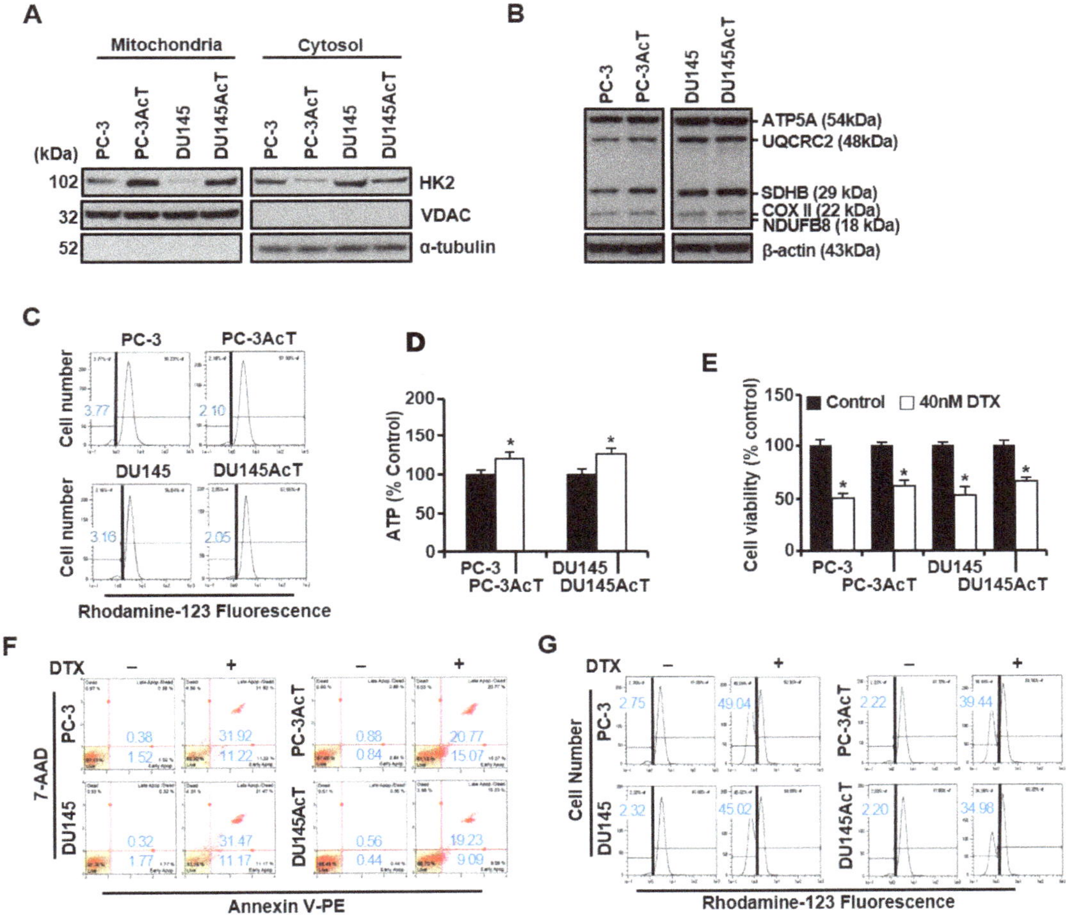

Figure 2. Mitochondrial localization of HK2 and effect of docetaxel treatment on PC-3AcT and DU145AcT cells. Cells were cultured in DMEM containing 3.8 μM lactic acid with or without docetaxel (40 nM) for 48 h. (**A**) Western blot analysis of HK2 in mitochondrial and cytosolic fractions. (**B**) Western blot analysis of complexes I–V in the mitochondrial electron transport chain. (**C**) Measurement of mitochondrial membrane potential after staining cells with rhodamine123. (**D**) Changes in intracellular ATP concentration. (**E**) Percent cell viability for cells treated with or without 40 nM docetaxel. (**F**) Annexin V-PE binding assay for cells treated with or without 40 nM docetaxel. (**G**) Measurements of mitochondrial membrane potential for cells treated with or without 40 nM docetaxel. Data are expressed as the mean ± standard deviation of three independent experiments. Statistical significance comparing respective PC-3 or DU145 cells was considered at * $p < 0.05$ using one-way ANOVA and Tukey's post hoc correction. HK2, hexokinase 2; VDAC, voltage-dependent anion channel; NDUFB8, NADH-ubiquinone oxidoreductase subunit B8 (complex I); SDHB, succinate dehydrogenase complex iron sulfur subunit B (complex II); UQCRC2, ubiquinone-cytochrome C reductase core protein 2 (complex III); COX II, mitochondrial cytochrome C oxidase subunit II (complex IV); ATP5A, ATP synthase F1 subunit alpha (complex V); DTX, docetaxel.

3.2. HK2-Targeting siRNA or Curcumin Inhibits Growth of Glycolytic and Docetaxel-Resistant PC Cells by Inducing Both Apoptosis and Necroptosis

In our previous paper, we showed that lactate-acclimated PC-3AcT cells (IC_{50} = 109.57 nM) were more resistant to docetaxel than parental PC-3 cells (IC_{50} = 49.83 nM), whereas the increased sensitivity to curcumin was more evident in PC-3AcT cells (IC_{50} = 42.19 μM) compared to PC-3 cells (IC_{50} = 80.51 μM) [21]. Furthermore, we also found that the preferential cytotoxicity of curcumin against PC-3AcT cells was associated with the inhibition of the glycolytic pathway [22]. To investigate the importance of HK2 as a critical modulator of glycolytic flux in the efficacy of curcumin to preferentially target PC-3AcT and Du145AcT cells, which exhibit a glycolytic and docetaxel-resistant phenotype, we transfected cells with HK2-targeting siRNA, after which cells were treated with vehicle (DMSO) or curcumin for 48 h. HK2 silencing alone induced a growth inhibition of approximately 43% and 40% in PC-3AcT and Du145AcT cells, respectively, compared with the siC group, and the addition of curcumin significantly induced a growth inhibition of approximately 62% and 58%, respectively ($p < 0.05$, Figure 3A). After HK2 was effectively knocked down, the expression level of HK2 decreased to approximately 35% and 37.8% in PC-3AcT and Du145AcT cells, respectively. After 48 h of culture, the expression levels of HK2 and PDH (Figure 3B) also decreased, along with decreased activities of HK and PDH (Figure 3C). Glucose concentration in the culture media remained increased by 14.9% and 21.6% in PC-3AcT and Du145AcT cells with HK2 knockdown, respectively, compared to the siC group (Figure 3D). In line with this, the amount of HK2 in the mitochondrial fraction was also reduced by HK2 silencing (Figure 3E).

HK2 silencing alone or in combination with curcumin treatment downregulated the expression of complexes I–V in the respiratory chain (Figure 4A) but increased the proportion of cells with $\Delta\Psi$ loss, indicative of mitochondrial dysfunction (Figure 4B). During this process, the ATP content of these cells was significantly reduced in the following order: HK2 silencing alone < curcumin < HK2 silencing/curcumin ($p < 0.05$, Figure 4C). Flow cytometric analysis of cells with HK2 knocked down using HK2-targeting siRNA showed an increase in the sub-G_0/G_1 peak, indicative of apoptosis (Figure 4D), accompanied by an increase in the proportion of apoptotic cells as determined by Annexin V-PE binding assay (Figure 4E). Consistently, HK2 silencing induced enhanced cleavage of procaspase-3 and its substrate PARP, and increased the phosphorylation levels of MLKL and RIP3 (Figure 4F) compared with the siC group. The effects of HK2 silencing alone were further enhanced by the addition of curcumin.

3.3. Combination Treatment with Curcumin and Docetaxel Inhibits Glycolysis but Increases Both Apoptosis and Necroptosis in 3D Spheroid Cultures and PC-3AcT Xenografts

To confirm the consistency of the results in 2D monolayer cultures and to assess whether co-treatment with docetaxel affected the efficacy of curcumin, we investigated the effect of combined treatment with docetaxel and curcumin in 3D spheroid cultures and a nude mouse xenograft model. In 2D monolayer cultures, curcumin treatment at concentrations minimally toxic to normal prostate epithelial cells (HPrEC and RWPE-1) reduced cell viability in a concentration-dependent manner, and the effect was further increased by combined treatment with docetaxel (Figure 5A). Curcumin (40 μM) alone or in combination with docetaxel (40 nM) exhibited growth inhibition of approximately 48% and 74% in PC-3AcT, and 38% and 63% in DU145AcT, respectively. The combination index calculated by treating curcumin (40 uM) and docetaxel (40 μM) was 0.711 in PC-3AcT and 0.715 DU145AcT, suggesting that combination treatment synergistically inhibited cell growth. Consistent with the 2D monolayer culture results, combined treatment with curcumin and docetaxel increased the red fluorescence of PI inside the spheroid, representing the necrotic core, but decreased the green fluorescence of FDA, representing surrounding viable cells, and inhibited spheroid growth (Figure 5B). Cell viability of 3D spheroids also decreased to 46.5% and 51.9% in PC-3AcT and Du145AcT cells, respectively, compared to the control (Figure 5B). In a xenograft mouse model of PC-3AcT cells, one week after subcutaneous inoculation of cancer cells (2 × 10^6) into male nude mice, curcumin (15 mg/kg) and docetaxel (0.5 mg/kg) were administered intratumorally every three days for a total of 24 days. PC-3AcT tumor volumes grew progressively in mice. However, the combination treatment with the agents significantly reduced tumor volume and weight during the experiments without apparent toxicity, as determined by body weight and appearance (posture, movement, and fur condition, etc.) of mice, indicating that the tumor-bearing mice tolerated treatment fairly well (Figure 5C).

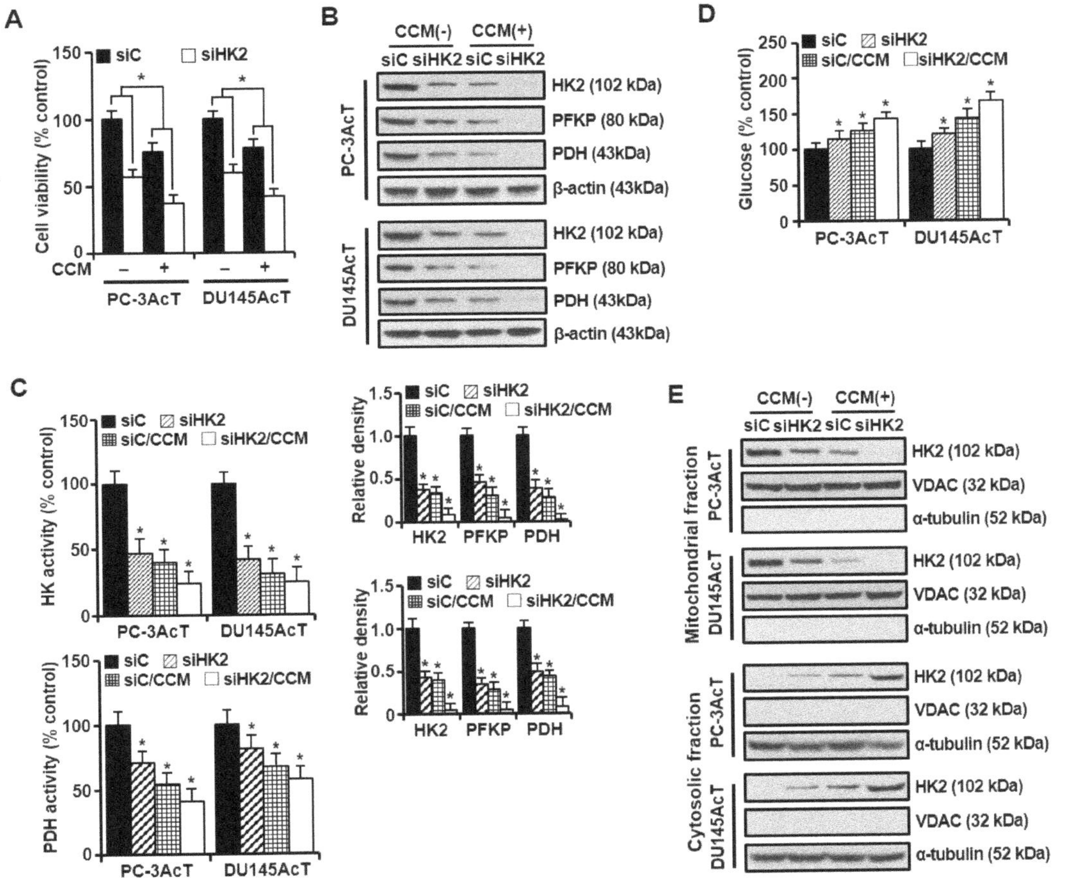

Figure 3. Effect of HK2 knockdown alone or in combination with curcumin on glucose metabolism in PC-3AcT and Du145AcT cells. Cells were transfected with 10 nM HK2-targeting siRNA (siHK2) or stealth RNAi control (siC) for 24 h. They were then treated with or without curcumin (40 μM) in DMEM containing 3.8 μM lactic acid for 48 h. (**A**) Percent cell viability. (**B**) Western blot analysis of key regulatory enzymes in glycolysis. (**C**) Activities of hexokinase and pyruvate dehydrogenase. (**D**) Changes in glucose concentration in culture medium. (**E**) Western blot analysis of HK2 in mitochondrial and cytosolic fractions. The bar graph represents densitometric analysis of Western blot images normalized to β-actin. Data are expressed as the mean ± standard deviation of three independent experiments. Statistical significance comparing the respective siC group was considered at * $p < 0.05$ using one-way ANOVA and Tukey's post hoc correction. CCM, curcumin; HK, hexokinase; PFKP, phosphofructokinase platelet; PDH, pyruvate dehydrogenase.

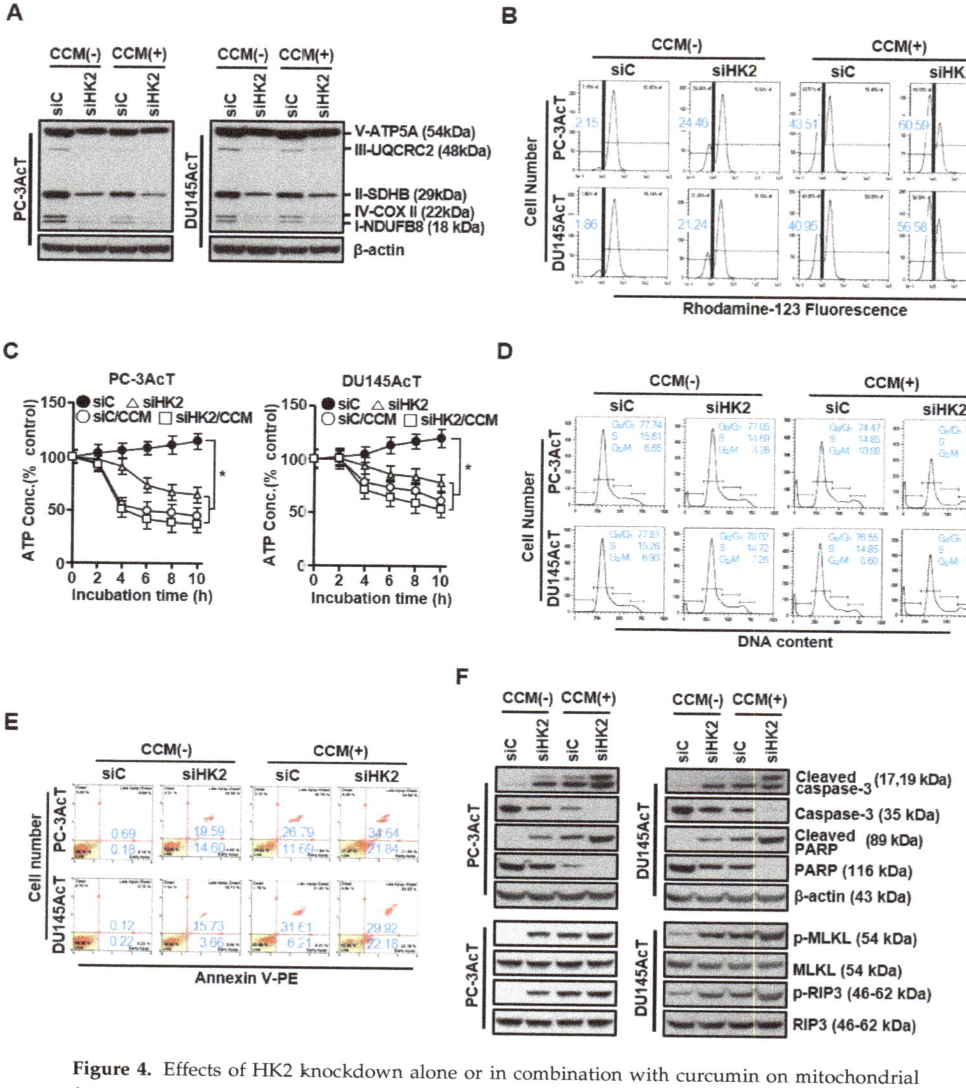

Figure 4. Effects of HK2 knockdown alone or in combination with curcumin on mitochondrial function and programmed cell death in PC-3AcT and Du145AcT cells. Cells were transfected with 10 nM HK2-targeting siRNA (siHK2) or stealth RNAi control (siC) for 24 h. They were then treated with or without curcumin (40 μM) in DMEM containing 3.8 μM lactic acid for 48 h. (**A**) Western blot analysis of complexes I–V in mitochondrial electron transport chain. (**B**) Measurements of mitochondrial membrane potential after staining cells with rhodamine123. (**C**) Changes in intracellular ATP concentration. (**D**) Cell cycle analysis. (**E**) Annexin V-PE binding assay. (**F**) Western blot analysis of apoptosis- and necroptosis-related proteins. Data are expressed as the mean ± standard deviation of three independent experiments. Statistical significance comparing the respective siC group was considered at * $p < 0.05$ using one-way ANOVA and Tukey's post hoc correction. CCM, curcumin; NDUFB8, NADH-ubiquinone oxidoreductase subunit B8 (complex I); SDHB, succinate dehydrogenase complex iron sulfur subunit B (complex II); UQCRC2, ubiquinone-cytochrome C reductase core protein 2 (complex III); COX II, mitochondrial cytochrome C oxidase subunit II (complex IV); ATP5A, ATP synthase F1 subunit alpha (complex V).

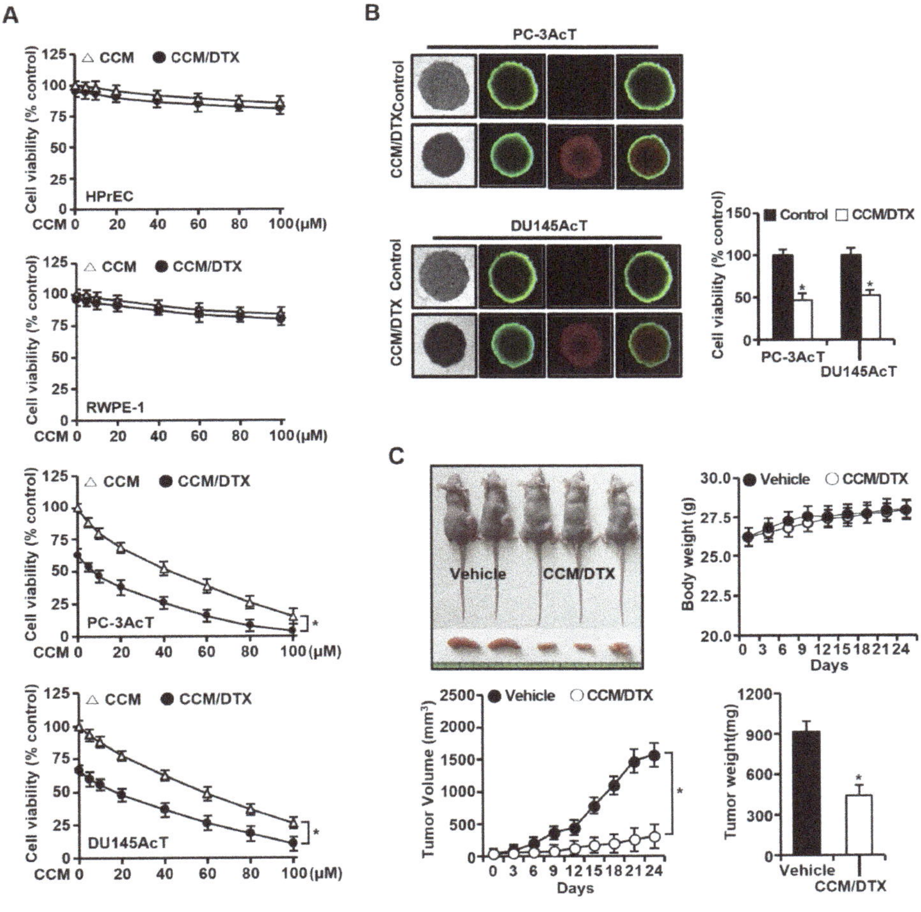

Figure 5. Growth-inhibiting effect of co-treatment with curcumin and docetaxel. (**A**) Cell viability in 2D monolayer culture. Cells were cultured in DMEM containing 3.8 µM lactic acid with or without curcumin (40 µM) and docetaxel (40 nM) for 48 h. (**B**) Vitality staining of spheroids: from left to right: (i) phase-contrast image, (ii) fluorescent images of fluorescein diacetate(+) living cells in green, (iii) propidium iodide(+) dead cells in red, and (iv) merged; and spheroid cell viability. Spheroids were then treated with or without curcumin (40 µM) and docetaxel (40 nM) for 48 h in DMEM containing 3.8 µM lactic acid. (**C**) Representative mice, body weight, tumor volume, and tumor weight in PC-3-xenografted nude mice model. Mice (0.3–0.4 cm wide and 0.3–0.4 cm long) were injected intratumorally with vehicle or curcumin (15 mg/kg) and docetaxel (0.5 mg/kg) three times per week for 24 days. Data are expressed as the mean ± standard deviation of three independent experiments. Statistical significance comparing the respective control group was considered at * $p < 0.05$ using one-way ANOVA and Tukey's post hoc correction. CCM/DTX, co-treatment with curcumin and docetaxel.

Next, we compared the effects of curcumin and docetaxel on the expression of key enzymes in glycolysis and programmed cell death. As shown in Figure 6A, downregulation of the expression levels of HK2, PFKP, and PDH, as well as the phosphorylation level of ERK1/2 was observed in both 2D and 3D cultures or tumor tissues in nude mouse xenograft models treated with the combination of two agents (Figure 6A). Additionally, along with an increase in the Bax/Bcl-2 ratio, cleaved caspase-3 and cleaved PARP, markers for apoptosis, and p-MLKL and p-RIP3, markers for necroptosis, were also upregulated by the combination treatment (Figure 6B). The above results indicate that our in vivo data reflect the in vitro results, and that the addition of docetaxel did not affect the antiglycolytic and cell killing effects of curcumin.

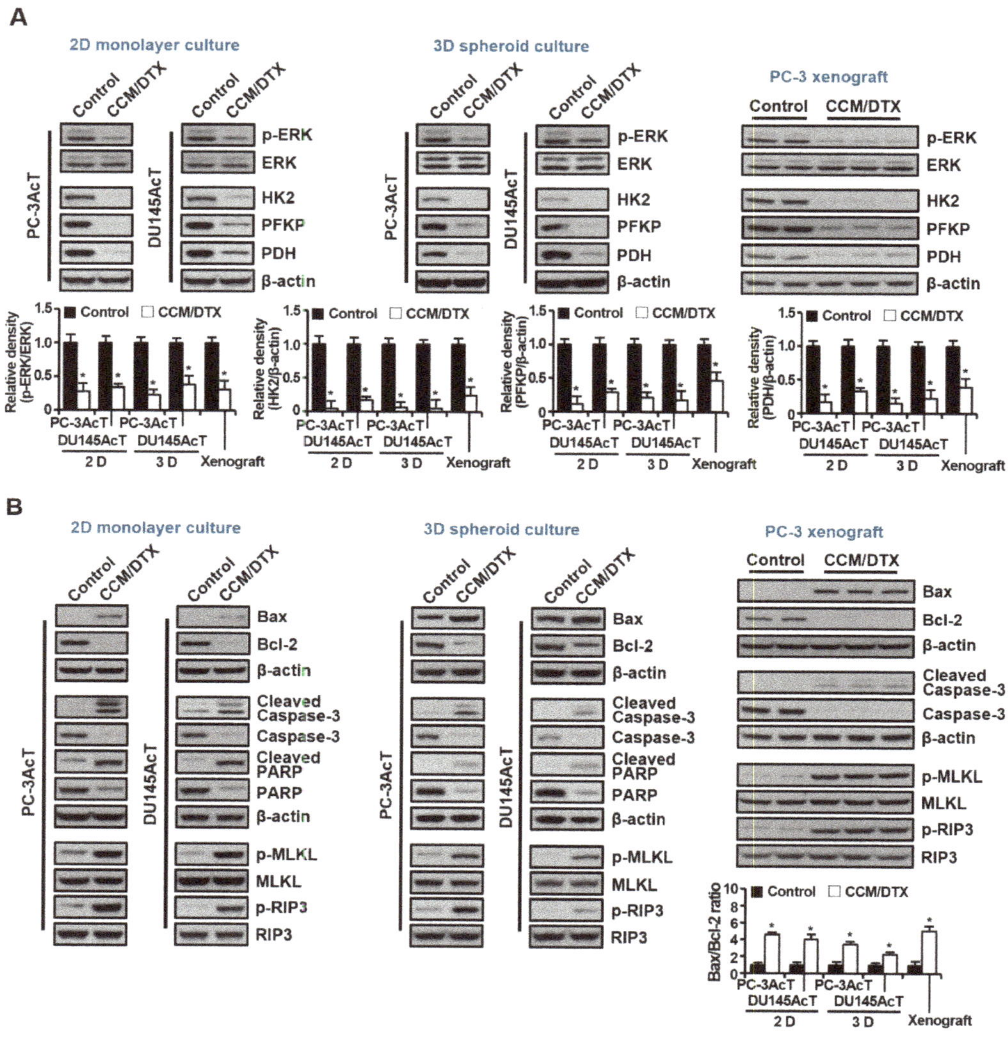

Figure 6. Effects of co-treatment with curcumin and docetaxel on expression of glycolysis-, apoptosis-, and necroptosis-related key proteins in 2D monolayer, 3D spheroid cultures, and nude mice xenograft models. Proteins were extracted from cells, spheroids, and tumors described in Figure 5, separated on 4–12% NuPAGE gels, and subjected to Western blot analysis. (**A**) Expression levels of key regulatory enzymes of glycolysis. (**B**) Expression levels of proteins related to apoptosis and necroptosis. The bar graph represents densitometric analysis of Western blot images normalized to β-actin. Data are expressed as the mean ± standard deviation of three independent experiments. Statistical significance comparing the respective control group was considered at * $p < 0.05$ using one-way ANOVA and Tukey's post hoc correction. CCM/DTX, co-treatment with curcumin and docetaxel.

4. Discussion

We have previously observed preferential cytotoxicity of curcumin against lactate-acclimated PC-3AcT cells, which showed a higher tolerance to docetaxel than parental PC-3 cells [20]. In this pre-adaption process, lactic acid might promote resistance to docetaxel, whereas curcumin was shown to induce ROS generation, DNA damage, and subsequent mitochondrial dysfunction, ultimately leading to apoptosis and necroptosis of PC-3AcT cells. In the present study, despite enhanced glycolysis in PC-3AcT and DU145AcT compared to parental PC-3 and DU145 cells, the basal levels of the five complexes of the mitochondrial respiratory chain and mitochondrial membrane potential were not significantly increased. This suggests that lactate-adapted PC cells have more metabolic dependence on glycolysis for ATP synthesis than on mitochondrial respiration. At basal levels, PC-3AcT and DU145AcT cells exhibited the following characteristics compared to PC-3 and Du145 cells: (i) increased cell growth with up-regulation of cyclin D1, cyclin B1, and p-cdc2^{Thr161} but down-regulation of p-cdc2^{Tyr15}, (ii) activation of the c-Raf/MEK/ERK pathway, (iii) increased glucose consumption along with increased levels and activities of key regulatory enzymes in glucose metabolism, including HK2, and (iv) increased tolerance to docetaxel.

Cell cycle progression is mediated by the sequential activation of Cdks in association with their regulatory cyclin subunits, in which phosphorylation or dephosphorylation by Cdk inhibitors is a major mechanism regulating the activity of Cdks [25]. Upregulation of cell cycle regulatory proteins cyclin D1 and cyclin B1 is vital in cell cycle progression in the G_0/G_1 phase and G_2/M transition, respectively. Activation of cdk1 (previously called cdc2) through phosphorylation of Thr161 and dephosphorylation of Thr14/Tyr15 also promotes subsequent mitotic entry in G_2 phase [26,27], ensuring faster proliferation of PC-3AcT and DU145AcT cells. The ERK1/2 pathway is activated by sequential reactions of upstream factors p-Raf and p-MEK1/2. In addition to its well-known role in regulating cell proliferation and survival, the involvement of ERK1/2 signaling in promoting the Warburg-like metabolism has also been reported by some researchers [28,29]. The MEK/ERK1/2 pathway not only increases the expression of glucose Transporter 1, lactate dehydrogenase A, and several enzymes in the glycolysis pathway through the role of the transcription factor c-Myc, but also cooperates with hypoxia-inducible factor-1α to induce HK2 [28]. Cui et al. have reported that HK2 upregulates cyclin A1 and downregulates p27 by activating ERK1/2 through the Raf/MEK signaling pathway, further promoting proliferation and tumor formation of cervical cancer cells [29]. Our previous study has shown that ERK1/2 inhibition by PD98059 (a synthetic inhibitor of MEK1/MEK2) or curcumin could reduce glucose consumption and downregulate the expression of key regulatory enzymes of glucose metabolism, including HK2, leading to apoptosis and necroptosis in PC-3AcT and Du145AcT cells [22]. These results demonstrated by us and others highlight the importance of the Raf/MEK/ERK pathways in promoting the Warburg effect.

In this study, docetaxel resistance in PC-3AcT and DU145AcT cells was manifested by improved cell viability, reduced apoptosis, and mitochondrial dysfunction compared to their parental cell lines PC-3 and Du145. Although multiple mechanisms are involved in the resistance of cancer cells to chemotherapy, our study suggests that increased aerobic glycolysis is associated with docetaxel resistance in lactate-acclimated PC cells. Aberrant expression of key regulators of glycolysis, including HK2, pyruvate kinase, PDH, and LDH, contributes to tumorigenesis and chemoresistance [30]. Additionally, activation of the pentose phosphate pathway through increased glycolytic flux provides reducing equivalents for protection against ROS [3], which may prevent or reduce oxidative damage caused by docetaxel in PC-3AcT and DU145AcT cells. Therefore, increased metabolic dependence of PC-3AcT and DU145AcT cells on glycolysis might prevent or reduce docetaxel-induced mitochondrial damage and ROS levels.

Overexpression of HK2 during tumor growth is associated with poor patient prognosis, disease progression, metastasis, and treatment resistance in various malignancies [31,32]. In particular, the localization and attachment of HK2 to the outer mitochondrial membrane allow tumor cells to cope with many stressful conditions by intersecting both metabolic and anti-apoptotic pathways [32]. Binding of HK to the VDAC can facilitate the release of mitochondrial-generated ATP, making it more readily available for glucose phosphorylation. It can also stabilize the mitochondrial permeability transition pore (MPTP), providing cells with protection against apoptotic stimuli [31,32]. Conversely, HK2 deficiency by knockdown or knockout of HK2 impaired tumor growth or increased treatment sensitivity. HK2 knockout can inhibit tumorigenesis in mouse models of KRAS-driven lung cancer [33], ErbB2-driven breast cancer [34], and PTEN-deficient PC [35]. In a mouse model of hepatocarcinoma, deletion or silencing of hepatic HK2 has resulted in reduced tumorigenesis and increased sensitivity to metformin or sorafenib [36]. Consistent with these reports, we found that HK2-targeting siRNAs clearly showed a significantly enhanced cell killing effect against both PC-3AcT and DU145AcT cells. A reduction in cellular ATP content due to the inhibition of both glycolysis and mitochondrial function appeared to be the main cause that led to induction of apoptosis and necroptosis. In this process, the effect of curcumin and HK2 silencing appear to be functionally additive, with curcumin's anti-glycolytic role further strengthening the effect of HK2 silencing on PC-3AcT and DU145AcT cells. These data demonstrate that HK2 has essential functions in regulating the survival and growth of PC-3AcT and DU145AcT cells, suggesting the potential significance of HK2 targeting by curcumin as a promising strategy to improve sensitivity to docetaxel.

The preferential cytotoxic effect of curcumin on PC-3AcT cells, which showed an increased tolerance to docetaxel in our previous study [21], and the better killing effect of combined treatment with docetaxel and curcumin than either docetaxel or curcumin observed in this study suggest the potential of curcumin as an adjunctive treatment to docetaxel. The chemo-potentiating effect of curcumin has been shown to be effective without increasing toxicity when used in combination with other established chemotherapeutic agents, such as docetaxel for the treatment of metastatic castration-resistant PC [37], cisplatin in bladder cancer lines [38], doxorubicin in Hodgkin's lymphoma-derived cell line L540 [39], 5-fluorouracil in colorectal cancer [40], and metformin in hepatocellular carcinoma and PC [41,42]. Prior to a full-scale preclinical evaluation of the combination therapy of curcumin and the anticancer drug docetaxel in animal models, we had the premise that the antiglycolytic efficacy of curcumin should not be affected by the addition of docetaxel. In this study, curcumin combined with docetaxel at concentrations that exhibited minimal cytotoxicity to normal prostate epithelial cells induced a significant cell death of PC-3AcT and DU145AcT, as evidenced by anti-glycolytic, apoptotic, and necroptotic effects. The response of cells to combined treatment observed in conventional monolayer cultures was similar in 3D spheroid cultures and nude mouse xenograft models. In particular, the antiglycolytic effect of curcumin in 3D spheroid and xenografts was not affected in the presence of docetaxel, as molecular analysis showed only minor or non-significant differences compared to the in vitro effect in monolayer culture. Three-dimensional (3D) spheroid cultures, which better mimic the in vivo microenvironment, generally tend to be more resistant to anticancer treatment than 2D monolayer cultures. Several factors that lead to different responses in 3D cultures relative to the 2D cultures include the accumulation of more quiescent cells in the center of the spheroid, resulting in increased resistance to chemotherapy [43], enhancement of signaling pathways that participate in drug resistance due to cell–cell or cell–matrix interactions [44], and poor accessibility of drugs inside the spheroid [45,46]. In addition, cells in the hypoxic core of spheroids (which are also seen in solid tumors) are more resistant to therapy and more dependent on anaerobic glycolysis, so oxygen availability may influence cell viability and expression of glycolytic enzymes in response to treatment. In this study, the anti-glycolytic and cytotoxic effects of curcumin and docetaxel in 3D spheroid cultures and xenograft models closely resembled their in vitro effects in monolayer cultures, with only minor or non-significant differences in molecular analysis. Our in vitro experimental conditions, which mimic the tumor microenvironment such as the slightly acidic nature of the lactic acid-containing medium (pH 6.8–7.0), might have minimized these differences. This result also supports a previous report showing that the microenvironment plays a significant role in cellular responses to drugs [47]. Therefore, studies using lactate-acclimated cell lines might be a useful strategy for understanding the role of lactic acid in the tumor microenvironment and developing drugs targeting it. To maintain consistency of drug responses between in vitro and in vivo experiments, it is necessary to introduce experimental conditions that mimic the tumor microenvironment, including a hypoxic condition. Together, we plan to conduct more intensive animal model experiments that take into account in vivo drug efficacy, dose optimization, administration route, toxicity testing, and safety testing, based on our validated in vitro experimental results.

5. Conclusions

Our results provide evidence that lactic acid may play a role in protecting cells against docetaxel through activation of glycolysis and the MEK/ERK pathways. Additionally, by mechanistically elucidating the role of curcumin in inhibiting these pathways, our results support the findings of a previous study revealing preferential cytotoxicity of curcumin against PC-3AcT cells showing increased tolerance to docetaxel. The chemo-potentiating effect of curcumin on PC cells displaying a glycolytic phenotype may help it exert profound cell killing effects by activating both apoptosis and necroptosis.

Author Contributions: D.C.; Writing—Review & Editing, Investigation, Validation, Methodology. J.G.L.; Validation, Investigation, Methodology, Writing—Review & Editing. S.-H.H.; Writing—Review & Editing, Investigation, Methodology. M.-K.C.; Writing—Review & Editing, Conceptualization, Software, Formal Analysis. H.-S.N.; Writing—Review & Editing, Methodology. S.-H.L.; Writing—Original Draft, Writing—Review & Editing, Investigation. Y.-J.L.; Writing—Original Draft, Writing—Review & Editing, Validation, Investigation, Resources, Funding Acquisition. All authors have read and agreed to the published version of the manuscript.

Funding: This research was supported by the Basic Science Research Program through the National Research Foundation (NRF) of Korea, funded by the Ministry of Education (No. NRF-2022R1F1A1069376), and supported by the Soonchunhyang University Research Fund of Soonchunhyang University (No. 2024-0046). We would like to thank the funders for their support of this research. The funders had no role in study design, data collection, analysis, the decision to publish, or the preparation of the manuscript.

Institutional Review Board Statement: Animal welfare and experimental procedures were performed strictly in accordance with high standards for animal welfare approved by the Institutional Animal Care and Use Committee of Soonchunhyang University (Approval No. SCH20-0060; date: 8 March 2021).

Informed Consent Statement: Not applicable.

Data Availability Statement: All data produced or assessed during this study are included in this article.

Conflicts of Interest: The authors declare no conflicts of interest.

References

1. Vaupel, P.; Multhoff, G. Revisiting the Warburg effect: Historical dogma versus current understanding. *J. Physiol.* **2021**, *599*, 1745–1757. [CrossRef]
2. Pfeiffer, T.; Schuster, S.; Bonhoeffer, S. Cooperation and competition in the evolution of ATP-producing pathways. *Science* **2001**, *292*, 504–507. [CrossRef]
3. Locasale, J.W.; Cantley, L.C. Altered metabolism in cancer. *BMC Biol.* **2010**, *25*, 88. [CrossRef]
4. de la Cruz-López, K.G.; Castro-Muñoz, L.J.; Reyes-Hernández, D.O.; García-Carrancá, A.; Manzo-Merino, J. Lactate in the regulation of tumor microenvironment and therapeutic approaches. *Front. Oncol.* **2019**, *1*, 1143. [CrossRef]
5. Chetta, P.; Sriram, R.; Zadra, G. Lactate as key metabolite in prostate cancer progression: What are the clinical implications? *Cancers* **2023**, *15*, 3473. [CrossRef]
6. Lin, C.; Salzillo, T.C.; Bader, D.A.; Wilkenfeld, S.R.; Awad, D.; Pulliam, T.L.; Dutta, P.; Pudakalakatti, S.; Titus, M.; McGuire, S.E.; et al. Prostate cancer energetics and biosynthesis. *Adv. Exp. Med. Biol.* **2019**, *1210*, 185–237.
7. Mah, C.Y.; Nassar, Z.D.; Swinnen, J.V.; Butler, L.M. Lipogenic effects of androgen signaling in normal and malignant prostate. *Asian J. Urol.* **2020**, *7*, 258–270. [CrossRef] [PubMed]

8. San-Millán, I.; Brooks, G.A. Reexamining cancer metabolism: Lactate production for carcinogenesis could be the purpose and explanation of the Warburg effect. *Carcinogenesis* **2017**, *38*, 119–133. [CrossRef] [PubMed]
9. Walenta, S.; Wetterling, M.; Lehrke, M.; Schwickert, G.; Sundfør, K.; Rofstad, E.K.; Mueller-Klieser, W. High lactate levels predict likelihood of metastases, tumor recurrence, and restricted patient survival in human cervical cancers. *Cancer Res.* **2000**, *60*, 916–921. [PubMed]
10. Fabbri, F.; Amadori, D.; Carloni, S.; Brigliadori, G.; Tesei, A.; Ulivi, P.; Rosetti, M.; Vannini, I.; Arienti, C.; Zoli, W.; et al. Mitotic catastrophe and apoptosis induced by docetaxel in hormone-refractory prostate cancer cells. *J. Cell. Physiol.* **2008**, *217*, 494–501. [CrossRef] [PubMed]
11. Sekino, Y.; Teishima, J. Molecular mechanisms of docetaxel resistance in prostate cancer. *Cancer Drug Resist.* **2020**, *3*, 676–685. [CrossRef]
12. Li, J.; Pan, J.; Liu, Y.; Luo, X.; Yang, C.; Xiao, W.; Li, Q.; Yang, L.; Zhang, X. 3-Bromopyruvic acid regulates glucose metabolism by targeting the c-Myc/TXNIP axis and induces mitochondria-mediated apoptosis in TNBC cells. *Exp. Ther. Med.* **2022**, *16*, 520. [CrossRef] [PubMed]
13. Saulle, E.; Spinello, I.; Quaranta, M.T.; Pasquini, L.; Pelosi, E.; Iorio, E.; Castelli, G.; Chirico, M.; Pisanu, M.E.; Ottone, T.; et al. Targeting lactate metabolism by inhibiting MCT1 or MCT4 Impairs leukemic cell proliferation, induces two different related death-pathways and increases chemotherapeutic sensitivity of acute myeloid leukemia cells. *Front. Oncol.* **2020**, *10*, 621458. [CrossRef] [PubMed]
14. Senthebane, D.A.; Rowe, A.; Thomford, N.E.; Shipanga, H.; Munro, D.; Mazeedi, M.; Almazyadi, H.A.M.; Kallmeyer, K.; Dandara, C.; Pepper, M.S.; et al. The role of tumor microenvironment in chemoresistance: To survive, keep your enemies closer. *Int. J. Mol. Sci.* **2017**, *18*, 1586. [CrossRef] [PubMed]
15. Cerezo, M.; Rocchi, S. Cancer cell metabolic reprogramming: A keystone for the response to immunotherapy. *Cell Death Dis.* **2020**, *11*, 964. [CrossRef] [PubMed]
16. Kooshan, Z.; Cárdenas-Piedra, L.; Clements, J.; Batra, J. Glycolysis, the sweet appetite of the tumor microenvironment. *Cancer Lett.* **2024**, *28*, 217156. [CrossRef]
17. Mokbel, K.; Wazir, U.; Mokbel, K. Chemoprevention of prostate cancer by natural agents: Evidence from molecular and epidemiological studies. *Anticancer Res.* **2019**, *39*, 5231–5259. [CrossRef]
18. Menon, V.P.; Sudheer, A.R. Antioxidant and anti-inflammatory properties of curcumin. *Adv. Exp. Med. Biol.* **2007**, *595*, 105–125. [PubMed]
19. Wong, S.C.; Kamarudin, M.N.A.; Naidu, R. Anticancer mechanism of curcumin on human glioblastoma. *Nutrients* **2021**, *13*, 950. [CrossRef]
20. Farghadani, R.; Naidu, R. Curcumin as an enhancer of therapeutic efficiency of chemotherapy drugs in breast cancer. *Int. J. Mol. Sci.* **2022**, *23*, 2144. [CrossRef]
21. Lee, Y.J.; Park, K.S.; Lee, S.H. Curcumin targets both apoptosis and necroptosis in acidity-tolerant prostate carcinoma cells. *Biomed. Res. Int.* **2021**, *2021*, 8859181. [CrossRef]
22. Lee, Y.J.; Lee, S.H. ERK1/2-dependent inhibition of glycolysis in curcumin-induced cytotoxicity of prostate carcinoma cells. *Biomed. Res. Int.* **2022**, *2022*, 7626405. [CrossRef] [PubMed]
23. Lee, Y.J.; Lee, Y.J.; Im, J.H.; Won, S.Y.; Kim, Y.B.; Cho, M.K.; Nam, H.S.; Choi, Y.J.; Lee, S.H. Synergistic anti-cancer effects of resveratrol and chemotherapeutic agent clofarabine against human malignant mesothelioma MSTO-211H cells. *Food Chem. Toxicol.* **2013**, *52*, 61–68. [CrossRef]
24. Chambers, K.F.; Mosaad, E.M.; Russell, P.J.; Clements, J.A.; Doran, M.R., 3rd. 3D cultures of prostate cancer cells cultured in a novel high-throughput culture platform are more resistant to chemotherapeutics compared to cells cultured in monolayer. *PLoS ONE* **2014**, *9*, e111029. [CrossRef]
25. Malumbres, M.; Barbacid, M. Mammalian cyclin-dependent kinases. *Trends Biochem. Sci.* **2005**, *30*, 630–641. [CrossRef]
26. Smits, V.A.; Medema, R.H. Checking out the G(2)/M transition. *Biochim. Biophys. Acta* **2001**, *1519*, 1–12. [CrossRef]
27. Dai, Q.S.; Liu, W.; Wang, X.B.; Lu, N.; Gong, D.D.; Kong, L.Y.; Guo, Q.L. NCPMF-60 induces G2/M cell cycle arrest and apoptosis in human hepatocellular carcinoma HepG2 cells. *Anticancer Drugs* **2011**, *22*, 46–57. [CrossRef]
28. Papa, S.; Choy, P.M.; Bubici, C. The ERK and JNK pathways in the regulation of metabolic reprogramming. *Oncogene* **2019**, *38*, 2223–2240. [CrossRef]
29. Cui, N.; Li, L.; Feng, Q.; Ma, H.M.; Lei, D.; Zheng, P.S. Hexokinase 2 promotes cell growth and tumor formation through the Raf/MEK/ERK signaling pathway in cervical cancer. *Front. Oncol.* **2020**, *10*, 581208. [CrossRef]
30. Liu, C.; Li, C.; Liu, Y. The role of metabolic reprogramming in pancreatic cancer chemoresistance. *Front. Pharmacol.* **2023**, *13*, 1108776. [CrossRef] [PubMed]
31. Mathupala, S.P.; Ko, Y.H.; Pedersen, P.L. The pivotal roles of mitochondria in cancer: Warburg and beyond and encouraging prospects for effective therapies. *Biochim. Biophys. Acta* **2010**, *1797*, 1225–1230. [CrossRef] [PubMed]
32. Ciscato, F.; Ferrone, L.; Masgras, I.; Laquatra, C.; Rasola, A. Hexokinase 2 in cancer: A prima donna playing multiple characters. *Int. J. Mol. Sci.* **2021**, *22*, 4716. [CrossRef] [PubMed]
33. Wiel, C.; Le Gal, K.; Ibrahim, M.X.; Jahangir, C.A.; Kashif, M.; Yao, H.; Ziegler, D.V.; Xu, X.; Ghosh, T.; Mondal, T.; et al. BACH1 Stabilization by antioxidants stimulates lung cancer metastasis. *Cell* **2019**, *178*, 330-345.e22. [CrossRef]

34. Patra, K.C.; Wang, Q.; Bhaskar, P.T.; Miller, L.; Wang, Z.; Wheaton, W.; Chandel, N.; Laakso, M.; Muller, W.J.; Allen, E.L.; et al. Hexokinase 2 is required for tumor initiation and maintenance and its systemic deletion is therapeutic in mouse models of cancer. *Cancer Cell* **2013**, *24*, 213–228. [CrossRef]
35. Wang, L.; Xiong, H.; Wu, F.; Zhang, Y.; Wang, J.; Zhao, L.; Guo, X.; Chang, L.J.; Zhang, Y.; You, M.J.; et al. Hexokinase 2-mediated Warburg effect is required for PTEN- and p53-deficiency-driven prostate cancer growth. *Cell Rep.* **2014**, *8*, 1461–1474. [CrossRef]
36. DeWaal, D.; Nogueira, V.; Terry, A.R.; Patra, K.C.; Jeon, S.M.; Guzman, G.; Au, J.; Long, C.P.; Antoniewicz, M.R.; Hay, N. Hexokinase-2 depletion inhibits glycolysis and induces oxidative phosphorylation in hepatocellular carcinoma and sensitizes to metformin. *Nat. Commun.* **2018**, *9*, 446. [CrossRef] [PubMed]
37. Banerjee, S.; Singh, S.K.; Chowdhury, I.; Lillard, J.W., Jr.; Singh, R. Combinatorial effect of curcumin with docetaxel modulates apoptotic and cell survival molecules in prostate cancer. *Front. Biosci.* **2017**, *9*, 235–245.
38. Park, B.H.; Lim, J.E.; Jeon, H.G.; Seo, S.I.; Lee, H.M.; Choi, H.Y.; Jeon, S.S.; Jeong, B.C. Curcumin potentiates antitumor activity of cisplatin in bladder cancer cell lines via ROS-mediated activation of ERK1/2. *Oncotarget* **2016**, *7*, 63870–63886. [CrossRef] [PubMed]
39. Guorgui, J.; Wang, R.; Mattheolabakis, G.; Mackenzie, G.G. Curcumin formulated in solid lipid nanoparticles has enhanced efficacy in Hodgkin's lymphoma in mice. *Arch. Biochem. Biophys.* **2018**, *648*, 12–19. [CrossRef]
40. Zhou, X.; Wang, W.; Li, P.; Zheng, Z.; Tu, Y.; Zhang, Y.; You, T. Curcumin enhances the effects of 5-fluorouracil and oxaliplatin in inducing gastric cancer cell apoptosis both in vitro and in vivo. *Oncol. Res.* **2016**, *23*, 29–34. [CrossRef]
41. Donadon, V.; Balbi, M.; Mas, M.D.; Casarin, P.; Zanette, G. Metformin and reduced risk of hepatocellular carcinoma in diabetic patients with chronic liver disease. *Liver Int.* **2010**, *30*, 750–758. [CrossRef]
42. Zaidi, S.; Gandhi, J.; Joshi, G.; Smith, N.L.; Khan, S.A. The anticancer potential of metformin on prostate cancer. *Prostate Cancer Prostatic Dis.* **2019**, *22*, 351–361. [CrossRef]
43. Lovitt, C.J.; Shelper, T.B.; Avery, V.M. Doxorubicin resistance in breast cancer cells is mediated by extracellular matrix proteins. *BMC Cancer* **2018**, *18*, 41. [CrossRef]
44. Samimi, H.; Sohi, A.N.; Irani, S.; Arefian, E.; Mahdiannasser, M.; Fallah, P.; Haghpanah, V. Alginate-based 3D cell culture technique to evaluate the half-maximal inhibitory concentration: An in vitro model of anticancer drug study for anaplastic thyroid carcinoma. *Thyroid Res.* **2021**, *14*, 27. [CrossRef]
45. Edmondson, R.; Adcock, A.F.; Yang, L. Influence of matrices on 3D-cultured prostate cancer cells' drug response and expression of drug-action associated proteins. *PLoS ONE* **2016**, *11*, e0158116. [CrossRef] [PubMed]
46. Sheta, R.; Bachvarova, M.; Plante, M.; Renaud, M.C.; Sebastianelli, A.; Gregoire, J.; Navarro, J.M.; Perez, R.B.; Masson, J.Y.; Bachvarov, D. Development of a 3D functional assay and identification of biomarkers, predictive for response of high-grade serous ovarian cancer (HGSOC) patients to poly-ADP ribose polymerase inhibitors (PARPis): Targeted therapy. *J. Transl. Med.* **2020**, *18*, 439. [CrossRef]
47. Wu, T.; Dai, Y. Tumor microenvironment and therapeutic response. *Cancer Lett.* **2017**, *387*, 61–68. [CrossRef] [PubMed]

nutrients

MDPI

Article

Tryptanthrin Down-Regulates Oncostatin M by Targeting GM-CSF-Mediated PI3K-AKT-NF-κB Axis

Na-Ra Han [1,2], Hi-Joon Park [3], Seong-Gyu Ko [2,4] and Phil-Dong Moon [5,*]

1 College of Korean Medicine, Kyung Hee University, Seoul 02447, Republic of Korea; nrhan@khu.ac.kr
2 Korean Medicine-Based Drug Repositioning Cancer Research Center, College of Korean Medicine, Kyung Hee University, Seoul 02447, Republic of Korea; epiko@khu.ac.kr
3 Department of Anatomy & Information Sciences, College of Korean Medicine, Kyung Hee University, Seoul 02447, Republic of Korea; acufind@khu.ac.kr
4 Department of Preventive Medicine, College of Korean Medicine, Kyung Hee University, Seoul 02447, Republic of Korea
5 Center for Converging Humanities, Kyung Hee University, Seoul 02447, Republic of Korea
* Correspondence: pdmoon@khu.ac.kr

Abstract: Background: Oncostatin M (OSM) is involved in several inflammatory responses. Tryptanthrin (TRYP), as a natural alkaloid, is a bioactive compound derived from indigo plants. Objectives/ Methods: The purpose of this study is to investigate the potential inhibitory activity of TRYP on OSM release from neutrophils using neutrophils-like differentiated (d)HL-60 cells and neutrophils from mouse bone marrow. Results: The results showed that TRYP reduced the production and mRNA expression levels of OSM in the granulocyte–macrophage colony-stimulating factor (GM-CSF)-stimulated neutrophils-like dHL-60 cells. In addition, TRYP decreased the OSM production levels in the GM-CSF-stimulated neutrophils from mouse bone marrow. TRYP inhibited the phosphorylation of phosphatidylinositol 3-kinase (PI3K), AKT, and nuclear factor (NF)-κB in the GM-CSF-stimulated neutrophils-like dHL-60 cells. Conclusions: Therefore, these results reveal for the first time that TRYP inhibits OSM release via the down-regulation of PI3K-AKT-NF-κB axis from neutrophils, presenting its potential as a therapeutic agent for inflammatory responses.

Keywords: tryptanthrin; oncostatin M; neutrophils; inflammation

1. Introduction

Inflammation is an immune reaction that results from a wide range of factors [1]. Acute inflammation is caused by infection or exposure to substances and is characterized by pain, redness, swelling, and heat. However, chronic inflammation can lead to serious and potentially life-threatening conditions [2,3]. Inflammation is also closely related to the development and malignant progression of a variety of cancers [4,5]. Oncostatin M (OSM) is well known to be a growth inhibitor of several types of tumor cells [6]. However, OSM is an inflammatory cytokine and implicated in the pathogenesis of inflammatory responses [7,8]. OSM has thus been identified as a therapeutic target for inflammatory responses as well as several types of cancers [9].

OSM is produced by neutrophils, osteoblasts, or bone marrow macrophages [7]. Neutrophils, as an important component of the innate immune response, are the first line of defense against pathogens arriving at sites of acute inflammation [10]. Neutrophils also contribute to the activation of other immune cells in sites of chronic inflammation [11]. Granulocyte macrophage–colony-stimulating factor (GM-CSF) functions as a differentiation factor for neutrophil precursors; stimulates mature neutrophils; and affects phagocytosis, degranulation, or transmigration of neutrophils [12]. GM-CSF leads to the release of OSM from neutrophil granules and augments inflammatory responses [12]. GM-CSF-induced OSM expression is regulated via the phosphatidylinositol 3-kinase (PI3K), AKT, and nuclear factor (NF)-κB signaling pathway in neutrophils [13].

Human promyelocytic leukemia (HL-60) is a commonly used surrogate cell line model of neutrophils [14]. Treatment of HL-60 cells with dimethyl sulfoxide (DMSO) induces differentiation into neutrophil-like cells [15,16]. The DMSO-induced neutrophils-like differentiated (d) HL-60 cells have already been applied in studies to elucidate neutrophil functions [15,17]. The bone marrow of mice serves as a reservoir for isolating large numbers of neutrophils [18]. The bone marrow-derived neutrophils have also been used in neutrophil research [19,20].

Tryptanthrin (TRYP), as a natural alkaloid, is a bioactive compound derived from medicinal indigo plants [21–23]. TRYP has been shown to exert anti-cancer [24], anti-atherosclerosis [25], anti-atopic dermatitis [26], and anti-neuroinflammatory activities [27]. Regarding neutrophils, there are reports that TRYP exerts pharmacological effects by regulating leukotriene formation in calcium ionophore or lipopolysaccharides-stimulated neutrophils [28,29]. However, no studies have investigated the regulatory effect of TRYP on OSM in GM-CSF-stimulated neutrophils. Considering the pharmacological effects of TRYP mentioned above, we hypothesized that TRYP may regulate OSM levels in the GM-CSF-stimulated neutrophils. Here, we demonstrate the effectiveness of TRYP on OSM in neutrophils-like dHL-60 cells and neutrophils from mouse bone marrow, and we explore mechanisms underlying these effects.

2. Materials and Methods

2.1. TRYP

TRYP (purity $\geq$ 99%) was bought from Sigma-Aldrich (St. Louis, MO, USA). It was dissolved in DMSO and then diluted with culture media.

2.2. Cells

HL-60 cells (Korean Cell Line Bank, Seoul, Republic of Korea) were differentiated into neutrophil-like dHL-60 cells by treating them with 1.3% v/v DMSO for 7 days. Bone marrow-derived neutrophils were isolated using the density gradient method according to an established protocol [18,30], which was approved by the Animal Care Committee (#KHSASP-24-623). Briefly, bone marrow from male C57BL/6 mice was extracted by flushing with RPMI 1640 (Gibco, Waltham, MA, USA). Neutrophils were enriched by density centrifugation using Histopaque 1077 (Sigma-Aldrich, Cat. No. 10771) and Histopaque 1119 (Sigma-Aldrich, Cat. No. 11191). Neutrophils were collected from the interphase of the two Histopaque layers. Both HL-60 cells and bone marrow-derived neutrophils were cultured in RPMI 1640 with 10% heat-inactivated fetal bovine serum (Merck Millipore, Burlington, MA, USA) and 1% penicillin/streptomycin antibiotics (Gibco) at 37 °C in 5% CO_2 and 95% air.

2.3. Cell Viability Assay

The cell viability was analyzed using a 3-(4,5-dimethylthiazol-2-yl)-2,5-diphenyltetrazolium bromide (MTT) assay after cells were incubated with TRYP for 1 h and then with recombinant GM-CSF (5 ng/mL, Cat. No. 215-GM (for HL-60 cells, *E. coli*-derived human GM-CSF protein Ala18-Glu144), Cat. No. 415-ML (for mouse neutrophils, *E. coli*-derived mouse GM-CSF protein Ala18-Lys141, with an N-terminal Met), R&D Systems, Minneapolis, MN, USA) for an additional 4 h.

3. Results

3.1. Effect of TRYP on OSM Release

The cell viability was first investigated at different concentrations of TRYP in GM-CSF-stimulated neutrophil-like dHL-60 cells using an MTT assay. Cells were incubated with TRYP for 1 h and then with recombinant GM-CSF for 4 h. The cell viability was suppressed at a concentration of 100 μM of TRYP (Figure 1a). The dose–response curve for cell viability clearly shows the concentration-dependent effects of TRYP on cell viability (Supplementary Figure S1). In subsequent experiments, we used TRYP at and below 10 μM less than

100 μM [26,31]. Additionally, we confirmed that TRYP (0.1 μM–10 μM) did not affect the survival rate at 12 h and 24 h after GM-CSF stimulation (Supplementary Figure S2). We next assessed the effects of TRYP on OSM release in the GM-CSF-stimulated neutrophil-like dHL-60 cells. Consistent with previous reports [12,13], the GM-CSF treatment augmented the OSM release from neutrophil-like dHL-60 cells. However, the treatment with TRYP dose-dependently reduced the OSM release compared to the GM-CSF-stimulated control group (Figure 1b). The dose–response curve for OSM release clearly demonstrates a concentration-dependent inhibitory effect of TRYP on OSM release (Supplementary Figure S3). The decreased expression levels of OSM by TRYP were visualized by immunofluorescence microscopy (Figure 1c). Furthermore, GM-CSF treatment resulted in a progressive release of OSM from bone marrow-derived neutrophils, with peak induction at 4 h (Supplementary Figure S4a). The treatment with TRYP dose-dependently reduced the OSM release from bone marrow-derived neutrophils (Supplementary Figure S4b), with no effect on neutrophil viability (Supplementary Figure S4c). In addition, Figure 2 shows that the GM-CSF-stimulation significantly increased mRNA expression of OSM. This effect caused by GM-CSF was clearly reversed by TRYP treatment.

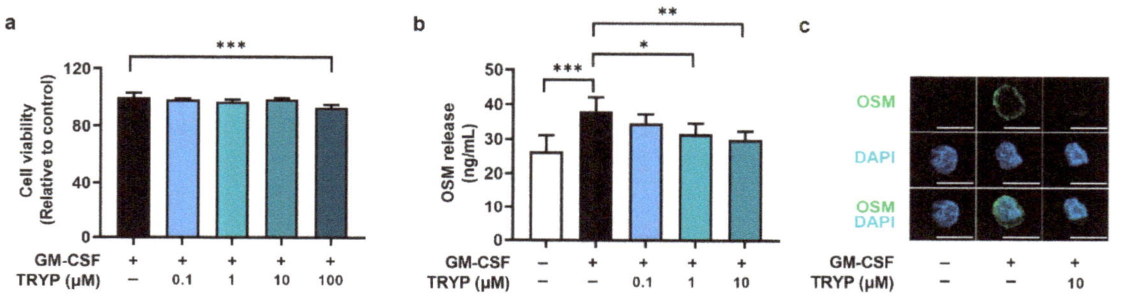

Figure 1. TRYP reduces OSM release. dHL-60 cells were stimulated with GM-CSF, with or without TRYP, for 4 h. (**a**) The cell viability was assessed using an MTT assay. (**b**) OSM production was examined using ELISA. (c) Representative images for OSM were obtained by confocal microscopy (scale bar, 10 μm). * $p < 0.05$; ** $p < 0.01$; *** $p < 0.001$.

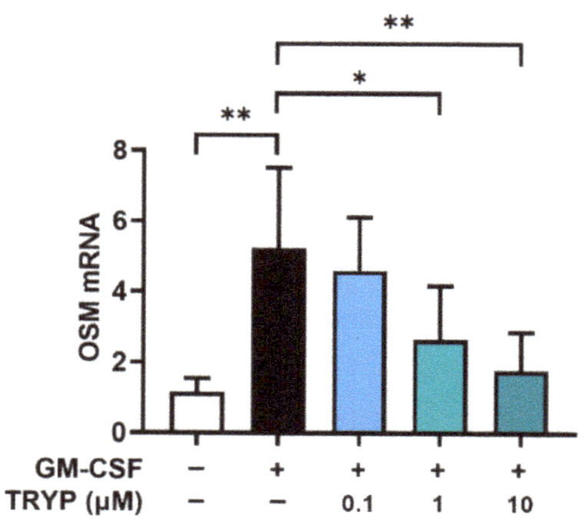

Figure 2. TRYP reduces the OSM mRNA levels. dHL-60 cells were stimulated with GM-CSF, with or without TRYP, for 30 min. OSM mRNA expression was assessed with qPCR. * $p < 0.05$; ** $p < 0.01$.

3.2. Effect of TRYP on Phosphorylation of PI3K

A PI3K inhibitor reduced the OSM expression in several cells, including neutrophils [13,32]. In addition, the authors' previous report revealed that wortmannin, a PI3K inhibitor, reduces the GM-CSF-induced OSM levels in neutrophil-like dHL-60 cells [13]. We thus performed Western blot analysis on the phosphorylation of PI3K in neutrophil-like dHL-60 cells to further elucidate the underlying mechanisms driving the regulatory effect of TRYP on GM-CSF-induced OSM production. As expected, TRYP significantly suppressed the phosphorylation levels of PI3K increased by GM-CSF (Figure 3).

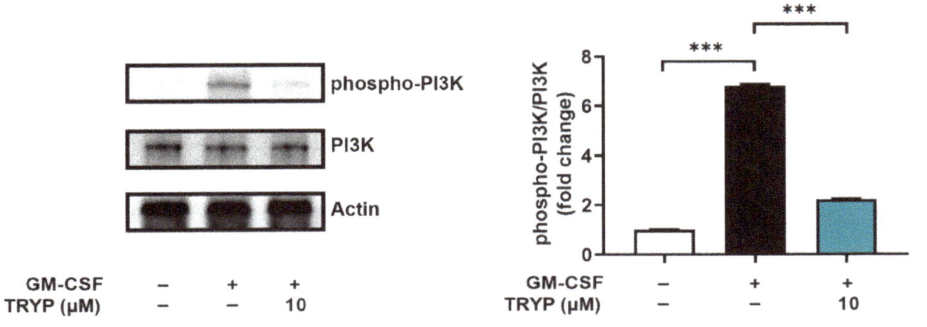

Figure 3. TRYP reduces the phosphorylation of PI3K. The phospho-PI3K levels were analyzed using immunoblots. Quantitative analysis of blots from three independent experiments is displayed in the right panel. *** $p < 0.001$.

3.3. Effect of TRYP on Phosphorylation of AKT

AKT, as a key downstream target of PI3K, is a critical component of signaling following PI3K activation [33]. In addition, MK 2206, an AKT inhibitor, decreased the GM-CSF-induced OSM levels in neutrophil-like dHL-60 cells [13]. WB analysis demonstrated that TRYP significantly inhibited the phosphorylation levels of AKT compared to the GM-CSF-stimulated control group (Figure 4).

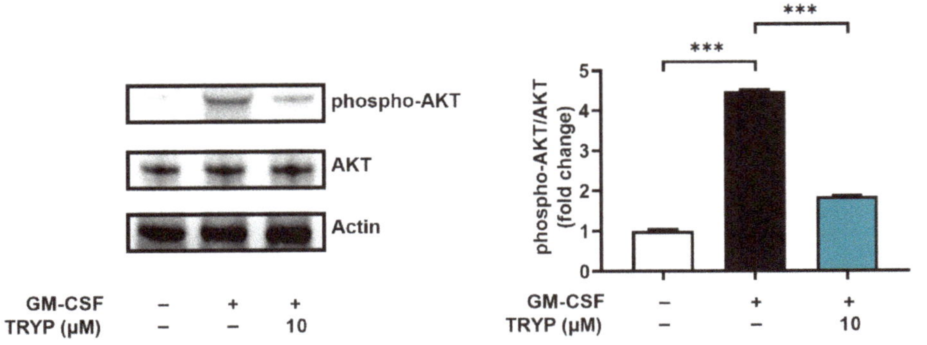

Figure 4. TRYP reduces the phosphorylation of AKT. The phospho-AKT levels were measured by WB analysis. Quantitative analysis of blots from three independent experiments is displayed in the right panel. *** $p < 0.001$.

3.4. Effect of TRYP on Phosphorylation of NF-κB

AKT induces phosphorylation of NF-κB and thus modulates the transcriptional activity of NF-κB [33]. PDTC, a NF-κB inhibitor, suppressed the GM-CSF-induced OSM levels in neutrophil-like dHL-60 cells [13]. Subsequently, we examined whether TRYP would regulate the phosphorylation of NF-κB. TRYP significantly inhibited the phospho-NF-κB levels increased by GM-CSF (Figure 5). These results (Figures 3–5) indicated that the anti-inflammatory effect of TRYP resulted from the inhibition of OSM levels regulated by PI3K-AKT-NF-κB signaling pathways in neutrophils.

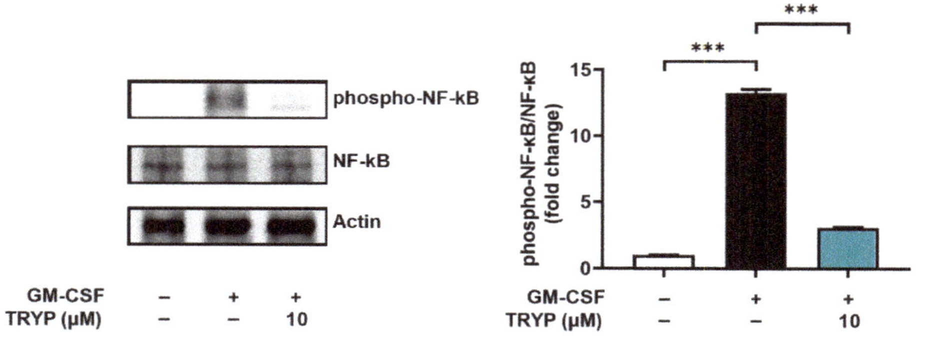

Figure 5. TRYP reduces the phosphorylation of NF-κB. The phospho-NF-κB levels were analyzed using immunoblots. Quantitative analysis of blots from three independent experiments is displayed in the right panel. *** $p < 0.001$.

4. Discussion

Medicinal plants are composed of bioactive compounds or secondary metabolites that possess biological activity [34]. Given the various side effects and drug resistance, medicinal plants may be a useful alternative treatment [34,35]. Bioactive compounds or phytonutrients, as health-promoting biologically active compounds found in medicinal plants or plant-based foods, have been actively researched scientifically for human health [36]. Phytonutrients include alkaloids, phenolics, and several other food components [36]. These have a variety of useful properties for human health, such as inhibition of inflammatory and oxidative reactions [37,38]. Indigo is commonly used to dye textile products, but it is also used as a dye in foods and pharmaceuticals [39]. Indigo also contains a significant amount of phytonutrients such as alkaloid, total phenols, tannins, saponins, and flavonoids [40] and has various pharmacological efficacy in the inhibition of oxidation, inflammation, and angiogenesis reactions [23,41]. Alkaloids are used in medicine, particularly for their anesthetic, cardioprotective, cytostatic, and anti-inflammatory effects [42]. TRYP is a natural alkaloid found in medicinal indigo plants [21]. This study revealed a novel pharmacological effect of TRYP by demonstrating that TRYP inhibits OSM production in neutrophils. This is the first work to demonstrate the regulatory effect of TRYP on neutrophil-derived OSM. However, additional experiments are needed to verify the effectiveness of TRYP against OSM in several inflammatory models.

Inflammation is a complex cellular process that involves immune cells and signaling molecules [43]. Several immune-related factors are involved in regulating both inflammation and cancer progression [44]. OSM, as a cytokine fulfilling several functions, is most closely associated with leukemia inhibitory factors [6]. However, a pro-tumorigenic role of OSM has also been reported in breast cancer or pancreatic cancer [45]. Interestingly, OSM in inflammatory responses plays opposing roles, suggesting that it may vary depending on the stage of inflammation and the inflammatory environment. The anti-inflammatory properties of OSM were established in experimental models of rheumatoid arthritis and lung inflammation [46,47]. In contrast, there is increasing evidence that OSM has pro-inflammatory properties [6,48,49]. Retrospective studies conducted in Hong Kong and Atlanta found that increased OSM was correlated with disease severity in COVID-19 infection [50]. OSM expression was increased in inflamed tissue from patients with Crohn's disease and ulcerative colitis compared to non-inflamed colonic lesions of these patients [51]. OSM expression was also increased in inflamed tissues of patients with inflammatory bowel disease, which was closely related to disease severity [52]. Subcutaneous injection of OSM induced an acute inflammatory response in mice [48]. There are several reports suggesting the possibility that TRYP's effects on OSM may influence current treatments for inflammatory diseases. OSM knockout mice with inflammatory bowel disease had reduced severity of overall pathology and disease features compared to wild-type mice [52]. The administration of anti-OSM antibodies to mouse models with arthritis significantly improved the arthritis severity [53]. In addition, a recent study has shown that a bioactive compound, berberine, attenuates chronic ulcerative colitis by inhibiting OSM production [54]. We demonstrated that OSM production was increased in the GM-CSF-stimulated neutrophil-like dHL-60 cells and neutrophils from mouse bone marrow, and TRYP decreased the increased OSM production, suggesting an anti-inflammatory effect of TRYP and its potential applications in various OSM-mediated inflammatory responses in this study. Nevertheless, further studies are warranted to study the efficacy of TRYP on the clinical significance of OSM in several OSM-mediated inflammatory models.

The AKT which functions as a critical downstream target of PI3K, and PI3K phosphorylate numerous protein targets that regulate several cellular processes [33,55]. In addition, the PI3K-AKT pathway is part of a signaling pathway required to induce key immune and inflammatory responses because PI3K-AKT functions as upstream kinases for NF-κB activation [56,57]. The NF-κB transcription factor is a critical mediator of the inflammatory responses, and several studies have demonstrated that NF-κB plays an important role in linking inflammation and cancer [58]. OSM has been reported to be expressed through the PI3K-AKT-NF-κB signaling pathway in osteoblasts [32]. In our previous report, we revealed that OSM expression was regulated via the PI3K-AKT-NF-κB signaling pathway in neutrophils [13]. Binding of GM-CSF to its receptor activates src-tyrosine kinase Lyn (LYN), which activate PI3K-AKT signaling in human neutrophils [59]. The serine/threonine protein kinase pim (PIM) and hematopoietic cell kinase (HCK, tyrosine protein kinase) interact with PI3K-AKT and induce PI3K-AKT phosphorylation [60–62]. Han et al. [63] indicated that indigo and TRYP potentially bind LYN, PIM1, and HCK and inhibit the expression of these proteins. We found that TRYP inhibits OSM levels via the PI3K-AKT-NF-κB signaling pathway in this study. Thus, we suggest that TRYP might down-regulate PI3K-AKT-NF-κB signaling by interacting with these kinase proteins. However, further studies are needed to elucidate the exact molecular mechanisms by analyzing the direct binding of TRYP to these proteins in GM-CSF-stimulated neutrophils.

5. Conclusions

Collectively, this study is the first to demonstrate that TRYP presented a significantly beneficial effect on neutrophils by regulating the OSM production through the PI3K, AKT, and NF-κB pathways. Therefore, TRYP may have the potential to treat OSM-mediated inflammatory diseases. However, this study has a limitation in that no in vivo experiments were conducted as part of the study. This study focused on the in vitro effects of TRYP on the OSM release from neutrophils. However, the findings of this study may provide foundational data and persuasive evidence to support the exploration of TRYP in future studies of animal models of OSM-mediated inflammatory responses. It also provides insight into the potential utility of TRYP in addressing OSM-mediated inflammatory diseases. However, in vivo studies clarifying functional OSM in several inflammation models are needed to demonstrate the anti-inflammatory effects of TRYP.

Supplementary Materials: The following supporting information can be downloaded at: https://www.mdpi.com/article/10.3390/nu16234109/s1, Figure S1: Dose-response curve for cell viability of TRYP; Figure S2: The effect of TRYP on survival rate; Figure S3: Dose-response curve for OSM release of TRYP; Figure S4: Effect of TRYP on OSM release from bone marrow-derived neutrophils. Table S1. PCR primer sequence.

Author Contributions: Conceptualization, N.-R.H., H.-J.P., S.-G.K. and P.-D.M.; methodology, H.-J.P. and S.-G.K.; formal analysis and data analysis, N.-R.H. and P.-D.M.; writing—original draft, N.-R.H.; funding acquisition, S.-G.K.; writing—review and editing, P.-D.M. All authors have read and agreed to the published version of the manuscript.

Funding: This work was supported by the National Research Foundation of Korea (NRF) grant funded by the Korea government (MSIT) (No. 2020R1A5A2019413).

Institutional Review Board Statement: Not applicable.

Informed Consent Statement: Not applicable.

Data Availability Statement: The data sets used and/or analyzed during the current study are available from the corresponding author due to legal reasons.

Conflicts of Interest: The authors declare no conflicts of interest.

References

1. Chen, L.; Deng, H.; Cui, H.; Fang, J.; Zuo, Z.; Deng, J.; Li, Y.; Wang, X.; Zhao, L. Inflammatory responses and inflammation-associated diseases in organs. *Oncotarget* **2017**, *9*, 7204–7218. [CrossRef] [PubMed]
2. Hannoodee, S.; Nasuruddin, D.N. Acute Inflammatory Response. In *StatPearls*; StatPearls Publishing: Treasure Island, FL, USA, 2024.
3. Pahwa, R.; Goyal, A.; Jialal, I. Chronic Inflammation. In *StatPearls*; StatPearls Publishing: Treasure Island, FL, USA, 2023.
4. Zhao, H.; Wu, L.; Yan, G.; Chen, Y.; Zhou, M.; Wu, Y.; Li, Y. Inflammation and tumor progression: Signaling pathways and targeted intervention. *Signal Transduct. Target. Ther.* **2021**, *6*, 263. [CrossRef] [PubMed]
5. Rutter, M.; Saunders, B.; Wilkinson, K.; Rumbles, S.; Schofield, G.; Kamm, M.; Williams, C.; Price, A.; Talbot, I.; Forbes, A. Severity of inflammation is a risk factor for colorectal neoplasia in ulcerative colitis. *Gastroenterology* **2004**, *126*, 451–459. [CrossRef] [PubMed]
6. Tanaka, M.; Miyajima, A. Oncostatin M, a multifunctional cytokine. *Rev. Physiol. Biochem. Pharmacol.* **2003**, *149*, 39–52. [CrossRef] [PubMed]
7. Sims, N.A.; Lévesque, J.P. Oncostatin M: Dual Regulator of the Skeletal and Hematopoietic Systems. *Curr. Osteoporos. Rep.* **2024**, *22*, 80–95. [CrossRef]
8. Verstockt, S.; Verstockt, B.; Machiels, K.; Vancamelbeke, M.; Ferrante, M.; Cleynen, I.; De Hertogh, G.; Vermeire, S. Oncostatin M Is a Biomarker of Diagnosis, Worse Disease Prognosis, and Therapeutic Nonresponse in Inflammatory Bowel Disease. *Inflamm. Bowel Dis.* **2021**, *27*, 1564–1575. [CrossRef]
9. Wolf, C.L.; Pruett, C.; Lighter, D.; Jorcyk, C.L. The clinical relevance of OSM in inflammatory diseases: A comprehensive review. *Front. Immunol.* **2023**, *14*, 1239732. [CrossRef]
10. Kraus, R.F.; Gruber, M.A. Neutrophils-From Bone Marrow to First-Line Defense of the Innate Immune System. *Front. Immunol.* **2021**, *12*, 767175. [CrossRef]
11. Herrero-Cervera, A.; Soehnlein, O.; Kenne, E. Neutrophils in chronic inflammatory diseases. *Cell. Mol. Immunol.* **2022**, *19*, 177–191. [CrossRef]
12. Elbjeirami, W.M.; Donnachie, E.M.; Burns, A.R.; Smith, C.W. Endothelium-derived GM-CSF influences expression of oncostatin M. *Am. J. Physiol. Cell Physiol.* **2011**, *301*, C947–C953. [CrossRef]
13. Han, N.R.; Ko, S.G.; Park, H.J.; Moon, P.D. Dexamethasone Attenuates Oncostatin M Production via Suppressing of PI3K/Akt/NF-κB Signaling in Neutrophil-like Differentiated HL-60 Cells. *Molecules* **2022**, *27*, 129. [CrossRef] [PubMed]
14. Babatunde, K.A.; Wang, X.; Hopke, A.; Lannes, N.; Mantel, P.Y.; Irimia, D. Chemotaxis and swarming in differentiated HL-60 neutrophil-like cells. *Sci. Rep.* **2021**, *11*, 778. [CrossRef] [PubMed]
15. Guo, Y.; Gao, F.; Wang, Q.; Wang, K.; Pan, S.; Pan, Z.; Xu, S.; Li, L.; Zhao, D. Differentiation of HL-60 cells in serum-free hematopoietic cell media enhances the production of neutrophil extracellular traps. *Exp. Ther. Med.* **2021**, *21*, 353. [CrossRef] [PubMed]
16. Wang, D.; Sennari, Y.; Shen, M.; Morita, K.; Kanazawa, T.; Yoshida, Y. ERK is involved in the differentiation and function of dimethyl sulfoxide-induced HL-60 neutrophil-like cells, which mimic inflammatory neutrophils. *Int. Immunopharmacol.* **2020**, *84*, 106510. [CrossRef] [PubMed]
17. Bhakta, S.B.; Lundgren, S.M.; Sesti, B.N.; Flores, B.A.; Akdogan, E.; Collins, S.R.; Mercer, F. Neutrophil-like cells derived from the HL-60 cell-line as a genetically-tractable model for neutrophil degranulation. *PLoS ONE* **2024**, *19*, e0297758. [CrossRef]
18. Wishart, A.L.; Swamydas, M.; Lionakis, M.S. Isolation of Mouse Neutrophils. *Curr. Protoc.* **2023**, *3*, e879. [CrossRef]
19. Evrard, M.; Kwok, I.W.H.; Chong, S.Z.; Teng, K.W.W.; Becht, E.; Chen, J.; Sieow, J.L.; Penny, H.L.; Ching, G.C.; Devi, S.; et al. Developmental Analysis of Bone Marrow Neutrophils Reveals Populations Specialized in Expansion, Trafficking, and Effector Functions. *Immunity* **2018**, *48*, 364–379.e8. [CrossRef]
20. Luo, Z.; Lu, Y.; Shi, Y.; Jiang, M.; Shan, X.; Li, X.; Zhang, J.; Qin, B.; Liu, X.; Guo, X.; et al. Neutrophil hitchhiking for drug delivery to the bone marrow. *Nat. Nanotechnol.* **2023**, *18*, 647–656. [CrossRef]

21. Liao, X.; Zhou, X.; Mak, N.K.; Leung, K.N. Tryptanthrin inhibits angiogenesis by targeting the VEGFR2-mediated ERK1/2 signalling pathway. *PLoS ONE* **2013**, *8*, e82294. [CrossRef]
22. Pinheiro, D.; Pineiro, M.; Pina, J.; Brandão, P.; Galvão, A.M.; Seixas de Melo, J.S. Tryptanthrin from indigo: Synthesis, excited state deactivation routes and efficient singlet oxygen sensitization. *Dye. Pigment.* **2020**, *175*, 108125. [CrossRef]
23. Chang, H.N.; Huang, S.T.; Yeh, Y.C.; Wang, H.S.; Wang, T.H.; Wu, Y.H.; Pang, J.H. Indigo naturalis and its component tryptanthrin exert anti-angiogenic effect by arresting cell cycle and inhibiting Akt and FAK signaling in human vascular endothelial cells. *J. Ethnopharmacol.* **2015**, *174*, 474–481. [CrossRef] [PubMed]
24. Yu, S.T.; Chen, T.M.; Tseng, S.Y.; Chen, Y.H. Tryptanthrin inhibits MDR1 and reverses doxorubicin resistance in breast cancer cells. *Biochem. Biophys. Res. Commun.* **2007**, *358*, 79–84. [CrossRef] [PubMed]
25. Zeng, Q.; Luo, C.; Cho, J.; Lai, D.; Shen, X.; Zhang, X.; Zhou, W. Tryptanthrin exerts anti-breast cancer effects both in vitro and in vivo through modulating the inflammatory tumor microenvironment. *Acta Pharm.* **2021**, *71*, 245–266. [CrossRef] [PubMed]
26. Han, N.R.; Moon, P.D.; Kim, H.M.; Jeong, H.J. Tryptanthrin ameliorates atopic dermatitis through down-regulation of TSLP. *Arch. Biochem. Biophys.* **2014**, *542*, 14–20. [CrossRef] [PubMed]
27. Kwon, Y.W.; Cheon, S.Y.; Park, S.Y.; Song, J.; Lee, J.H. Tryptanthrin Suppresses the Activation of the LPS-Treated BV2 Microglial Cell Line via Nrf2/HO-1 Antioxidant Signaling. *Front. Cell. Neurosci.* **2017**, *11*, 18. [CrossRef]
28. Pergola, C.; Jazzar, B.; Rossi, A.; Northoff, H.; Hamburger, M.; Sautebin, L.; Werz, O. On the inhibition of 5-lipoxygenase product formation by tryptanthrin: Mechanistic studies and efficacy in vivo. *Br. J. Pharmacol.* **2012**, *165*, 765–776. [CrossRef]
29. Danz, H.; Stoyanova, S.; Thomet, O.A.; Simon, H.U.; Dannhardt, G.; Ulbrich, H.; Hamburger, M. Inhibitory activity of tryptanthrin on prostaglandin and leukotriene synthesis. *Planta Med.* **2002**, *68*, 875–880. [CrossRef]
30. Hackert, N.S.; Radtke, F.A.; Exner, T.; Lorenz, H.M.; Müller-Tidow, C.; Nigrovic, P.A.; Wabnitz, G.; Grieshaber-Bouyer, R. Human and mouse neutrophils share core transcriptional programs in both homeostatic and inflamed contexts. *Nat. Commun.* **2023**, *14*, 8133. [CrossRef]
31. Kaur, R.; Manjal, S.K.; Rawal, R.K.; Kumar, K. Recent synthetic and medicinal perspectives of tryptanthrin. *Bioorg. Med. Chem.* **2017**, *25*, 4533–4552. [CrossRef]
32. Su, C.M.; Lee, W.L.; Hsu, C.J.; Lu, T.T.; Wang, L.H.; Xu, G.H.; Tang, C.H. Adiponectin Induces Oncostatin M Expression in Osteoblasts through the PI3K/Akt Signaling Pathway. *Int. J. Mol. Sci.* **2015**, *17*, 29. [CrossRef]
33. Bai, D.; Ueno, L.; Vogt, P.K. Akt-mediated regulation of NFkappaB and the essentialness of NFkappaB for the oncogenicity of PI3K and Akt. *Int. J. Cancer* **2009**, *125*, 2863–2870. [CrossRef] [PubMed]
34. Abubakar, A.R.; Haque, M. Preparation of Medicinal Plants: Basic Extraction and Fractionation Procedures for Experimental Purposes. *J. Pharm. Bioallied Sci.* **2020**, *12*, 1–10. [CrossRef] [PubMed]
35. Sasidharan, S.; Chen, Y.; Saravanan, D.; Sundram, K.M.; Yoga Latha, L. Extraction, isolation and characterization of bioactive compounds from plants' extracts. *Afr. J. Tradit. Complement. Altern. Med.* **2011**, *8*, 1–10. [CrossRef] [PubMed]
36. Kussmann, M.; Abe Cunha, D.H.; Berciano, S. Bioactive compounds for human and planetary health. *Front. Nutr.* **2023**, *10*, 1193848. [CrossRef] [PubMed]
37. Hoang, T.; Kim, J. Phytonutrient supplements and metabolic biomarkers of cardiovascular disease: An umbrella review of meta-analyses of clinical trials. *Phytother. Res.* **2021**, *35*, 4171–4182. [CrossRef]
38. Gupta, C.; Prakash, D. Phytonutrients as therapeutic agents. *J. Complement. Integr. Med.* **2014**, *11*, 151–169. [CrossRef]
39. Gunun, N.; Kaewpila, C.; Khota, W.; Polyorach, S.; Kimprasit, T.; Phlaetita, W.; Cherdthong, A.; Wanapat, M.; Gunun, P. The Effect of Indigo (*Indigofera tinctoria* L.) Waste on Growth Performance, Digestibility, Rumen Fermentation, Hematology and Immune Response in Growing Beef Cattle. *Animals* **2022**, *13*, 84. [CrossRef]
40. Sharma, V.; Agarwal, A. Physicochemical and Antioxidant Assays of Methanol and Hydromethanol Extract of Ariel Parts of Indigofera tinctoria Linn. *Indian. J. Pharm. Sci.* **2015**, *77*, 729–734. [CrossRef]
41. Yang, Q.-Y.; Zhang, T.; He, Y.-N.; Huang, S.-J.; Deng, X.; Han, L.; Xie, C.-G. From natural dye to herbal medicine: A systematic review of chemical constituents, pharmacological effects and clinical applications of indigo naturalis. *Chin. Med.* **2020**, *15*, 127. [CrossRef]
42. Kukula-Koch, W.A.; Widelski, J. Chapter 9-Alkaloids. In *Pharmacognosy Fundamentals, Applications and Strategies*; Simone, B., Rupika, D., Eds.; Academic Press: San Diego, CA, USA, 2017; pp. 163–198. [CrossRef]
43. Kiss, A.L. Inflammation in Focus: The Beginning and the End. *Pathol. Oncol. Res.* **2022**, *27*, 1610136. [CrossRef]
44. Mantovani, A.; Allavena, P.; Sica, A.; Balkwill, F. Cancer-related inflammation. *Nature* **2008**, *454*, 436–444. [CrossRef] [PubMed]
45. Geethadevi, A.; Ku, Z.; Tsaih, S.W.; Parashar, D.; Kadamberi, I.P.; Xiong, W.; Deng, H.; George, J.; Kumar, S.; Mittal, S.; et al. Blocking Oncostatin M receptor abrogates STAT3 mediated integrin signaling and overcomes chemoresistance in ovarian cancer. *NPJ Precis. Oncol.* **2024**, *8*, 127. [CrossRef] [PubMed]
46. Wahl, A.F.; Wallace, P.M. Oncostatin M in the anti-inflammatory response. *Ann. Rheum. Dis.* **2001**, *60* (Suppl. 3), iii75–iii80. [CrossRef]
47. Boutten, A.; Venembre, P.; Seta, N.; Hamelin, J.; Aubier, M.; Durand, G.; Dehoux, M.S. Oncostatin M is a potent stimulator of alpha1-antitrypsin secretion in lung epithelial cells: Modulation by transforming growth factor-beta and interferon-gamma. *Am. J. Respir. Cell Mol. Biol.* **1998**, *18*, 511–520. [CrossRef]

48. Modur, V.; Feldhaus, M.J.; Weyrich, A.S.; Jicha, D.L.; Prescott, S.M.; Zimmerman, G.A.; McIntyre, T.M. Oncostatin M is a proinflammatory mediator. In vivo effects correlate with endothelial cell expression of inflammatory cytokines and adhesion molecules. *J. Clin. Investig.* **1997**, *100*, 158–168. [CrossRef]
49. O'Connell, J.; Doherty, J.; Buckley, A.; Cormican, D.; Dunne, C.; Hartery, K.; Larkin, J.; MacCarthy, F.; McCormick, P.; McKiernan, S.; et al. Colonic oncostatin M expression evaluated by immunohistochemistry and infliximab therapy outcome in corticosteroid-refractory acute severe ulcerative colitis. *Intest. Res.* **2022**, *20*, 381–385. [CrossRef]
50. Arunachalam, P.S.; Wimmers, F.; Mok, C.K.P.; Perera, R.A.P.M.; Scott, M.; Hagan, T.; Sigal, N.; Feng, Y.; Bristow, L.; Tak-Yin Tsang, O.; et al. Systems biological assessment of immunity to mild versus severe COVID-19 infection in humans. *Science* **2020**, *369*, 1210–1220. [CrossRef]
51. Beigel, F.; Friedrich, M.; Probst, C.; Sotlar, K.; Göke, B.; Diegelmann, J.; Brand, S. Oncostatin M mediates STAT3-dependent intestinal epithelial restitution via increased cell proliferation, decreased apoptosis and upregulation of SERPIN family members. *PLoS ONE* **2014**, *9*, e93498. [CrossRef]
52. West, N.R.; Hegazy, A.N.; Owens, B.M.J.; Bullers, S.J.; Linggi, B.; Buonocore, S.; Coccia, M.; Görtz, D.; This, S.; Stockenhuber, K.; et al. Oncostatin M drives intestinal inflammation and predicts response to tumor necrosis factor-neutralizing therapy in patients with inflammatory bowel disease. *Nat. Med.* **2017**, *23*, 579–589. [CrossRef]
53. Plater-Zyberk, C.; Buckton, J.; Thompson, S.; Spaull, J.; Zanders, E.; Papworth, J.; Life, P.F. Amelioration of arthritis in two murine models using antibodies to oncostatin M. *Arthritis Rheum.* **2001**, *44*, 2697–2702. [CrossRef]
54. Li, H.; Feng, C.; Fan, C.; Yang, Y.; Yang, X.; Lu, H.; Lu, Q.; Zhu, F.; Xiang, C.; Zhang, Z.; et al. Intervention of oncostatin M-driven mucosal inflammation by berberine exerts therapeutic property in chronic ulcerative colitis. *Cell Death Dis.* **2020**, *11*, 271. [CrossRef] [PubMed]
55. He, Y.; Sun, M.M.; Zhang, G.G.; Yang, J.; Chen, K.S.; Xu, W.W.; Li, B. Targeting PI3K/Akt signal transduction for cancer therapy. *Signal. Transduct. Target. Ther.* **2021**, *6*, 425. [CrossRef] [PubMed]
56. Ozes, O.N.; Mayo, L.D.; Gustin, J.A.; Pfeffer, S.R.; Pfeffer, L.M.; Donner, D.B. NF-kappaB activation by tumour necrosis factor requires the Akt serine-threonine kinase. *Nature* **1999**, *401*, 82–85. [CrossRef]
57. Sun, X.; Wang, X.; Chen, T.; Li, T.; Cao, K.; Lu, A.; Chen, Y.; Sun, D.; Luo, J.; Fan, J.; et al. Myelin activates FAK/Akt/NF-kappaB pathways and provokes CR3-dependent inflammatory response in murine system. *PLoS ONE* **2010**, *5*, e9380. [CrossRef]
58. DiDonato, J.A.; Mercurio, F.; Karin, M. NF-κB and the link between inflammation and cancer. *Immunol. Rev.* **2012**, *246*, 379–400. [CrossRef]
59. Pintard, C.; Ben Khemis, M.; Liu, D.; Dang, P.M.; Hurtado-Nedelec, M.; El-Benna, J. Apocynin prevents GM-CSF-induced-ERK1/2 activation and -neutrophil survival independently of its inhibitory effect on the phagocyte NADPH oxidase NOX2. *Biochem. Pharmacol.* **2020**, *177*, 113950. [CrossRef]
60. Aziz, A.U.R.; Farid, S.; Qin, K.; Wang, H.; Liu, B. PIM Kinases and Their Relevance to the PI3K/AKT/mTOR Pathway in the Regulation of Ovarian Cancer. *Biomolecules* **2018**, *8*, 7. [CrossRef]
61. Roversi, F.M.; Bueno, M.L.P.; da Silva, J.A.F.; Assis-Mendonça, G.R.; Torello, C.O.; Shiraishi, R.N.; Pericole, F.V.; Ferro, K.P.; Duarte, A.S.S.; Rego, E.M.; et al. Novel inhibitor of hematopoietic cell kinase as a potential therapeutic agent for acute myeloid leukemia. *Cancer Immunol. Immunother.* **2022**, *71*, 1909–1921. [CrossRef]
62. Roversi, F.M.; Pericole, F.V.; Machado-Neto, J.A.; da Silva Santos Duarte, A.; Longhini, A.L.; Corrocher, F.A.; Palodetto, B.; Ferro, K.P.; Rosa, R.G.; Baratti, M.O.; et al. Hematopoietic cell kinase (HCK) is a potential therapeutic target for dysplastic and leukemic cells due to integration of erythropoietin/PI3K pathway and regulation of erythropoiesis: HCK in erythropoietin/PI3K pathway. *Biochim. Biophys. Acta Mol. Basis Dis.* **2017**, *1863*, 450–461. [CrossRef]
63. Han, Z.; Song, L.; Qi, K.; Ding, Y.; Wei, M.; Jia, Y. Deciphering the Key Pharmacological Pathways and Targets of Yisui Qinghuang Powder That Acts on Myelodysplastic Syndromes Using a Network Pharmacology-Based Strategy. *Evid. Based Complement. Alternat. Med.* **2020**, *2020*, 8877295. [CrossRef]

nutrients MDPI

Article

Phytochemical, Cytoprotective Profiling, and Anti-Inflammatory Potential of *Colchicum luteum* in Rheumatoid Arthritis: An Experimental and Simulation Study

Huda Abbasi [1], Maria Sharif [1], Peter John [1,*], Attya Bhatti [1], Muhammad Qasim Hayat [1] and Qaisar Mansoor [2]

1 Atta ur Rahman School of Applied Biosciences, National University of Sciences and Technology, Sector H-12, Islamabad 44000, Pakistan; habbasi.phdabs14asab@asab.nust.edu.pk (H.A.); msharif.phdabs22asab@student.nust.edu.pk (M.S.); attyabhatti@asab.nust.edu.pk (A.B.); m.qasim@asab.nust.edu.pk (M.Q.H.)

2 Institute of Biomedical and Genetic Engineering (IBGE), Sector G-9/4, Islamabad 44000, Pakistan; qmibge@gmail.com

* Correspondence: pjohn@asab.nust.edu.pk; Tel.: +92-051-90856151

Abstract: Background: Rheumatoid arthritis (RA) is a chronic autoimmune disorder characterized by severe pain, inflammation, and joint deformity. Currently, it affects 1% of the population, with a projection to exceed 23 million cases by 2030. Despite significant advancements, non-steroidal anti-inflammatory drugs (NSAIDs), the first line of treatment, are associated with a range of adverse effects. Consequently, plant-based derivatives are being utilized as an effective alternative. This study evaluates the anti-inflammatory and safety profile of *Colchicum luteum* hydroethanolic extract (CLHE) in comparison to NSAIDs, with a focus on COX-2 and TNFα inhibition. Methods: CLHE potential was evaluated by phytochemical screening and in vitro bioactivity assays. Toxicity profile was conducted in Human Colon Epithelial Cells (HCEC) and Balb/c mice. Anti-inflammatory potential was explored in a collagen-induced arthritic (CIA) mice model. Bioactive compounds were identified computationally from GCMS data and subjected to docking and simulation studies against COX2 and TNFα. Results: CLHE demonstrated significant antioxidant (IC-50 = 6.78 μg/mL) and anti-inflammatory (IC-50 = 97.39 μg/mL) activity. It maintained 50% cell viability at 78.5 μg/μL in HCEC cells and exhibited no toxicity at a dose of 5000 mg/kg in mice. In the CIA model, CLHE significantly reduced paw swelling, arthritic scoring, C-reactive protein levels, and spleen indices, outperforming ibuprofen. Expression analysis confirmed the downregulation of COX-2, TNFα, and MMP-9. Histopathological analysis indicated the superior efficacy of CLHE compared to ibuprofen in reducing inflammation, synovial hyperplasia, and bone erosion. Computational studies identified compound-15 (CL15), (4-(4,7-dimethoxy-1,3-benzodioxol-5-yl)-2-oxo pyrrolidine-3-carboxylic acid), a non-toxic compound with strong binding affinities to COX-2 (−12.9 KJ/mol), and TNF-α (−5.8 KJ/mol). Conclusions: The findings suggest the potential of *Colchicum luteum* as a safer, anti-inflammatory, and multi-targeted alternative to NSAIDs for RA treatment.

Keywords: plant extract; anti-inflammatory; NSAIDs; acute toxicity; phytochemicals; bioactive compound compounds; simulations

1. Introduction

Rheumatoid arthritis (RA) is a progressive chronic disorder affecting bones and cartilage, leading to joint deformity and loss of function. It impacts 1% of the global population and ranks among the top 10 causes of disability worldwide. Furthermore, the trends of rheumatic diseases in Pakistan have shown an increase in prevalence, deaths, and disability-adjusted life years (DALYs) over the past 30 years, emphasizing the growing burden of rheumatic conditions in the country [1]. The onset and progression of RA are influenced by genetic predisposition, environmental factors, and lifestyle choices. The disabilities caused by chronic RA not only impair individual functioning and productivity but also place a significant economic burden on healthcare systems. Effective management strategies for RA involve early clinical diagnosis, lifestyle modifications, patient education, and advancements in therapeutic interventions [2]. Current treatments for inflammation in rheumatoid arthritis (RA) include disease-modifying antirheumatic drugs (DMARDs) and non-steroidal anti-inflammatory drugs (NSAIDs). However, both drug classes are associated with significant adverse effects, such as gastric perforation, renal and liver damage, and pancytopenia, which limit their long-term use in chronic illness patients [3]. Approximately 20 to 40% of patients experience NSAID-induced abdominal pain and diarrhea, and 15% of long-term users develop gastrointestinal ulcers and perforations, with 67% showing elevated bilirubin levels (>2.5 mg/dL). In the past decade, 0.01% of hospitalizations due to hepatotoxicity have been linked to NSAIDs [4]. Developing novel therapeutic agents involves a multi-step screening process to identify pharmacologically active compounds that inhibit biological targets while minimizing harm to healthy cells. Identifying therapeutic targets is crucial in drug discovery, and more than 1200 receptors and enzymes have been explored as potential targets for RA [5].

Cyclooxygenase-2 (COX-2), an inducible enzyme and the primary source of prostaglandins, is considered pathologic due to its role in mediating pain and inflammation [6]. Tumor necrosis factor-alpha (TNFα) is a key inflammatory cytokine that orchestrates the immune response in chronic inflammatory disorders such as RA [7]. Both COX-2 and TNFα are central to the initiation, progression, and inflammation seen in RA, with evidence suggesting that TNFα can induce COX-2 expression and vice versa (Figure 1) [8]. This highlights the importance of targeting these molecules for therapeutic inhibition.

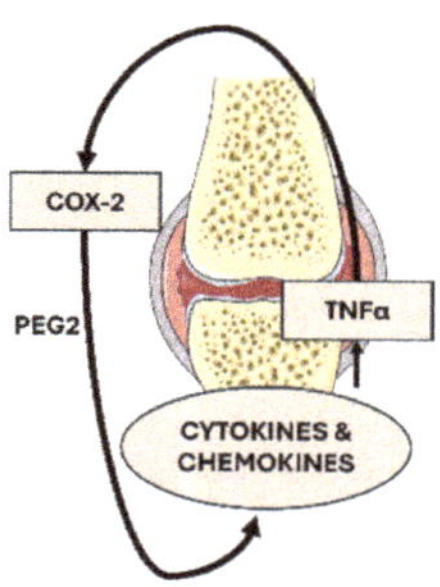

Figure 1. Crosstalk interaction between COX-2 and TNFα in a rheumatoid arthritis joint. COX-2 leads to TNFα activation through PGE_2 stimulation, while TNFα simultaneously enhances COX-2 expression, creating a feedback loop that amplifies inflammation.

Plant-derived compounds, known for their diverse biological activities and unique chemical structures, are being investigated as treatments for chronic diseases. Phytoderivatives from traditional medicinal herbs, particularly those used in Chinese medicine, are often employed as complementary therapies in managing inflammatory conditions. However, the potential toxic effects of these compounds on healthy tissues remain inadequately studied [9].

Colchicum luteum is a medicinal herb well-known for its anti-inflammatory and analgesic properties. *C. luteum* belongs to the Colchicaceae family, which is native to China, Pakistan, India, Himalayan regions, and regions along the Mediterranean coast. Commonly known as autumn crocus or meadow saffron, this herb is identified by its characteristic yellow-colored flowers, alternate or whorled leaves, and corms or starchy rhizomes. The aerial and root parts of *C. luteum* are mentioned in Greek, Indian, and Chinese traditional medicine for their diverse medicinal applications. The corms of *C. luteum* are extensively used to treat gastric, hematological, and rheumatic diseases. *Colchicum* species have been used in traditional Chinese medicine for their antiproliferative, anti-rheumatic, antifungal, and antipyretic characteristics, and several compounds have been identified from their extracts [10–13].

Despite its extensive use in traditional medicine for the treatment of rheumatism and gout, the efficacy and safety of *Colchicum luteum* as an individual therapeutic agent for RA remains underexplored. Previous studies have shown that the methanolic extract of *C. luteum* significantly inhibits lipoxygenase activity in vitro [11], demonstrating its potential anti-inflammatory effects. Additionally, polyherbal formulations containing *C. luteum* have been investigated in clinical trials for managing joint deformities [14]. This study aims to evaluate the toxicity and anti-inflammatory potential of *C. luteum* hydroethanolic extract by targeting key RA mediators, particularly COX-2 and TNF-α. By identifying safer bioactive constituents such as CL15, we seek to establish *C. luteum* as a viable alternative to conventional NSAIDs and biologics, offering a promising therapeutic option for the management of RA.

2. Materials and Methods

2.1. The Phytochemical Analysis and Characterization of the Extract

2.1.1. Identification of *Colchicum luteum* Herb and Extract Preparation

C. luteum was collected from Islamabad, Pakistan (33°42′35″ N 73°5′45″ E), during the fall season, from October to November 2022, as this is its flowering season. The plant was verified by taxonomists from NUST Islamabad, Pakistan. The specimen was compared to the herbarium vouchers 26,049 (RAW), 2522 (RAW), and 8457 (RAW) and confirmed to be a *Colchicum luteum* Baker (Colchicaceae). The herbarium number for *Colchicum luteum* was HUP0001096 and the taxonomy ID was 225785. The morphological and botanical information is provided on eFolras.org. For extract preparation, the corms of *Colchicum luteum* were dried and ground into a fine powder for hydroethanolic extraction (1:1 v/v), following a previously reported method with slight modifications. The mixture was macerated in the dark for two weeks and subsequently filtered using Whatman filter paper no. 1. The filtrate was then air-dried in a biosafety cabinet for 48 h [15]. The yield of the plant extract was calculated with the following formula:

$$Yield(\%) = weight\ of\ pure\ extract/weight\ of\ dried\ plant\ part \times 100$$

2.1.2. Phytochemical Screening

Phytochemical analysis of the crude extract was conducted using a previously reported protocol with slight modifications [15]. An additional step involving chloroform removal through N-hexane separation was added to reduce the color intensity of the extract. The colorimetric method was used for the qualitative identification of alkaloids, phenols, flavonoids, anthocyanins, leucoanthocyanins, tannins, phlobatannins, coumarins, terpenoids, steroids, saponins, and emodin.

2.1.3. Total Phenolic and Flavonoid Content

Total phenolic content was calculated using the Folin–Ciocalteu (FC) method [16]. A mixture of FC reagent (2.5 mL), $NaHCO_3$ (2.5 mL), and the extract (0.5 mL) was incubated at room temperature for 30 min. Gallic acid served as the standard, and absorbance was measured at 765 nm using a UV-vis spectrophotometer. Results were expressed as milligrams of gallic acid equivalent (GAE) per gram of dry sample.

The total flavonoid content of CLHE was quantified by the aluminum chloride ($AlCl_3$) method [16]. After serial dilution of the extract, 5% sodium nitrite was added and incubated for 5 min at 25 °C. Then, 10% $AlCl_3$ was added, followed by sodium hydroxide. A calibration curve was prepared using rutin as the standard, and absorbance was measured at 510 nm. The results were expressed as milligrams of rutin equivalent per gram of dry extract.

2.1.4. Chromatographic Characterization

The dried extract was dissolved in the methanol in the ratio of 1:1, which was injected into a capillary column fused with 1,4-bis (dimethyl-siloxy) phenylene dimethyl polysiloxane (0.25 μm × 20 m × 0.25 mm). The gas chromatograph was coupled with an SH-Rxi-5Sil mass spectrometer (QP-2020, SHIMADZU (Kyoto, Japan). The system was run with 70 eV ionization energy for 38 min at 1 mL/min gas flow rate and 100 °C final oven temperature. Mass spectrometry data was verified by the NIST (2017) library.

2.2. Evaluation of the Biological Activity of CLHE

2.2.1. Inhibition of Protein Denaturation

The protein denaturation inhibition assay was performed with albumin [17]. Albumin was dissolved in distilled water at 1:1 *w/v* concentration and mixed with 2.8 mL phosphate-buffered saline (pH 6.4). The extract was serially diluted (50, 100, 150, 200, and 250 μL) and added to the albumin–PBS mixture, followed by a 15 min incubation at 37 °C. The solution was heated to 70 °C for 5 min and then cooled to room temperature. The commercially prescribed anti-inflammatory agent ibuprofen was used as a control and processed similarly to CHLE. The absorbance was measured at 660 nm using a UV-vis spectrophotometer, and percentage denaturation was calculated with the following formula:

$$Denaturation\ (\%) = 1 - (Absorbance\ of\ control / Absorbance\ of\ sample) \times 100 \quad (1)$$

2.2.2. Free Radical Scavenging Activity

Radical scavenging or antioxidant activity was established by free radical scavenging activity using DPPH. A previously reported methodology was used with slight modifications [17]. CLHE concentrations of 10, 30, 50, 70, 90, and 110 μL were tested against identical dilutions of ibuprofen. The absorbance was measured at 570 nm using a UV-vis spectrophotometer. The percentage scavenging was calculated with the following formula:

$$Scavenging\ (\%) = 1 - (Absorbance\ of\ control / Absorbance\ of\ sample) \times 100 \quad (2)$$

2.3. Experimental Animals

Female BALB/c mice (8–12 weeks old) were obtained and housed at the animal house laboratory of ASAB, NUST. Mice weighing 30–35 g were kept in metal cages. All the obtained animals, i.e., experimental and control groups, were provided with a temperature- (25 °C ± 2) and humidity-regulated, pathogen-free environment. The acclimatization period was ten days. The Institutional Review Board (IRB No. 11-2020-01/04) of ASAB, NUST approved the study protocol. All experimental methods were carried out per the standards established by the Institute of Laboratory Animal Research, Division on Earth and Life Sciences, National Institute of Health, United States (Guide for the Care and Use of Laboratory Animals). All the mice included in the study were carefully examined for any pathological anomalies; initial inspections focused on characteristics like hair and coat color as well as the lack of any tissue damage.

2.4. Cell Lines

The Human Colon Epithelial Cells (HCEC) were provided by the Institute of Biotechnology and Genetic Engineering (IBGE), Islamabad. The cell lines were grown in Dulbecco's Modified Eagle Media (DMEM) (Gibco) with 10% FBS and 0.1% Penicillin/Streptomycin (Sigma Aldrich, Taufkirchen, Germany) at 35 °C in 5% CO_2.

2.5. Toxicology Profile of CLHE

2.5.1. In Vitro Toxicity Studies

To determine the cytotoxicity of plant extract MTT (3-(4,5-dimethyl thiazolyl-2)-2,5-diphenyltetrazolium bromide) assay (Sigma Aldrich, Germany) was performed to evaluate cell growth and viability. In a 96-well plate, 100 μL HCEC were cultured, and serially diluted CLHE extract was added followed by incubation. After 48 h, 20 μL MTT solution and 50 μL solubilization solution were mixed in by pipetting. The plate was incubated in the dark for 30 min and absorbance was measured at 570 nm using a UV-vis spectrophotometer.

2.5.2. In Vivo Toxicity Studies

Acute toxicity was measured with the Enegide method in healthy, 3–6-week-old, female Balb/c mice [18]. CLHE was orally administered in three phases in gradually increasing concentrations. After each phase, the mice were subjected to a 12 h fasting period to excrete the previous dose from the system. After each administration, the mice were observed for up to 6 h for signs of acute toxicity. After 24 h, mice were sacrificed, and their blood was collected via cardiac puncture to evaluate serum bilirubin, urea, and creatinine levels.

2.6. Analysis of Anti-Inflammatory Activity in Arthritic Mice Model

2.6.1. Collagen Induced Arthritis (CIA) Model Development

Female mice were divided into 4 groups (1: healthy control; 2: disease control; 3: CLHE-treated; and 4: ibuprofen-treated). A CIA mice model was developed by the administration of type II collagenase, Freud Adjuvant, and bovine serum albumin via transdermal injection. At the end of week 2, the paws of immunized mice were observed for signs of edema and inflammation [19]. The mice showing arthritic indexes of 3 and 4 were selected for further study. Groups 3 and 4 were given CLHE (5000 mg/kg) and ibuprofen solution (636 mg/kg), respectively, as a treatment for 10 days. The selected dose of CLHE (5000 mg/kg) was based on previous acute toxicity studies, which demonstrated no significant adverse effects at this concentration, making it suitable for evaluating the extract's therapeutic and safety profile [20]. The ibuprofen solution (636 mg/kg) was chosen to correspond to its established therapeutic dose in animal models, allowing for a comparative analysis of anti-inflammatory effects between CLHE and a standard NSAID.

2.6.2. Arthritis Index

Inflammatory edema and arthritic index were used as markers of localized inflammation. Edema was assessed via paw volume measured using a Vernier caliper (Mitutoyo, Aurora, IL, USA). The arthritis index was measured by observing the paws of groups 1–4 and graded according to the digital arthritic index [19].

2.6.3. Spleen Indices

For spleen indices, the weight of the spleen was divided by the body weight of the mice.

2.6.4. Serum Antibody Analysis

C-reactive protein (CRP) was used as a marker for systemic inflammation. Mouse blood was drawn using cardiac puncture and collected in EDTA tubes. The test was performed by the ASAB Diagnostic Lab (NUST, Islamabad, Pakistan) by employing commercial ELISA kits (Elabscience) according to the manufacturer's protocol. The levels of antibodies were examined to determine the extent of the inflammation caused by arthritis and the efficacy of the extracts in alleviating these levels.

2.6.5. Quantitative Real-Time PCR Analysis

Gene expression was carried out via qPCR (Applied Biosystems, Thermo Fischer Scientific, Waltham, MA, USA). GAPDH was used as the housekeeping gene, and the relative expression of TNFα, COX-2, and MMP-9 were analyzed and recorded as fold change. The RNA was isolated by the TRIzol (Thermo Fischer Scientific, USA) method, and the cDNA was synthesized according to previously reported protocols [19].

2.6.6. Histological Analysis

Hematoxylin and eosin (H&E) staining was employed for the histopathology analysis of the joints. The paw and tarsal joints were collected and stored in a 10% Formalin solution. The specimens were prepared according to the previously reported protocol. Samples were observed under the light microscope at 10× and 40× resolution. The parameters of inflammation, membrane infiltration, and bone erosion were studied and scored [19].

2.7. *In Silico Analysis of* C. luteum *Bioactive Compound*

2.7.1. ADMET Screening of Bioactive Compounds

Canonical SMILES (Simplified Molecular Input Line Entry System) of GC–MS data and the structure of all the phyto-compounds were retrieved from the PubChem database. The bioactive compounds were shortlisted based on physicochemical parameters of molecular mass, blood–brain barrier permeability, and druggability using SwissADME (2017) and ADMET Lab 3.0 [21].

2.7.2. Toxicology Profiling of Shortlisted Compounds

The virtual lab ProTox 3.0 was used to predict hepatotoxicity, immunotoxicity, cytotoxicity, and lethal dose (LD_{50}). The toxicity levels were used to categorize shortlisted compounds into toxicological classes I, II (fatal), III (toxic), IV (harmful), and V (non-toxic) [22].

2.7.3. Target Preparation

The 3D crystal structures of target proteins COX-2 (PDB ID: 5F19) and TNFα (PDB ID: 2AZ5) were retrieved from the RCSB-protein databank. The proteins were prepared in BIOVIA discovery studio v. 21.1.0.20298 (2020) by removing water molecules, steric clashes, and pre-docked ligands. The polar hydrogens and Kollman charges were added.

2.7.4. Molecular Docking

Molecular docking was performed on AutoDock Vina v.4.2.0 [23]. The Lamarckian genetic algorithm was used, and results were analyzed by docking score (Gibbs Free energy). The protein targets COX-2 and TNFα were used as macromolecules. The protein–ligand complex with the lowest RMSD and binding energy from the top 10 poses were selected for molecular dynamics simulation (MDS).

2.7.5. Molecular Dynamic Simulation

The MDS was performed on the GROMACS (2020.4) [24]. The protein–ligand interaction was observed for 100 ns using CHARMM36m forcefield (2020). The trajectory and energy files were written every 10 ps. The production run for simulation was carried out at a constant temperature of 300 K and a pressure of 1 atm (NPT). The MDS results were analyzed based on root mean square deviation (RMSD), the radius of gyration (RoG), and the number and strength of H-bonds. The conformational change of ligand–protein complexes was analyzed on a time scale of 0, 50, and 100 ns.

2.7.6. Binding Free Energy Calculation

The binding free energies (DG) were calculated by the MMGBSA approach. The net DG of the system was determined by finding the difference in DG between the ligand only, the protein only, and their complex, as expressed in the following equation:

$$\Delta G_{bind} = \Delta G_{complex} - \Delta G_{receptor} - \Delta G_{ligand}$$

This DG represents Gibb's free energy, which is measured via MMGBSA, as shown in the following equation:

$$\Delta G = \Delta E_{gas} + \Delta G_{Solv} - \Delta TS_{solute}$$

The above equation represents the DG calculation, with E_{gas} representing the energy from the molecular mechanics force field and "T" and "S" representing the temperature and entropy of ligand binding, respectively. The E_{gas} term encompasses electrostatic energies, internal energy, and van der Waals interactions.

2.8. Statistical Analysis

All data were expressed as mean ± standard deviation (SD). The data from the antioxidant and protein stability assays were analyzed via the nonlinear regression method. The data for paw volume, spleen size, blood CRP, histology scores, and cell viability were analyzed in GraphPad Prism v.8.0.1 by one-way and two-way ANOVA. The level of significance was $p < 0.05$.

3. Results

3.1. CLHE Phytochemical Screening, Quantification and Characterization

The identification of *C. luteum* was confirmed through its characteristic yellow flowers (Figure 2a), and the corms were selected for extract preparation (Figure 2b). This process yielded a 21% dried extract from 315 g of corms, reflecting efficient extraction of bioactive constituents from the corms. The yield indicates the richness of the corms in potentially active compounds, making them suitable for further biochemical and pharmacological evaluation.

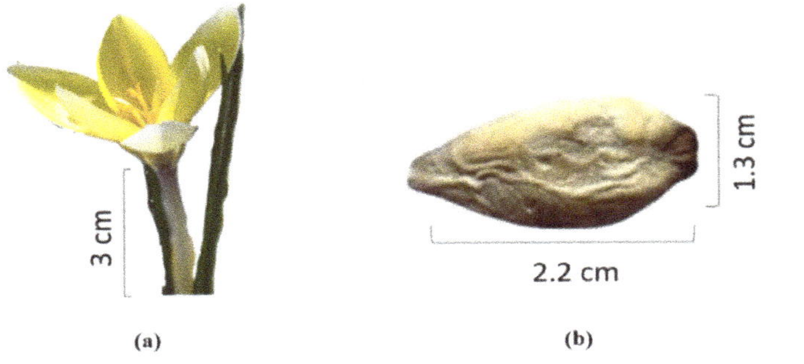

Figure 2. *Colchicum luteum* identification by (**a**) flower and stem, (**b**) corm.

A qualitative analysis of the secondary metabolites present in the CLHE of the corms is summarized in Table 1. The results revealed an abundance of phenols, alongside the presence of alkaloids, anthocyanins, leucoanthocyanin, coumarins, saponins, emodins, sterols, and glycosides. In contrast, tannins, phlobatannins, terpenoids, steroids, and amino acids were absent in the extract. The presence of these bioactive compounds underscores the medicinal potential of the corm extract.

The total phenolic content of CLHE was calculated by analyzing the absorbance of the extract on the standard gallic acid curve. The total phenolic content was 4.91 ± 0.085 mg of GAE/gram of extract. Total flavonoid content was calculated using the rutin calibration curve. The corms of *C. luteum* were estimated to have a flavonoid content of 2.01 ± 0.0424 mg ($R^2 = 0.98$).

Table 1. Phytochemical constituents of *C. luteum* corms extract: (+) present, ++ (abundant), and (-) absent.

S. No.	Secondary Metabolites	*C. luteum* Hydroalcoholic Extract
1	Alkaloids	+
2	Phenols	++
3	Flavonoids	+
4	Anthocyanins	+
5	Leucoanthocyanins	+
6	Tannins	-
7	Phlobatannins	-
8	Coumarins	+
9	Terpenoids	-
10	Steroids	-
11	Saponins	+
12	Emodins	+
13	Amino acids	-
14	Sterols	+
15	Glycosides	+

The GC-MS chromatographic analysis of CLHE separated 600 volatile compounds, among which phenolics, flavonoids, alkaloids, and sequesterpine hydrocarbons were notably abundant, comprising 10.8%, 10%, 8.5%, and 3% of the extract, respectively. From the total pool, select compounds with previously reported medicinal properties were highlighted. For phenolics, 2,3-dihydrobenzoic acid, thymol TBDMS derivative, quinol, and mandelic acid were identified, each known for antioxidant, antimicrobial, and antitumor effects [25–28]. Alkaloid analysis revealed N-alpha-methylhistamine, 1-(5-fluoro-2-nitrophenyl)piperidine, and tetraponerine T4, compounds linked to neurotherapeutic, anti-inflammatory, and anticancer activities [29–31]. Flavonoids such as 2-formyl-9-[β-d-ribofuranosyl]hypoxanthine, 6-chloro-2-cyclohexyl quinazolin-4(3h)-one, and 12-cinnolinedicarboxylic acid were detected, known for their anti-neurodegenerative, sedative, and antimicrobial effects [32–35]. Additionally, the sequesterpine hydrocarbon ginsenol, with antiviral and antifungal properties [36], was noted. The full list of identified compounds, along with their retention times and peak areas, has been provided in the Supplementary Table S1 for further reference. These selected compounds were discussed to illustrate the therapeutic potential of the CLHE extract.

3.2. CLHE Biological Potential

The plant extract prevents the denaturation of the protein by heat. The percentage of inhibition increases with the increase in concentration, exhibiting extract anti-inflammatory potential. The percentage inhibition at the highest concentration of 550 was 53% ± 0.007 and 60% ± 0.006 for CLHE and aspirin (Figure 3a). IC_{-50} for CLHE was calculated as 97.39 (R^2 = 0.99), while for aspirin, it was 292.2 (R^2 = 0.99).

DPPH was utilized to detect the presence of antioxidants in the plant extracts. The higher the percentage of inhibition, the higher the antioxidant properties exhibited by the plant. The percentage of inhibition showed that the plant extract scavenged free radicals in a dose-dependent manner (10–90 μg/mL). The antioxidant capacity of CLHE was recorded as higher than ascorbic acid (Figure 3b). The IC_{50} was for CLHE was calculated as 6.78 (R^2 = 0.86), while for ascorbic acid, it was 99.85 (R^2 = 0.80).

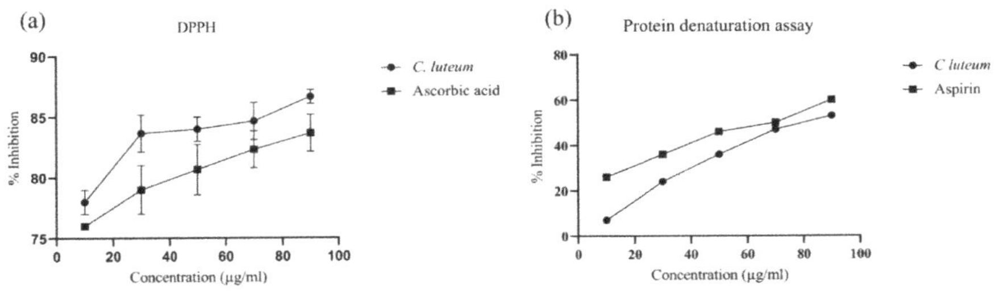

Figure 3. Biological potential of CLHE expressed as (**a**) DPPH assay: The radical scavenging potential of CLHE shows a concentration-dependent increase comparable to ibuprofen. (**b**) Protein denaturation assay: Protein denaturation inhibition activity is significantly increased with extract concentration. CLHE is a significant inhibitor of protein denaturation at 250 μg/mL ($n = 3$) ($R^2 = 0.96$).

3.3. *Invitro Cytotoxicity Effect of CLHE*

The potential cytotoxic effect of CLHE was evaluated on HCEC cell lines via MTT assay for 48 h. CLHE was tested at concentrations ranging from 2 to 20 μg/mL, with results depicted in Figure 4. Cell viability was significantly reduced with increasing concentrations ($p < 0.0001$), with CLHE exhibiting toxicity at doses greater than 10 μg/μL. The concentration of CLHE responsible for a 50% reduction in cell viability (IC50) was calculated to be 78.5 μg/mL for the HCEC cell line, highlighting the significant safety profile of CLHE. Control cells, treated with the same solvent without CLHE, demonstrated 100% viability, providing a baseline for comparison.

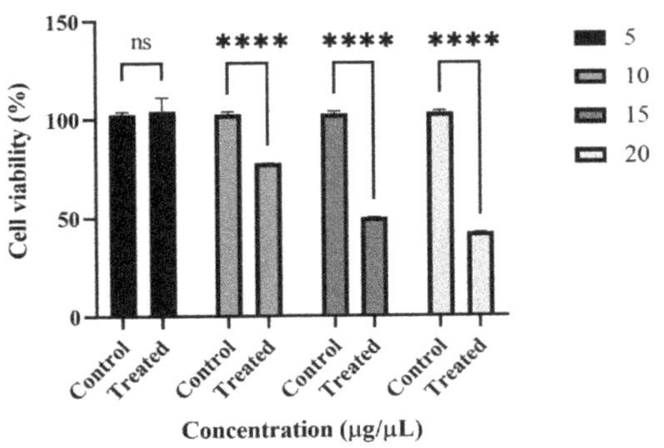

Figure 4. Cytoprotective activity of CLHE expressed as cell viability % in HCEC cells $R^2 = 0.9$ Statistical significance was determined by one-way ANOVA, followed by Bonferroni multiple comparison test where ns = non-significant and **** $p < 0.0001$.

3.4. *In Vivo Acute Toxicity Effect of CLHE*

The acute lethal toxicity results show that CLHE does not cause any death in any of the phases. Even at the highest dose of 5000 mg/kg, no death or noticeable physical or behavioral changes were observed, suggesting that the extract is safe for oral administration. Except for increased motor activity in the Dose II group, none showed abnormal physical and behavioral changes (Table 2). Moreover, no significant difference was detected in the creatinine, urea, and total bilirubin levels of mice treated with CLHE, as shown in Table 3.

Table 2. Acute toxicity evaluation of CLHE.

Signs of Acute Toxicity	Dose I: 800 mg/kg	Dose II: 2000 mg/kg	Dose III: 5000 mg/kg
Sedation	-	-	-
Respiratory distress	-	-	-
Salivation	-	-	-
Hyperesthesia	-	-	-
Diarrhea	-	-	-
Blanching	-	-	-
Increased motor activity	-	+	-
Writhing/twisting	-	-	-
Straub reaction	-	-	-
Tremors	-	-	-
Arching and rolling	-	-	-
Tonic convulsions	-	-	-
Tonic extension	-	-	-
Lacrimation	-	-	-
Cyanosis	-	-	-
Number of deaths	0	0	0

+ indicates presence of symptoms and - indicates absence of symptoms

Table 3. Creatinine, urea, and total bilirubin levels of CLHE treated mice.

Test Name	Control	CLHE
T. Bilirubin	0.6	0.5
Urea	36	45
Creatinine	0.33	0.20

3.5. *Effect of CHLE on Paw Swelling and Arthritic Index*

A CIA model was developed to evaluate the therapeutic effect of *C luteum*. Immunization with CII leads to the development of CIA models with significant paw swelling and inflammation (Figure 5a). There was a significant increase in the paw size from week 1 to 4 ($p < 0.0001$) in group 2 as compared to the healthy control (Figure 5b). A significant thickness in the paws of mice was observed between 1.5 and 2 weeks. The paw volume increased with time in all groups. However, after the treatment, the paw volume significantly decreased for both CLHE and ibuprofen as compared to the arthritic control ($p < 0.0001$).

The arthritis score was determined after regular intervals of 7 days. The scoring ranges from 0 to 4 and is linked to clinical observations. According to this criterion, the mice with maximum scores of 3 and 4 were selected for further experimentation. All three groups showed visible swelling on the entire paw extending to the tarsal joint. Moreover, the selected mice were unable to hold cage wires with the swollen paw, indicating restriction in paw function. The joint swelling and damage were significant on day 7 and boosted substantially for the arthritic control throughout the study ($p < 0.0001$). However, a significant reduction was observed in the treatment groups, i.e., fever clinical signs of inflammation. The extract-treated group showed a greater reduction in arthritic index ($p < 0.0001$) than the standard ibuprofen-treated group ($p < 0.001$) (Figure 5c).

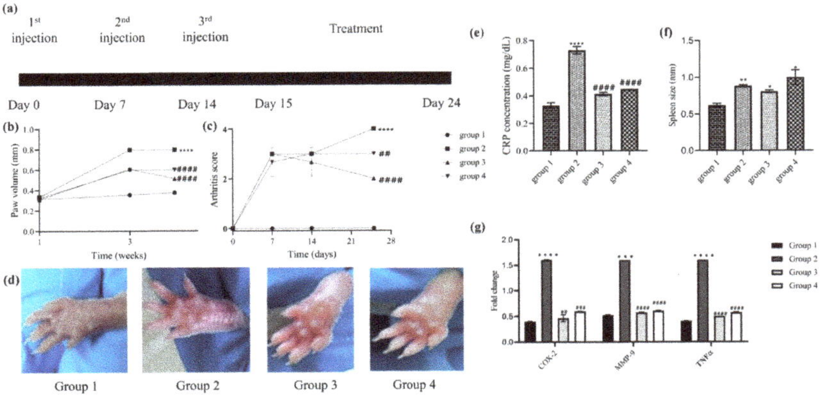

Figure 5. Anti arthritic activity of CLHE. (**a**) Experimental design, (**b**) paw edema, (**c**) arthritic index, (**d**) paw at the end of the experiment, (**e**) blood CRP levels, (**f**) spleen indices, (**g**) expression analysis of COX2, TNFα, and MMP9. Statistical significance was determined by two-way ANOVA or one-way ANOVA, wherever applicable, followed by Bonferroni multiple comparison test where * $p < 0.01$, ** $p < 0.001$, *** $p = 0.0001$ **** $p < 0.0001$ represents control group vs. disease control group and ## $p < 0.001$, ### $p = 0.0001$ and #### $p < 0.0001$ represents disease control group vs. treatment groups.

3.6. Effect of CHLE on C-Reactive Protein

CLHE reduces CIA-induced inflammation by decreasing the serum levels of CRP. Results showed that the arthritic mice model had elevated levels of CRP as compared to the healthy control ($p < 0.0001$). Treatment with the extract and ibuprofen significantly reduced the level of CRP as compared to the arthritic group $p < 0.0001$, i.e., both ibuprofen and extract showed comparable results in reducing the levels of CRP (Figure 5e).

3.7. Effect of CHLE on Spleen Indices

An enlarged spleen is indicative of an inflated immune response and inflammation. To evaluate the severity of arthritis in animal models, spleen indices were conducted. Spleen indices were significantly increased in the CIA model ($p < 0.001$). No significant difference was found between the CLHE- and ibuprofen-treated groups in comparison to the arthritic group. However, spleen indices were significantly more increased for ibuprofen ($p < 0.0001$) than extract ($p < 0.01$) as compared to the healthy mice (Figure 5f).

3.8. Effect of CLHE on Inflammatory Biomarkers

The expression of TNFα, COX-2, and MMP-9 genes was analyzed by qPCR. Group 1 showed basal level expression while group 2 showed a significant upregulation of COX2, TNFα, and MMP9 ($p < 0.0001$) compared to the healthy mice. The expressions of COX2, TNFα, and MMP9 significantly decreased in both CLHE-treated and ibuprofen-treated groups. Interestingly both extract and ibuprofen showed comparable results (Figure 5g).

3.9. Effect of CLHE on Histopathological Changes

Histopathological analysis of the arthritic mice showed visible signs of inflammation, immunocyte infiltration, synovial hyperplasia, and bone erosion. However, treatment with extracts alleviated the arthritic symptoms significantly (Figure 6). Enlarged and effused joints indicate hyperplastic and hypertrophic synovium, which was observed in the arthritic group. The joint enlargement was reduced in the CHLE joint, where relatively smoother membrane boundaries were observed. Treatment with the extract significantly reduced inflammation ($p < 0.001$), immune infiltration ($p < 0.0001$), and synovial hyperplasia ($p < 0.0001$) as compared to ibuprofen ($p < 0.01$). Similarly, in the CLHE-treated group, a significant reduction in the reversal of bone erosion was also recorded ($p < 0.001$), whereas the ibuprofen-treated group showed a non-significant reduction as compared to the arthritic control (Figure 6i–l).

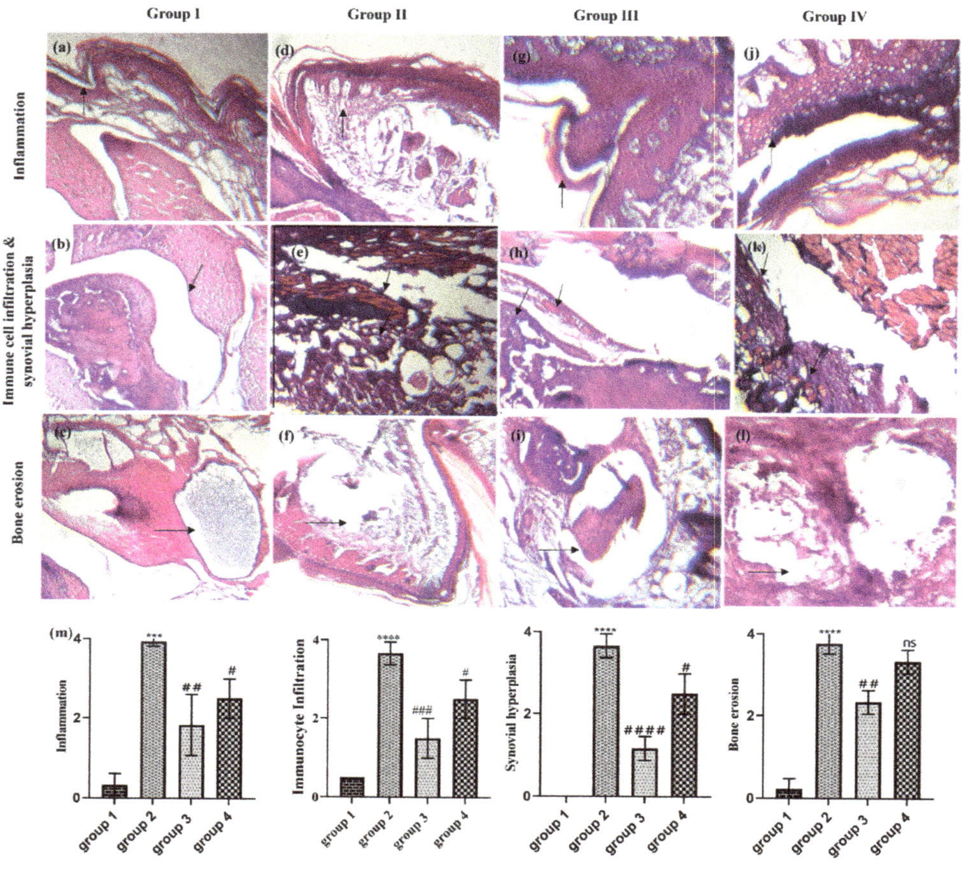

Figure 6. H&E-stained tissue of the tarsal joint of CIA Balb/c mice. (**a**–**c**) Group 1: (**a**) inflammation, (**b**) immune cell infiltration and synovial hyperplasia, (**c**) bone erosion represented by black arrows. (**d**–**f**) Group 2: (**d**) inflammation, (**e**) immune cell infiltration and synovial hyperplasia, (**f**) bone erosion represented by black arrows. (**g**–**i**) Group 3: (**g**) inflammation, (**h**) immune cell infiltration and synovial hyperplasia, (**i**) bone erosion represented by black arrows. (**j**–**l**). Group 4: (**j**) inflammation, (**k**) immune cell infiltration and synovial hyperplasia, (**l**) bone erosion represented by black arrows. Figures were scaled to 100 μm and original magnifications were 20× and 40×. (**m**) Histopathological scoring; statistical significance was determined by one-way ANOVA, followed by Bonferroni multiple comparison test where *** $p = 0.0001$, **** $p < 0.0001$ represents control group vs. disease control group and # $p < 0.01$, ## $p < 0.001$, ### $p = 0.0001$ and #### $p < 0.0001$ represents disease control group vs. treatment groups where ns = non-significant.

3.10. *In Silico Analysis of C. luteum Bioactive Compounds*

3.10.1. Screening of Bioactive Compounds

GCMS analysis identified 600 phytocompounds. Out of the 600 CLHE-derived natural compounds, pharmacokinetic screening identified 15 phytoconstituents (CL01 to CL15) that fulfilled the parameters of absorption, distribution, metabolism, and excretion (Figure 7). Out of these fifteen compounds, CL-1, -4, -5, -10, -11, and -13 presented a Lipinski violation (molecular weight > 350 g/mol). CL-2 presented low GI absorption. CL-3 was identified as a natural toxin. CL-6 was an interfering or "promiscuous" compound with potential off-target effects identified by pan-assay interference structure (PAINS). CL- 7, -8, -9, and -14 presented lower Log S values, rendering them moderately soluble. CL-12 was a chemically reactive and metabolically unstable moiety identified by Brenk alert (Supplementary Table S2). However, compound 15 (CL15) was screened as an ideal candidate for evaluation as it fulfilled the ideal physicochemical profile of absorption, distribution, metabolism, excretion, and toxicity (Table 4).

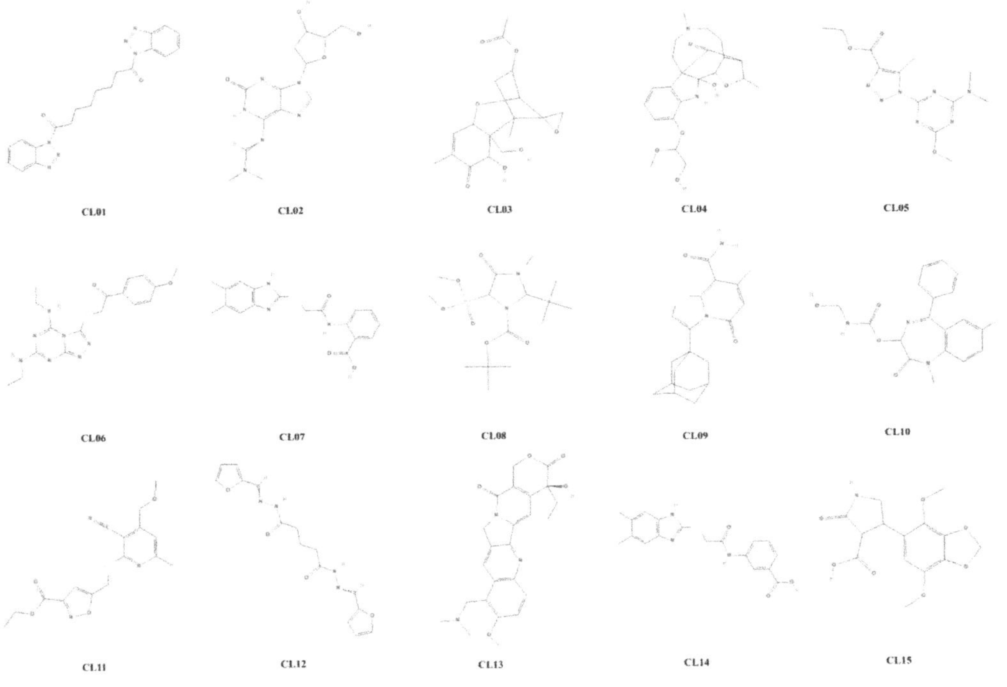

Figure 7. Bioactive natural compounds identified in CHLE through GC-MS from CL01 to CL15.

Table 4. Pharmacokinetic profile of CL15 compared to the accepted values of ADMET.

PK Category	Parameters	CL15	Accepted Value
Absorption	HIA	0.1	$0 \geq 30\%$ $1 \leq 30\%$
Distribution	Volume distribution	0.247	0.04–20 L/kg
	BBB penetration	0.28	The value corresponds to the probability
Metabolism	CYP1A2	0.496	>0.0
	CYP2C19	0.214	>0.0
	CYP2D6	0.005	>0.0
	CYP3A4	0.100	>0.0
Excretion	Clearance	1.34	5–15 mL/min/kg
	Half-life	1.58	0–3 h
Drug-likeness	Molecular weight	309.08	100–600
	Polar surface area	103.32	0–140
	H-bond donors	2	0–7
	H-bond acceptors	8	0–12
	No. of rotatable bonds	4	0–11

3.10.2. Toxicity Profiling of Bioactive Compound

The toxicity analysis of CL15 classified it as non-toxic, placing it within the class IV toxicity category according to the Globally Harmonized System (GHS) for chemical classification and labeling. Compounds in this category are considered non-toxic but may pose a risk if ingested. The predicted lethal oral dose for CL15 was determined to be 450 mg/kg, with a 0.7 probability of causing immunotoxicity (Figure 8).

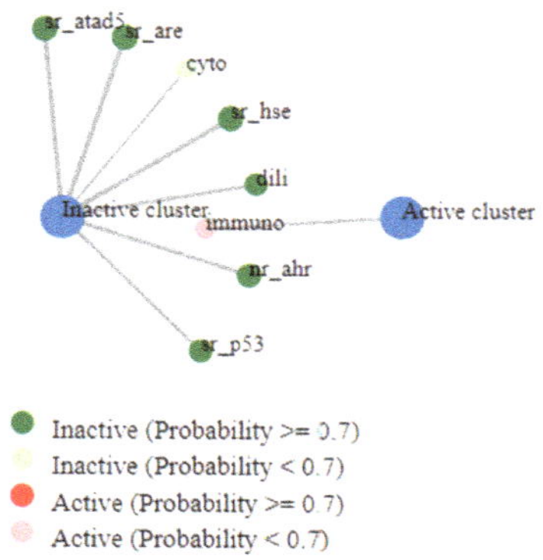

Figure 8. ProTox 3.0 indicating safety of CL15 in all parameters except slight immunotoxicity ($p = 0.7$).

3.10.3. Molecular Docking

Molecular docking analysis revealed a strong binding affinity of CL15 with COX-2 (−12.5 Kcal/mol) and TNFα (−5.8 Kcal/mol). CL15 interacts with COX-2 with four H-bonds at ARG^{120}, SER^{119,} and LYS^{83} residues (Figure 9a), while with TNFα, it interacts with seven H-bonds at PRO^{91}, ARG^{94}, PRO^{104}, THR^{96}, and LYS^{103} residues (Figure 9b).

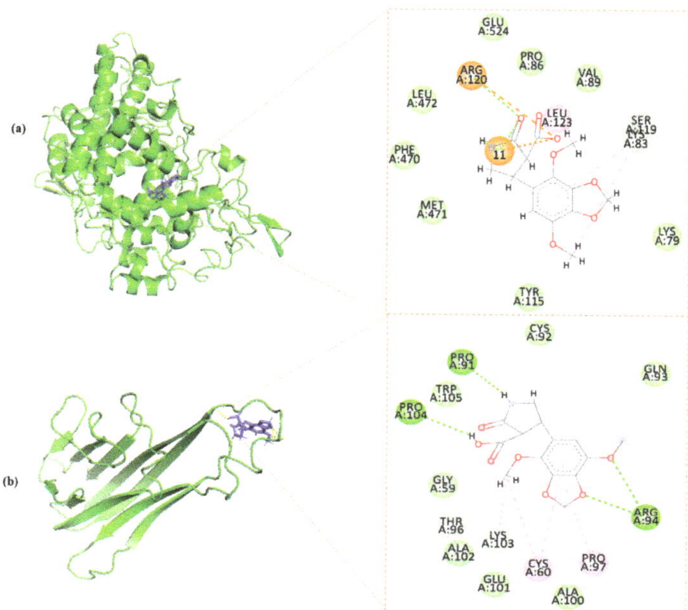

Figure 9. Molecular interaction of CL15 with (**a**) COX-2 and (**b**) TNFα.

3.10.4. Molecular Dynamics Simulation

Protein–ligand complexes of CL15 with COX2 (complex 1) and TNF α (complex 2) were further evaluated for 100 ns simulation. For complex 1, the mean RMSD was 0.28 $\pm$ 0.03 nm, with a rising trend after 30 ns. Complex 1 underwent a conformational change from 70 to 90 ns; however, the changes remained within the acceptable values (0.12 nm). For complex 2, the average RMSD was 0.16 $\pm$ 0.02 nm, with minimum fluctuation throughout the simulation. The complex showed minor fluctuations at the beginning of the simulation; however, the complex remained stable after 7 ns (Figure 10a).

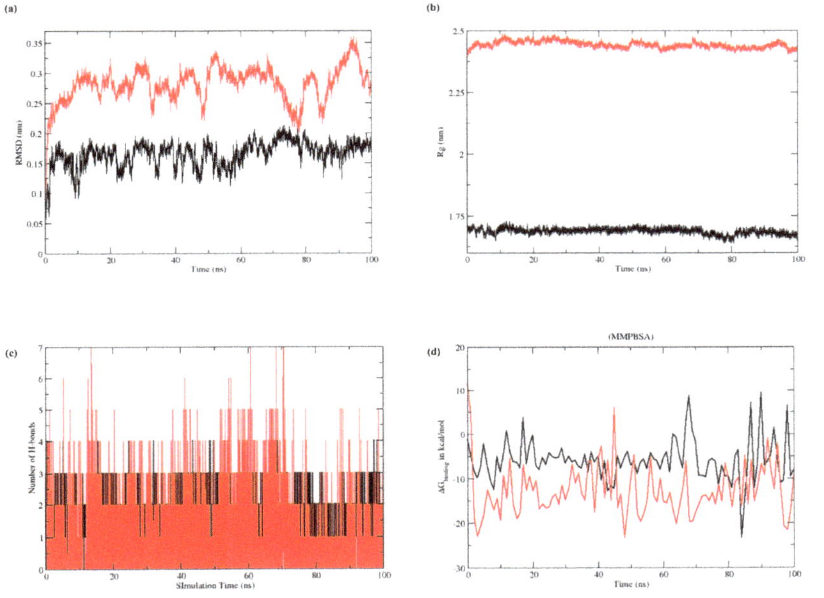

Figure 10. Molecular dynamics simulation graphically representing (**a**) RMSD, (**b**) RoG, (**c**) H-bond, and (**d**) MMGBPSA, where red represents complex 1 and black represents complex 2.

The RoG for complex 1 was 2.44 $\pm$ 0.01 nm, and no significant changes were observed in the compactness of the complex. The RoG for complex 2 was 1.68 $\pm$ 0.01 nm. A slight decrease in complex 2 radii was observed at 80 ns; however, the compactness of the complex was not affected (Figure 10b).

The H-bond strength was calculated as the average number of bonds within the complexes. Complex 1 shows consistent bond formation throughout the simulation, valued at 1.70 $\pm$ 0.67. The density of the graph indicates the strength of H-bonds. For complex 2, consistent, but low-strength, H-bonds were observed throughout the simulation after 5 ns. The average number of H-bonds in complex 2 was 1.66 $\pm$ 0.5 (Figure 10c).

Binding free energies were estimated by employing MMGBSA methods to better understand the complexes' binding abilities with target proteins. Stable complexes were generated because all the binding interactions were energetically favorable, and Table 5 displays the results of these experiments. The net energy in MMGBSA for COX2-CL15 and TNFα-CL15 were calculated as -12.72 (5.98 $\pm$ 0.59) and -14.42 (8.12 $\pm$ 0.25) kcal/mol, respectively. Moreover, the ΔG graph remained stable throughout the simulation (Figure 10d).

Table 5. Binding free energies (Kcal/mol) and the individual energetic terms for the systems using the MMPBSA method.

Parameters	COX-2	TNFα
	CL15 Avg. Binding Energy (Std. Dev ± Std. Err. of Mean	CL15 avg. Binding Energy (Std. Dev ± Std. Err. of Mean
Van der Waals (EVDW)	31.91 (2.99 ± 0.29)	27.11 (8.68 ± 0.27)
Electrostatic (EEL)	11.07 (8.19 ± 0.81)	15.94 (8.63 ± 0.27)
Polar (EPB)	33.89 (7.62 ± 0.75)	31.57 (9.36 ± 0.29)
Non-polar (ENPOLAR)	−3.62 (0.13 ± 0.01)	−2.94 (0.44 ± 0.01)
EDISPER	0.00	0.00
Delta G (gas)	−42.98 (9.63 ± 0.95)	−43.06 (13.95 ± 0.44)
Delta G (sol)	30.26 (7.56 ± 0.75)	28.63 (9.02 ± 0.28)
Delta Total	−12.72 (5.98 ± 0.59)	−14.42 (8.12 ± 0.25)

The conformation of the complexes was observed from 0 to 100 ns. An *N*-terminal shift was observed in complex 1; however, CL15 remained stably bound to the substrate-binding domain of COX-2 (Figure 11a). Conformation changes of complex 2 also showed the stable binding of CL15 with the binding pocket of TNFα (Figure 11b).

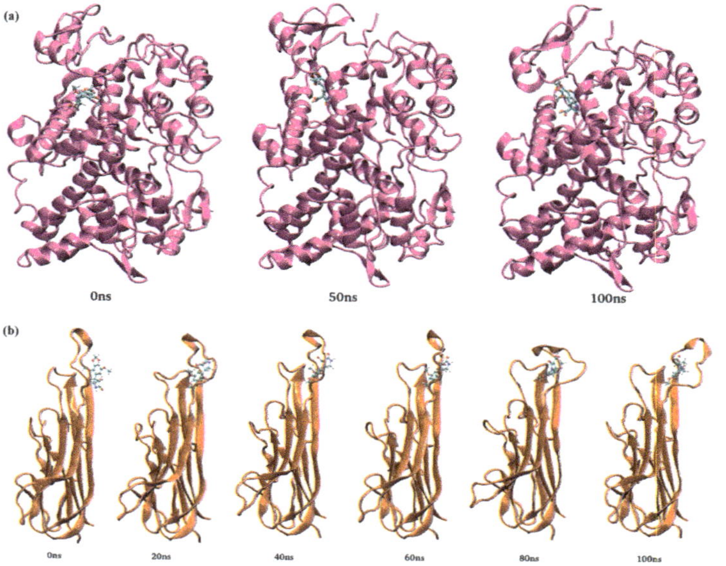

Figure 11. Conformational change and structural rotation of (**a**) complex 1 and (**b**) complex 2.

4. Discussion

RA is a chronic autoimmune disorder marked by severe pain, inflammation, and progressive joint deterioration. Its global incidence is rising rapidly, yet current treatment options remain limited. NSAIDs, commonly used as the first line of treatment, are associated with significant side effects such as gastrointestinal bleeding and cardiovascular risks. Advanced therapies, including biologics, are costly, target only specific pathways, and also carry the risk of adverse effects [37]. As a result, there is a growing shift toward alternative therapeutic strategies to address these limitations. Medicinal plants have long been explored as potential remedies for RA. However, their widespread use, often regarded as safe, is frequently based on incomplete knowledge of their chemical makeup and a lack of understanding about proper dosing and toxicity risks. To identify viable drug candidates, it is crucial to thoroughly examine the chemical composition, safe dosage levels, and toxicity profiles of these plants. This study aims to evaluate the safety and anti-inflammatory effects of *C. luteum* while identifying safer and more effective bioactive compounds for RA treatment through in vitro, in vivo, and in silico methodologies.

C. luteum extract was analyzed for secondary metabolites, revealing the presence of pharmacologically important compounds such as flavonoids, phenols, and emodin (Table 1). Nearly 20% of the metabolites identified through GC-MS analysis were phenolics and flavonoids, indicating a strong antioxidant profile. Additionally, 8.5% of the identified compounds were alkaloids and their derivatives. Notably, colchicine was not detected in the extract, which is significant given its high toxicity that limits its therapeutic use, particularly as an anti-tumor agent [38]. This absence suggests a safer pharmacological profile for CLHE, enhancing its therapeutic potential while mitigating the risks associated with colchicine itself, thereby making CLHE a more favorable option for therapeutic applications.

Both phenols and flavonoids play a key role in providing antioxidant and anti-inflammatory effects [39]. CLHE demonstrated substantial concentrations of these phytochemicals, which aligned with its biological activity in antioxidant and anti-inflammatory assays. The DPPH assay, used in this study, specifically measures the radical scavenging activity of the extract. While the assay does not directly quantify antioxidant capacity, radical scavenging is a key mechanism through which antioxidants function, as it neutralizes free radicals that contribute to oxidative stress. Thus, the DPPH assay provides valuable insight into the antioxidant potential of CLHE. Previous studies have validated the use of DPPH as an indicator of antioxidant properties in biological samples [40], supporting its relevance to the current study.

Notably, CLHE demonstrated superior effectiveness in inhibiting protein denaturation compared to ibuprofen, suggesting its better potential to protect cells from inflammation-induced damage. Furthermore, its enhanced ability to scavenge and stabilize free radicals beyond that of the standard control highlights its promising role in reducing oxidative stress and preventing cellular harm.

In drug design and development, toxicology is as crucial as efficacy. The cytotoxicity of CLHE was assessed using the HCEC cell line, which originates from a healthy adult's colonic biopsy and is widely used as an in vitro model for studying intestinal absorption and toxicology studies [41]. After 48 h of treatment with CLHE, 48% cell viability was observed at the highest concentration (20 μg/mL) (Figure 5a). These findings suggest that CLHE is non-toxic to healthy organs and gastrointestinal tissues. The acute toxicity assessment, using the Enegide method, provided a reliable and reproducible approach with minimal animal use, reducing the need for excessive animal testing [42]. Oral administration of CLHE did not result in any behavioral or neurological abnormalities, and its high LD50 (5000 mg/kg) confirms its safety at elevated doses. Additionally, fasting for 12 h prior to dosing ensures no interference from previous feed intake (Table 2). The lack of significant changes in serum urea, bilirubin, or creatinine levels, compared to healthy controls, further supports the non-toxic profile of CLHE [43]. Nasir et al. previously conducted an acute toxicity study of *C. luteum* on mice, with a maximum dose of 2000 mg/kg, reporting no adverse effects [44]. Our findings extend this, demonstrating that even at a dose of 5000 mg/kg, CLHE remains safe, validating the earlier study.

Once the safety of CHLE was established, its anti-inflammatory potential was evaluated in a CIA mice model, using ibuprofen as a reference NSAID. Previous studies have explored the effects of *C. luteum* in arthritis models, but its comparison against any NSAID has not been established [45]. In this study, oral administration of CLHE resulted in a significant reduction in both systemic and localized inflammation in the arthritic mice. Peripheral edema, a key indicator of inflammation, directly correlates with disease severity and progression [46]. In the post-treatment groups, the reduction in paw volume in group 3 highlights the ability of CLHE to effectively reduce edema. Interestingly, CLHE demonstrated a greater reduction in arthritic scores compared to ibuprofen, indicating its superior efficacy in reducing both inflammation and arthritis-related symptoms.

At the organ level, spleen size is an important indicator of inflammation. During inflammation, the spleen is enlarged to cater to the increased circulation of cytokines [47]. In the disease model, the spleen size increased to maximum of 1 mm, which was significantly reduced in the post-treatment groups. Notably, spleen indices were markedly higher in the ibuprofen-treated group ($p < 0.0001$) than in the CLHE-treated group ($p < 0.01$), further emphasizing CLHE's enhanced anti-inflammatory potency. CRP is a systemic inflammatory marker whose concentration increases in response to tissue damage and inflammation [48]. While CRP levels were significantly elevated during the inflammatory phase, the post-treatment groups showed marked reductions in CRP concentrations. The observed decrease in CRP in groups 3 and 4 suggests that the anti-inflammatory effects of CLHE are comparable to those of ibuprofen.

Further assessment of the anti-inflammatory effects of CLHE was conducted via the expression of key inflammation-related genes. CLHE significantly downregulated the expression of COX-2, TNFα, and MMP-9, all of which play critical roles in RA-induced inflammation [49]. TNFα, produced by T-lymphocytes and macrophages, is involved in joint damage and immune cell activation [50]. Its upregulation leads to increased COX-2 expression, which promotes prostaglandin synthesis. MMP-9, activated by both TNFα and COX-2, is a key enzyme responsible for cartilage degradation and bone erosion [51,52]. The comparable reduction of COX-2, TNFα, and MMP-9 by both CLHE and ibuprofen suggests that CLHE effectively reduces immune cell activation and offers protection against joint damage. Similar results were confirmed by histopathological analysis of the paw, where the immunomodulatory potential of the CLHE-treated group showed reversal of bone erosion and alleviation of arthritic-induced inflammation, immunocyte infiltration, and synovial hyperplasia to a greater degree than ibuprofen. Therefore, CHLE can be considered as a therapeutic with a comparatively safer profile as compared to NSAIDs with severe cytotoxic side effects.

The use of in silico studies to evaluate the toxicity of drug or plant-based compounds has become increasingly popular due to their cost- and time-effectiveness [53]. Following GC–MS analysis, an in silico approach is commonly employed for the initial screening of phytochemicals from medicinal plants [54]. To explore the mechanism of action for safer, non-toxic bioactive compounds, the library of CLHE constituents identified via GC-MS was subjected to ADMET screening. This computational tool assesses the pharmacokinetic profiles of compounds, focusing on absorption, distribution, metabolism, and excretion, which are direct predictors of biological activity. Among the natural compounds derived from CLHE, fifteen met the ADMET criteria, but only one compound, CL15, satisfied all the parameters for drug-likeness.

Further toxicity analysis of CL15, conducted through the Protox 3.0 tool, revealed its safety across various toxicological endpoints, including hepatic, neurological, cardiac, and respiratory systems, characterizing it as non-toxic. To evaluate its potential as an alternative to NSAIDs, CL15 was docked with COX-2 and TNFα, two key targets in inflammation. COX-2 is the primary target for NSAIDs in reducing inflammatory symptoms, while TNFα induces COX-2 expression [37]. CL15 exhibited significant pharmacological and anti-inflammatory potential through its strong binding affinity with both COX-2 and TNFα, which was further validated by stable simulations of these complexes. In the case of TNFα, CL15 binds at positions 91 and 94, which is closer to a structurally important residue at position 90. Position 90 is a key residue that is involved in maintaining the TNFα loop structure and contributes to receptor binding activity, as shown in amino acid substitution models [55]. Hydrogen bond formation at residues 91, 94, 96, and 104 with sufficient stability within the protein structure potentially exerts anti-inflammatory effects, as observed in the in vivo evaluations. The interaction between CL15 and TNFα remained stable throughout the simulation, suggesting that CL15 may modulate TNFα activity effectively. Similarly, in the case of COX-2, CL15 demonstrated a very stable interaction throughout the simulation. Moreover, low ΔG for both the complex suggested high stability in the molecular environment and minimal conformational changes over the 0–100 ns MD period.

In COX-2, ARG^{120} is one of the three conserved residues within the active site, responsible for binding the physiological substrate, arachidonic acid, as well as NSAIDs [56]. CL15 binds to ARG^{120} through both covalent (H-bond) and ionic (salt bridge) bonds (Figure 9a). These salt bridges serve as "molecular clips" that stabilize the conformation of the protein–ligand complex, a critical factor in rational drug design [57]. This dual interaction, combined with an additional H-bond at SER^{119}, allows CL15 to occupy much of the COX-2 active site, consistent with the number and strength of H-bonds. Notably, SER^{119}, located at the entrance of the active site, is unique to COX-2, as COX-1 has a VAL^{119} residue instead. The targeted interaction of CL15 with SER^{119} contributes to its selective inhibition of COX-2 [56]. Thus, this study suggests that CL15 has the potential to overcome the limitations of current RA treatments. NSAIDs, which are commonly used as the first line of therapy, carry significant risks, while biologics, though effective in targeting TNFα, are expensive and often cause side effects. CL15, with its targeting of both COX-2 and TNFα, offers a more comprehensive and safer alternative; however, further wet lab experiments are needed to quantify and validate its therapeutic potential.

5. Conclusions

Our study demonstrates the therapeutic potential of CLHE in the management of RA. Through a combination of in vitro, in vivo, and computational analyses, we identified CLHE's anti-inflammatory and antioxidant properties, along with its safety profile at high doses. Specifically, we found that CLHE significantly reduced inflammation and arthritic symptoms in a collagen-induced arthritis model without inducing toxicity. The identification of CL15 as a selective inhibitor of COX-2 and TNFα, key mediators in RA, further underscores the therapeutic promise of *Colchicum luteum*. These findings suggest that CLHE could serve as a safer alternative to NSAIDs, offering multi-targeted efficacy for RA management. However, further clinical studies are required to validate its effectiveness in humans.

Supplementary Materials: The following supporting information can be downloaded at: https://www.mdpi.com/article/10.3390/nu16234020/s1, Table S1: GC-MS of C. luteum extract; Table S2: ADMET screening data of CL01-CL15.

Author Contributions: Conceptualization, P.J.; formal analysis, H.A. and M.S.; investigation, H.A., M.S. and Q.M.; methodology, H.A. and M.Q.H.; resources, P.J., A.B. and Q.M.; supervision, P.J. and A.B.; validation, M.Q.H.; writing—original draft, H.A. and M.S.; writing—review and editing, P.J. and A.B. All authors have read and agreed to the published version of the manuscript.

Funding: This research received no external funding.

Institutional Review Board Statement: Approval for experimentation on mice model was acquired from institutional review board committee with Performa number 01-2020-01/04 at Atta-ur-Rahman School of Applied Biosciences, National University of Sciences and technology; approve date: 1 November 2020 (meeting 01 case number 04).

Informed Consent Statement: Not applicable.

Data Availability Statement: All data generated or analyzed during this study are included in this article and Supplementary Information Files.

Acknowledgments: We would like to thank ASAB technical staff for the smooth running of the experiments.

Conflicts of Interest: The authors declare no conflicts of interest.

Abbreviations

Arg	Arginine
CLHE	*Colchicum luteum* hydroethanolic extract
COX-2	Cyclooxygenase 2
CRP	C-reactive protein
DMARDs	Disease-modifying anti-rheumatic drugs
DMEM	Dulbecco's modified Eagle medium
DPPH	2,2-diphenyl-1-picrylhydrazyl
FBS	Fetal bovine serum
GAPDH	Glyceraldehyde-3-phosphate dehydrogenase
GC-MS	Gas chromatography-mass spectrometry
GHS	Globally harmonized system
H&E	Hematoxylin and eosin
H-bond	Hydrogen bond
HCEC	Human colon epithelial cells
IC_{50}	Half maximal inhibitory concentration
LD_{50}	Lethal dose 50%
MDS	Molecular dynamics simulation
MMP-9	Matrix metalloproteinase 9
MTT	3-(4,5-dimethylthiazolyl-2)-2,5-diphenyltetrazolium bromide
NSAIDs	Non-steroidal anti-inflammatory drugs
Pro	Proline
qPCR	Quantitative polymerase chain reaction
RA	Rheumatoid arthritis
RMSD	Root mean square deviation
RMSF	Root mean square fluctuation
RNA	Ribose nucleic acid
RoG	Radius of gyration
Ser	Serine
TNFα	Tumor necrosis factor-alpha
UV-vis	Ultraviolet-visible

References

1. Khan, M.N.; Ahmed, B.; Majeed, H.; Tareen, I.; Hassan, M.; Shehzad, M.; Raheem, A.; ur Rehman, Z. Thirty Years Trend of Rheumatic Heart Diseases, Pakistan Chapter: Insights from the Global Burden of Disease Study. *Pakistan Heart J.* **2022**, *55*, 231–235. [CrossRef]
2. Radu, A.-F.; Bungau, S.G. Management of rheumatoid arthritis: An overview. *Cells* **2021**, *10*, 2857. [CrossRef] [PubMed]
3. Lubrano, E.; Scarpa, R. Psoriatic arthritis: Treatment strategies using anti-inflammatory drugs and classical DMARDs. *Reumatismo* **2012**, *64*, 107–112. [CrossRef] [PubMed]
4. Sriuttha, P.; Sirichanchuen, B.; Permsuwan, U. Hepatotoxicity of nonsteroidal anti-inflammatory drugs: A systematic review of randomized controlled trials. *Int. J. Hepatol.* **2018**, *2018*, 5253623. [CrossRef]
5. Katiyar, C.; Gupta, A.; Kanjilal, S.; Katiyar, S. Drug discovery from plant sources: An integrated approach. *AYU (An Int. Q. J. Res. Ayurveda)* **2012**, *33*, 10–19. [CrossRef]
6. Ju, Z.; Li, M.; Xu, J.; Howell, D.C.; Li, Z.; Chen, F.-E. Recent development on COX-2 inhibitors as promising anti-inflammatory agents: The past 10 years. *Acta Pharm. Sin. B* **2022**, *12*, 2790–2807. [CrossRef]
7. van Loo, G.; Bertrand, M.J.M. Death by TNF: A road to inflammation. *Nat. Rev. Immunol.* **2023**, *23*, 289–303. [CrossRef]
8. Nakao, S.; Ogtata, Y.; Shimizu, E.; Yamazaki, M.; Furuyama, S.; Sugiya, H. Tumor necrosis factor α (TNF-α)-induced prostaglanding E 2 release is mediated by the activation of cyclooxygenase-2 (COX-2) transcription via NFκB in human gingival fibroblasts. *Mol. Cell. Biochem.* **2002**, *238*, 11–18. [CrossRef]
9. Fürst, R.; Zündorf, I. Plant-derived anti-inflammatory compounds: Hopes and disappointments regarding the translation of preclinical knowledge into clinical progress. *Mediat. Inflamm.* **2014**, *2014*, 146832. [CrossRef]
10. Siddiqui, M.Z.; Akhtar, S. Suranjan Talkh (Colchicum luteum): A review of an anti-arthritic Unani drug. *Int. J. Res. Anal. Rev.* **2019**, *6*, 328–332.
11. Akbar, S.; Akbar, S. Colchicum luteum Baker (Colchicaceae). In *Handbook of 200 Medicinal Plants*; Springer: Cham, Switezrland, 2020; pp. 691–694.
12. Reeta, M.; Ravindra, S.; Sharma, T.; Sumit, N.; Kotecha, M. SURANJANA (COLCHICUM LUTEUM BAKER.)-A RHIZOMATIC PLANT. *Sci. Res. J.* **2015**, *2*.

13. Ahmad, W.; Ahmad, M.R.; Rahman, M.N.; Alam, M.T. Therapeutic Indication of Suranjan Shirin (Colchicum luteum). *Am. J. PharmTech Res.* **2020**, *10*, 268–274. [CrossRef]
14. Joshi, V.R.; Lele, R.D.; Kulkarni, R.D. Treatment of rheumatoid arthritis with rumalaya. *Probe* **1973**, *13*, 22–24.
15. Ahmed, S.; John, P.; Paracha, R.Z.; Bhatti, A.; Guma, M. Docking and molecular dynamics study to identify novel phytobiologics from Dracaena trifasciata against metabolic reprogramming in rheumatoid arthritis. *Life* **2022**, *12*, 1148. [CrossRef]
16. Aryal, S.; Baniya, M.K.; Danekhu, K.; Kunwar, P.; Gurung, R.; Koirala, N. Total Phenolic Content, Flavonoid Content and Antioxidant Potential of Wild Vegetables from Western Nepal. *Plants* **2019**, *8*, 96. [CrossRef]
17. Enechi, O.C.; Okeke, E.S.; Nwankwo, N.E.; Nweze, J.E.; Obilor, C.P.; Okoye, C.I.; Awoh, O.E. Membrane Stabilization, Albumin Denaturation, Protease Inhibition, and Antioxidant Activity as Possible Mechanisms for the Anti-Inflammatory Effects of Flavonoid-Rich Extract of Peltophorum pterocarpum (DC.) K. Heyne (FREPP) Stem Bark. *Trop. J. Nat. Prod. Res.* **2020**, *4*, 812–816. [CrossRef]
18. Erhirhie, E.O.; Ihekwereme, C.P.; Ilodigwe, E.E. Advances in acute toxicity testing: Strengths, weaknesses and regulatory acceptance. *Interdiscip. Toxicol.* **2018**, *11*, 5–12. [CrossRef]
19. Jannat, A.; John, P.; Bhatti, A.; Hayat, M.Q. Tomorou attenuates progression of rheumatoid arthritis through alteration in ULK-1 independent autophagy pathway in collagen induced arthritis mice model. *Cell Death Discov.* **2019**, *5*, 142. [CrossRef]
20. Hor, S.Y.; Ahmad, M.; Farsi, E.; Yam, M.F.; Hashim, M.A.; Lim, C.P.; Sadikun, A.; Asmawi, M.Z. Safety assessment of methanol extract of red dragon fruit (Hylocereus polyrhizus): Acute and subchronic toxicity studies. *Regul. Toxicol. Pharmacol.* **2012**, *63*, 106–114. [CrossRef]
21. Dong, J.; Wang, N.-N.; Yao, Z.-J.; Zhang, L.; Cheng, Y.; Ouyang, D.; Lu, A.-P.; Cao, D.-S. ADMETlab: A platform for systematic ADMET evaluation based on a comprehensively collected ADMET database. *J. Cheminform.* **2018**, *10*, 29. [CrossRef]
22. Banerjee, P.; Kemmler, E.; Dunkel, M.; Preissner, R. ProTox 3.0: A webserver for the prediction of toxicity of chemicals. *Nucleic Acids Res.* **2024**, *52*, W513–W520. [CrossRef] [PubMed]
23. Trott, O.; Olson, A.J. AutoDock Vina: Improving the speed and accuracy of docking with a new scoring function, efficient optimization and multithreading. *J. Comput. Chem.* **2010**, *31*, 455–461. [CrossRef] [PubMed]
24. Abraham, M.J.; Murtola, T.; Schulz, R.; Páll, S.; Smith, J.C.; Hess, B.; Lindah, E. GROMACS: High performance molecular simulations through multi-level parallelism from laptops to supercomputers. *SoftwareX* **2015**, *1–2*, 19–25. [CrossRef]
25. Orozco, M.N.; Solomons, N.W.; Schümann, K.; Friel, J.K.; de Montenegro, A.L.M. Antioxidant-rich oral supplements attenuate the effects of oral iron on in situ oxidation susceptibility of human feces. *J. Nutr.* **2010**, *140*, 1105–1110. [CrossRef]
26. Kwon, T.-H.; Chao, D.L.; Malloy, K.; Sun, D.; Alessandri, B.; Bullock, M.R. Tempol, a novel stable nitroxide, reduces brain damage and free radical production, after acute subdural hematoma in the rat. *J. Neurotrauma* **2003**, *20*, 337–345. [CrossRef]
27. Sahoo, C.R.; Paidesetty, S.K.; Padhy, R.N. The recent development of thymol derivative as a promising pharmacological scaffold. *Drug Dev. Res.* **2021**, *82*, 1079–1095. [CrossRef]
28. Berry, J.M.; Bradshaw, T.D.; Fichtner, I.; Ren, R.; Schwalbe, C.H.; Wells, G.; Chew, E.-H.; Stevens, M.F.G.; Westwell, A.D. Quinols as Novel Therapeutic Agents. 2. 4-(1-Arylsulfonylindol-2-yl)-4-hydroxycyclohexa-2,5-dien-1-ones and Related Agents as Potent and Selective Antitumor Agents. *J. Med. Chem.* **2005**, *48*, 639–644. [CrossRef]
29. Bosque, I.; Gonzalez-Gomez, J.C.; Loza, M.I.; Brea, J. Natural Tetraponerines: A General Synthesis and Antiproliferative Activity. *J. Org. Chem.* **2014**, *79*, 3982–3991. [CrossRef]
30. Frolov, N.A.; Vereshchagin, A.N. Piperidine Derivatives: Recent Advances in Synthesis and Pharmacological Applications. *Int. J. Mol. Sci.* **2023**, *24*, 2937. [CrossRef]
31. Konturek, P.C.; Nikiforuk, A.; Brzozowski, T.; Pawlik, M.; Raithel, M.; Hahn, E.G.; Konturek, S.J. Effect of N-alpha-methyl histamine on ulcer healing in rats. *Inflamm. Res.* **2004**, *53*, S27–S28. [CrossRef]
32. Ongtanasup, T.; Prommee, N.; Jampa, O.; Limcharoen, T.; Wanmasae, S.; Nissapatorn, V.; Paul, A.K.; Pereira, M. de L.; Wilairatana, P.; Nasongkla, N.; et al. The Cholesterol-Modulating Effect of the New Herbal Medicinal Recipe from Yellow Vine (Coscinium fenestratum (Goetgh.)), Ginger (Zingiber officinale Roscoe.), and Safflower (*Carthamus tinctorius* L.) on Suppressing PCSK9 Expression to Upregulate LDLR Expression in HepG2 Cells. *Plants* **2022**, *11*, 1835. [CrossRef]
33. Kapri, A.; Pant, S.; Gupta, N.; Nain, S. Recent Advances in the Biological Significance of Xanthine and its Derivatives: A Review. *Pharm. Chem. J.* **2022**, *56*, 461–474. [CrossRef]
34. Hosseinzadeh, L.; Aliabadi, A.; Rahnama, M.; Sadeghi, H.M.M.; Khajouei, M.R. Synthesis and cytotoxic evaluation of some new 3-(2-(2-phenylthiazol-4-yl) ethyl)-quinazolin-4(3H) one derivatives with potential anticancer effects. *Res. Pharm. Sci.* **2017**, *12*, 290–298. [CrossRef] [PubMed]
35. Lewgowd, W.; Stanczak, A. Cinnoline Derivatives with Biological Activity. *Arch. Pharm.* **2007**, *340*, 65–80. [CrossRef] [PubMed]
36. Volobueva, A.S.; Yarovaya, O.I.; Kireeva, M.V.; Borisevich, S.S.; Kovaleva, K.S.; Mainagashev, I.Y.; Gatilov, Y.V.; Ilyina, M.G.; Zarubaev, V.V.; Salakhutdinov, N.F. Discovery of New Ginsenol-Like Compounds with High Antiviral Activity. *Molecules* **2021**, *26*, 6794. [CrossRef]
37. Nash, P.; Clegg, D.O. Psoriatic arthritis therapy: NSAIDs and traditional DMARDs. *Ann. Rheum. Dis.* **2005**, *64* (Suppl. S2), ii74–ii77. [CrossRef]
38. Sapra, S.; Bhalla, Y.; Nandani; Sharma, S.; Singh, G.; Nepali, K.; Budhiraja, A.; Dhar, K.L. Colchicine and its various physicochemical and biological aspects. *Med. Chem. Res.* **2013**, *22*, 531–547. [CrossRef]

39. Zhang, L.; Ravipati, A.S.; Koyyalamudi, S.R.; Jeong, S.C.; Reddy, N.; Smith, P.T.; Bartlett, J.; Shanmugam, K.; Münch, G.; Wu, M.J. Antioxidant and anti-inflammatory activities of selected medicinal plants containing phenolic and flavonoid compounds. *J. Agric. Food Chem.* **2011**, *59*, 12361–12367. [CrossRef]
40. Gulcin, İ.; Alwasel, S.H. DPPH Radical Scavenging Assay. *Processes* **2023**, *11*, 2248. [CrossRef]
41. Steensma, A.; Noteborn, H.P.J.M.; Kuiper, H.A. Comparison of Caco-2, IEC-18 and HCEC cell lines as a model for intestinal absorption of genistein, daidzein and their glycosides. *Environ. Toxicol. Pharmacol.* **2004**, *16*, 131–139. [CrossRef]
42. Creton, S.; Dewhurst, I.C.; Earl, L.K.; Gehen, S.C.; Guest, R.L.; Hotchkiss, J.A.; Indans, I.; Woolhiser, M.R.; Billington, R. Acute toxicity testing of chemicals—Opportunities to avoid redundant testing and use alternative approaches. *Crit. Rev. Toxicol.* **2010**, *40*, 50–83. [CrossRef] [PubMed]
43. Njinga, N.S.; Kola-Mustapha, A.T.; Quadri, A.L.; Atolani, O.; Ayanniyi, R.O.; Buhari, M.O.; Amusa, T.O.; Ajani, E.O.; Folaranmi, O.O.; Bakare-Odunola, M.T. Toxicity assessment of sub-acute and sub-chronic oral administration and diuretic potential of aqueous extract of Hibiscus sabdariffa calyces. *Heliyon* **2020**, *6*, e04853. [CrossRef] [PubMed]
44. Nair, V.; Singh, S.; Gupta, Y.K. Evaluation of the disease modifying activity of Colchicum luteum Baker in experimental arthritis. *J. Ethnopharmacol.* **2011**, *133*, 303–307. [CrossRef] [PubMed]
45. Nair, V.; Kumar, R.; Singh, S.; Gupta, Y.K. Investigation into the Anti-inflammatory and Antigranuloma Activity of Colchicum luteum Baker in Experimental Models. *Inflammation* **2012**, *35*, 881–888. [CrossRef]
46. Luan, J.; Hu, Z.; Cheng, J.; Zhang, R.; Yang, P.; Guo, H.; Nan, G.; Guo, N.; Gou, X. Applicability and implementation of the collagen-induced arthritis mouse model, including protocols (Review). *Exp. Ther. Med.* **2021**, *22*, 939. [CrossRef]
47. Teixeira, J.H.; Silva, A.M.; Almeida, M.I.; Bessa-Gonçalves, M.; Cunha, C.; Barbosa, M.A.; Santos, S.G. The Systemic Immune Response to Collagen-Induced Arthritis and the Impact of Bone Injury in Inflammatory Conditions. *Int. J. Mol. Sci.* **2019**, *20*, 5436. [CrossRef]
48. Jimenez, R.V.; Szalai, A.J. Therapeutic Lowering of C-Reactive Protein. *Front. Immunol.* **2020**, *11*, 619564. [CrossRef]
49. Lianxu, C.; Hongti, J.; Changlong, Y. NF-κBp65-specific siRNA inhibits expression of genes of COX-2, NOS-2 and MMP-9 in rat IL-1β-induced and TNF-α-induced chondrocytes. *Osteoarthr. Cartil.* **2006**, *14*, 367–376. [CrossRef]
50. Mease, P. TNFα therapy in psoriatic arthritis and psoriasis. *Ann. Rheum. Dis.* **2004**, *63*, 755–758. [CrossRef]
51. Abramson, S.B. The role of COX-2 produced by cartilage in arthritis. *Osteoarthr. Cartil.* **1999**, *7*, 380–381. [CrossRef]
52. Ahmed, E.A.; Ahmed, O.M.; Fahim, H.I.; Ali, T.M.; Elesawy, B.H.; Ashour, M.B. Potency of Bone Marrow-Derived Mesenchymal Stem Cells and Indomethacin in Complete Freund's Adjuvant-Induced Arthritic Rats: Roles of TNF-α, IL-10, iNOS, MMP-9, and TGF-β1. *Stem Cells Int.* **2021**, *2021*, 6665601. [CrossRef] [PubMed]
53. Sarkar, S.; Modak, D.; Roy, S.K.; Biswas, A.; Islam, M.; Baishya, R.; Bose, S.; Georrge, J.J.; Bhattacharjee, S. In silico, in vitro, and in vivo acute and sub-acute toxicity profiling of whole plant methanol extract of Equisetum diffusum D. Don from the sub-Himalayan West Bengal, India, having ethnobotanical uses. *BMC Complement. Med. Ther.* **2024**, *24*, 324. [CrossRef] [PubMed]
54. Rajkumar, P.; Sundari, S.; Selvaraj, S.; Natarajan, A.; Suganya, R.; Jayaprakash, R.; Kasthuri, K.; Kumaresan, S. GC-MS, Phytochemical Analysis and In Silico Approaches of a Medicinal Plant Acalypha indica. *J. Sci. Res.* **2022**, *14*, 671–684. [CrossRef]
55. Shibata, H.; Kamada, H.; Kobayashi-Nishibata, K.; Yoshioka, Y.; Nishibata, T.; Abe, Y.; Nomura, T.; Nabeshi, H.; Minowa, K.; Mukai, Y.; et al. Role of amino acid residue 90 in bioactivity and receptor binding capacity of tumor necrosis factor mutants. *Biochim. Biophys. Acta Proteins Proteom.* **2007**, *1774*, 1029–1035. [CrossRef]
56. Oniga, S.D.; Pacureanu, L.; Stoica, C.I.; Palage, M.D.; Crăciun, A.; Rusu, L.R.; Crisan, E.-L.; Araniciu, C. COX inhibition profile and molecular docking studies of some 2-(trimethoxyphenyl)-thiazoles. *Molecules* **2017**, *22*, 1507. [CrossRef]
57. Spassov, D.S.; Atanasova, M.; Doytchinova, I. A role of salt bridges in mediating drug potency: A lesson from the N-myristoyltransferase inhibitors. *Front. Mol. Biosci.* **2023**, *9*, 1066029. [CrossRef]

nutrients

MDPI

Article

Lysimachia mauritiana Lam. Extract Alleviates Airway Inflammation Induced by Particulate Matter Plus Diesel Exhaust Particles in Mice

Yoon-Young Sung [1], Seung-Hyung Kim [2], Won-Kyung Yang [2], Heung Joo Yuk [1], Mi-Sun Kim [1] and Dong-Seon Kim [1,*]

[1] KM Science Research Division, Korea Institute of Oriental Medicine, 1672 Yuseongdae-ro, Yuseong-gu, Daejeon 34054, Republic of Korea; yysung@kiom.re.kr (Y.-Y.S.); yukhj@kiom.re.kr (H.J.Y.); misun210@gmail.com (M.-S.K.)

[2] Institute of Traditional Medicine and Bioscience, Daejeon University, 62 Daehak-ro, Dong-gu, Daejeon 34520, Republic of Korea; sksh518@dju.kr (S.-H.K.); ywks1220@dju.kr (W.-K.Y.)

* Correspondence: dskim@kiom.re.kr; Tel.: +82-42-868-9639

Abstract: Exposure to air pollution poses a risk to human respiratory health, and a preventive and therapeutic remedy against fine dust-induced respiratory disease is needed. Background/Objectives: The respiratory-protective effects of *Lysimachia mauritiana* (LM) against airway inflammation were evaluated in a mouse model exposed to a fine dust mixture of diesel exhaust particles and particulate matter with a diameter of less than 10 μm (PM10D). Methods: To induce airway inflammation, PM10D was intranasally injected into BALB/c mice three times a day for 12 days, and LM extracts were given orally once per day. The immune cell subtypes, histopathology, and expression of inflammatory mediators were analyzed from the bronchoalveolar lavage fluid (BALF) and lungs. Results: LM alleviated the accumulation of neutrophils and the number of inflammatory cells in the lungs and the BALF of the PM10D-exposed mice. LM also reduced the release of inflammatory mediators (MIP-2, IL-17, IL-1α, CXCL1, TNF-α, MUC5AC, and TRP receptor channels) in the BALF and lungs. Lung histopathology was used to examine airway inflammation and the accumulation of collagen fibers and inflammatory cells after PM10D exposure and showed that LM administration improved this inflammation. Furthermore, LM extract inhibited the MAPK and NF-κB signaling pathway in the lungs and improved expectoration activity through an increase in phenol red release from the trachea. Conclusions: LM alleviated PM10D-exposed neutrophilic airway inflammation by suppressing MAPK/NF-κB activation. This study indicates that LM extract may be an effective therapeutic agent against inflammatory respiratory diseases.

Keywords: airway inflammation; lung; neutrophil; PM10D; respiratory disease

1. Introduction

The presence of fine particulate matter (PM), a type of air pollution, poses a danger to human health by damaging the respiratory system, including the airway and lungs [1]. PM with a diameter of 2.5–10 μm includes diverse chemical constituents, such as sulfates, nitrates, ammonium, organic and elemental carbon, biological compounds, organic compounds (e.g., polycyclic aromatic hydrocarbons), and metals (e.g., copper, nickel, vanadium, zinc, and cadmium) [2]. Diesel exhaust particles (DEPs), consisting of a combination of elemental carbon, organic compounds (including polycyclic aromatic hydrocarbons), sulfates, nitrates, and metals, are the main constituent of PM with a diameter of less than 2.5 μm (PM2.5) and are associated with airway inflammation and remodeling as well as heart dysfunction [3]. Because this fine PM can cause chronic respiratory diseases, it is crucial to investigate ways to prevent and treat respiratory disorders caused by air pollution [4].

Lysimachia mauritiana (LM) is a dicotyledonous plant found in coastal rocky areas in the southern region of South Korea, including Jeju Island, Dokdo Island, and Ulleung Island [5,6]. LM-containing *Lysimachia* plants, known as seagrass, pearls vegetables, and beach pearls grass, live in relatively dry conditions, such as rocky crevices along the coast, and are considered to be medical plants due to their antioxidant, anticancer, antibacterial, and antiviral activities from the large amounts of flavonol glycosides (quercetin, kaempferol, and myricetin types) they contain [7–10]. Flavonol glycosides of hyperin and kaempferol-3-O-rhamnosyl-galactosides have been isolated from the whole plant of LM [7]. The young leaves and shoots of LM are eaten as vegetables, and the plant is also used for ornamental purposes. In oriental herbal medicine, LM is mainly used as a diuretic and for urinary diseases, menstrual irregularities, and labor pains. It is also known to be effective for trauma, high blood pressure, diabetes, constipation, swelling, bruising, and sore throat [11,12]. However, although LM has been used for respiratory diseases, the effect of LM on airway inflammation has not been examined. Thus, this study investigated the possible effects of LM extract on mice with airway inflammation induced by exposure to a fine dust mixture: a mixture of PM with a diameter of less than 10 μm (PM10) and DEP (PM10D).

2. Materials and Methods

2.1. Preparation of *Lysimachia mauritiana* and UPLC-QTof MS Analysis

LM extract was provided by Dongkook Pharmaceutical (Seoul, Republic of Korea). The LM extract was extracted from air-dried aerial parts (leaves) with 50% ethanol for 5-h. The extract was filtered, concentrated under reduced pressure, and then after mixing the food-grade maltodextrin, the mixture was spray-dried to obtain a powdered sample (code name DKB-139, batch No. 240425-001, S&D Co., Ltd, Cheongju-si, Chungcheongbuk-do, Republic of Korea). The 50% ethanol extract from *L. mauritiana* was analyzed using an AQUITYTM UPLC system (Waters Corp., Milford, MA, USA) equipped with a binary gradient system, an auto-injector, and a UV-Visible detector. The sample (2.0 μL) was separated on a BEH C18 column (2.1 × 100 mm, 1.7 μm) at a flow rate of 0.4 mL/min and eluted using a linear gradient of two mobile phases containing 0.1% formic acid (A: water; B: acetonitrile). A chromatographic gradient was optimized as follows: 0 min, 10% B; 0–8 min, 10–30% B; 8–11 min, 30–90% B; 11–12 min, 90–100% B; 12–13.3 min, 100% B; and at 13.4 min, it returned to 10% B and was maintained until the 15 min mark. Mass spectrometry analysis was conducted using a quadrupole time-of-flight mass spectrometer (Xevo G2 QToF, Waters Corp., Milford, MA, USA) with an electrospray ionization (ESI) interface operating in negative ion mode. The system was configured with the following settings: a cone voltage of 40 V, a capillary voltage of 2500 V, a source temperature at 110 °C, and a desolvation temperature at 350 °C. Leucine-enkephalin ([M−H]− *m*/*z* 554.2615) was used as the lock mass with a sprayer reference solution. All solvents used for extraction and chromatography were of a LC/GC-MS grade (J. T. Baker, Phillipsburg, NJ, USA).

2.2. Animal Experiments

Experiment 1: Seven-week-old male BALB/c mice (Orient Bio, Seongnam, Republic of Korea) were maintained in the specific pathogen-free facility at 60% ± 10% humidity and 21 °C ± 2 °C. The experiment was performed according to the Guide for the Care and Use of Laboratory Animals and approved by the Committee for Animal Welfare at Daejeon University (DJUARB2022-041). Respiratory damage was induced by intranasal injection of PM10D (MilliporeSigma, Burlington, MA, USA) in aluminum hydroxide (1%) gel adjuvant, which included PM10 (ERMCZ120; 3 mg/mL) and DEP (NIST2975; 0.6 mg/mL), on days 4, 7, and 10 [13]. The mice were divided into five groups (n = 6/group): normal, PM10D control, PM10D and 3 mg dexamethasone/kg, PM10D and 50 mg LM extract/kg, and PM10D and 100 mg LM extract/kg [13]. The doses were determined from preliminary dose-dependent experiments. Dexamethasone (as a positive control) or LM extract was orally administered every day for 12 days. After completing the experiment, blood, bronchoalveolar lavage fluid (BALF), and tissues were isolated from the mice of each group under euthanasia. Figure 1A shows the schedule for determining the preventive effects of LM using an animal model of respiratory damage.

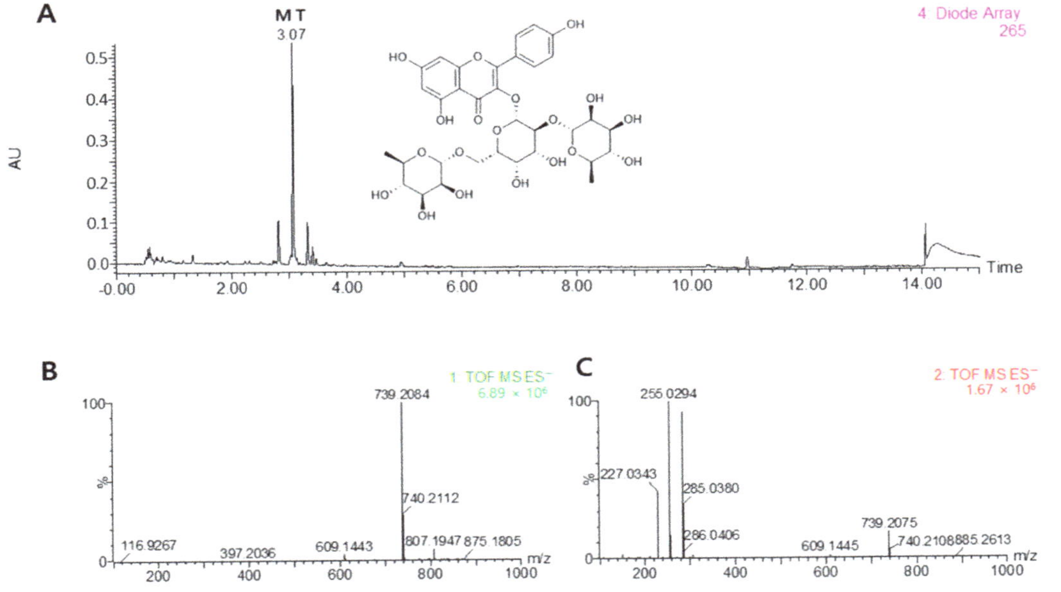

Figure 1. Chemical structure of mauritianin (MT). Comparison of UPLC DAD chromatograms of the 50% ethanol extract from *Lysimachia mauritiana* (**A**), MS (**B**), and MS/MS (**C**) data for the qualitative analysis of major chemical constituents. The UPLC chromatogram was acquired at 265 nm.

Experiment 2: The study of phenol red secretion for expectorant activity was carried out as previously reported [14]. The experiment was approved by the Animal Ethics Committee for the Korea Institute of Oriental Medicine (approval code 23-054). Seven-week-old male ICR mice (Orients Bio, Seongnam-Si, Republic of Korea) were divided into five groups (n = 12): normal, phenol red control, phenol red and 200 mg Levosol/kg (PharmGen Science, Seoul, Republic of Korea), phenol red and 50 mg LM extract/kg, and phenol red and 100 mg LM extract/kg. Levosol or LM extract was administered orally once a day for 3 days. The vehicle was administered to normal and control mice. Except for the normal group, phenol red (5%) was injected intraperitoneally in each mouse on day 3. The trachea was removed after 60 min and incubated in saline (1 mL) for 1 h to extract phenol red and then treated with sodium hydroxide (0.1 mL) to stop the reaction. The amount of secreted phenol red was quantified by measuring the absorbance at 546 nm.

2.3. Collection of Cells from BALF and Lung

The BALF was collected by trachea cannulation and aspiration. The differential cell count was examined in a cytospin with Diff-Quick staining. The lungs were treated with collagenase IV (1 mg/mL), then filtered and centrifuged, and the lung cells were collected [4].

2.4. Flow Cytometry Analysis

The lung cells or BALF cells were incubated with individual fluorescent-conjugated antibodies against lymphocytes, T cells, and B cells, and the cells were analyzed on a FACSCalibur (BD, Seoul, Republic of Korea) as performed in a previous study [14].

2.5. Release of Cytokines

The secretion levels of IL-17, IL-1α, macrophage inflammatory protein-2 (MIP-2), CXCL-1, and TNF-α in the BALF were measured using an enzyme-linked immunosorbent assay (R&D Systems, Minneapolis, MN, USA), and the absorbance at 450 nm was determined (Molecular Devices, San Jose, CA, USA).

2.6. Histopathological Analysis

The removed lungs were fixed, paraffinized, sectioned to a 5 μm thickness, and stained with Masson's trichrome solution to examine collagen fiber formation or hematoxylin and eosin (H and E) solution to examine inflammation. The inflammatory severity was determined in a double-blind manner and rated on a subjective scale of 0–2 [13].

2.7. Quantitative Reverse Transcription-Polymerase Chain Reaction

Total RNA was isolated from the removed lungs using a HiGene precipitation assay (BIOFACT, Daejeon, Republic of Korea). The gene expression was quantified by quantitative reverse transcription-polymerase chain reaction with an SYBR Green Master Mix and primers using an Applied Biosystems 7500 Fast (Thermo Fisher Scientific, Waltham, MA, USA). The sequence of the primers is shown in Table 1 [13]. The transcript was expressed as ΔΔCt, normalized to β-actin.

Table 1. Primers' sequence used in qRT-PCR analysis.

Gene	Primer	Oligonucleotide Sequence (5′-3′)
Actin	F	TGGAATCCTGTGGCATCCAT
	R	TAAAACGCAGCTCGTAACAG
TNF-α	F	CCTGTAGCCCACGTCGTAGC
	R	TTGACCTCAGCGCTGAGTTG
MIP-2	F	ATGCCTGAAGACCCTGCCAAG
	R	GGTCAGTTAGCCTTGCCTTTG
CXCL1	F	CCGAAGTCATAGCCACAC
	R	GTGCCATCAGAGCAGTCT
MUC5AC	F	AGAATATCTTTCAGGACCCCT
	R	ACACCAGTGCTGAGCATACTT
TRPV1	F	CATCTTCACCACGGCTGCTTAC
	R	CAGACAGGATCTCTCCAGTGAC
TRPA1	F	TGAGATCGACCGGAGT
	R	TGCTGAAGGCATCTTG

Abbreviations: F, forward; R, reverse.

2.8. Western Blot

Proteins from the lungs were extracted using PRO-PREP solution (Intron, Seongnam, Republic of Korea), and gel electrophoresis and membrane transfer were performed using a Bio-Rad Trans-Blot transfer system (Hercules, CA, USA). The membrane was blocked using a blocking buffer (EzBlock Chemi, ATTO, Daejeon, Republic of Korea) and then treated with phospho-NF-κB, -JNK, -p38, or -ERK and total-NF-κB, -ERK, -p38, or -JNK antibodies (Cell Signaling Technology, Danvers, MA, USA, 1:1000) for 24 h. The band was detected with chemiluminescence (Thermo Fisher Scientific, Waltham, MA, USA) and evaluated by ImageJ 7 software. The protein expression was expressed relative to β-actin.

2.9. Statistical Analysis

The data are expressed as the mean ± standard error of the mean. Statistical testing was performed by one-way analysis of variance and Duncan's multiple comparison test using GraphPad Prism 7.0 software. p-values less than 0.05 were considered to demonstrate significant differences.

3. Results

3.1. Effects of LM Extract on Neutrophil Accumulation in PM10D-Exposed Mice

As shown in Figure 1, the major phytochemical from LM was identified by UPLC-QTof MS analysis. The details for the identification were as follows. The peak had an [M–H]− at m/z 739.2084 and fragment ions at m/z 285 for the aglycon kaempferol (loss of 454 amu for di-rhamnosyl-galactoside). On the basis of this information, the peak was assigned to kaempferol-3-O-(2,6-di-O-α-rhamnopyranosyl-β-galactopyranoside), a well-known compound in *L. mauritiana*, and was tentatively identified as mauritianin (MT).

The effect of LM on airway inflammation was investigated in PM10D-exposed mice. Body weight change and food intake were not significantly different among groups. All mice survived and there were no other abnormal symptoms during the experiment. Airway neutrophilia, a common feature of chronic respiratory inflammation disease, is associated with disease progression [15]. Figure 2B–D shows the number of neutrophils in the BALF and the total numbers of BALF cells and lung cells after administering the LM extract in an animal model of respiratory damage. The exposure of the mice to PM10D for 12 days increased the number of neutrophils in the BALF, and this neutrophil infiltration was limited following the administration of LM extract (Figure 2B). Similarly, the total numbers of BALF and lung cells increased following exposure to PM10D, and the increased cell numbers decreased in LM extract–treated mice (Figure 2C,D).

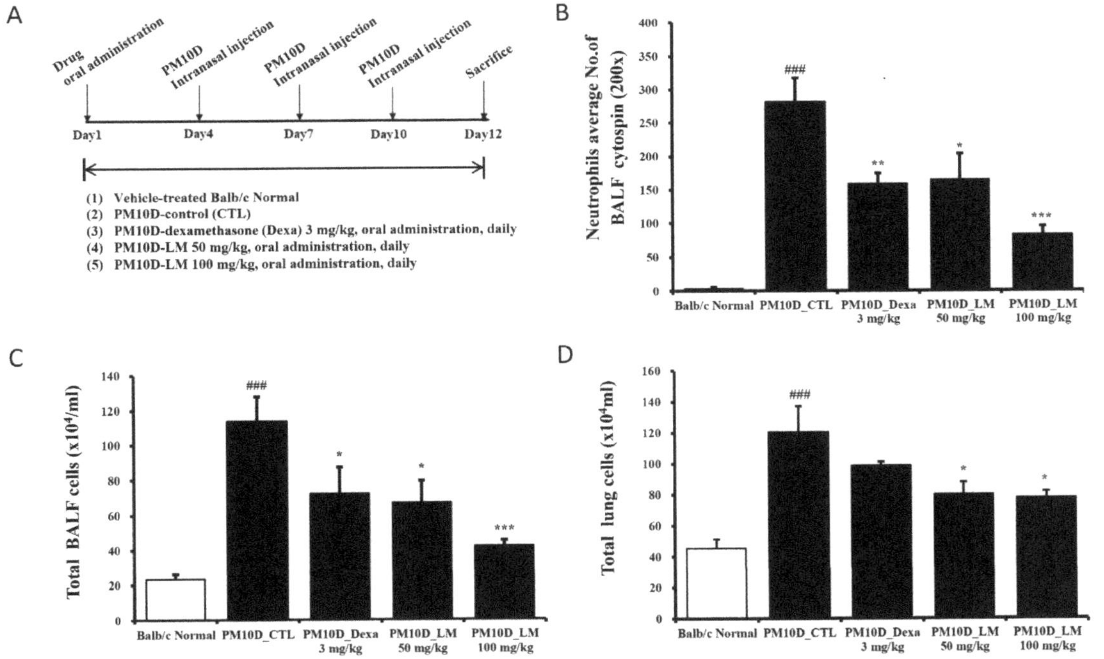

Figure 2. Experimental setup and the effect of *Lysimachia mauritiana* extract on total and immune cell numbers in a model of airway inflammation induced by particulate matter with a diameter less than 10 μm plus diesel exhaust particles (PM10D) [13]. (**A**) Experimental setup; (**B**) neutrophils in bronchoalveolar lavage fluid (BALF) cytospin (magnification: 200×); total numbers of (**C**) BALF cells and (**D**) lung cells. N = 6/group. ### $p < 0.001$ vs. normal. * $p < 0.05$, ** $p < 0.01$, and *** $p < 0.001$ vs. PM10D control (CTL).

3.2. Effects of LM Extract on the Number of White Blood Cells

As immune cells such as CD4 T cells migrate to lung tissue due to the lung inflammation caused by PM10D, the hematological analysis of white blood cells showed a reduced cell number following PM10D exposure. However, these levels recovered following administration of dexamethasone and LM extract (Figure 3A). WBC differential counting results indicate the percentages of each type of leukocytes (neutrophils, lymphocytes, monocytes, eosinophils, and basophils) that are present in the blood. The number of neutrophils in particular increased in PM10D-exposed mice and significantly decreased following the administration of dexamethasone or LM extract (Figure 3B). These results are consistent with an increase in neutrophils in BALF as seen in Figure 1B. Furthermore, the decreased number of lymphocytes in PM10D-exposed mice recovered following LM administration (Figure 3B). The levels of other white blood cells (i.e., eosinophils, monocytes, and basophils) did not change (Figure 3C).

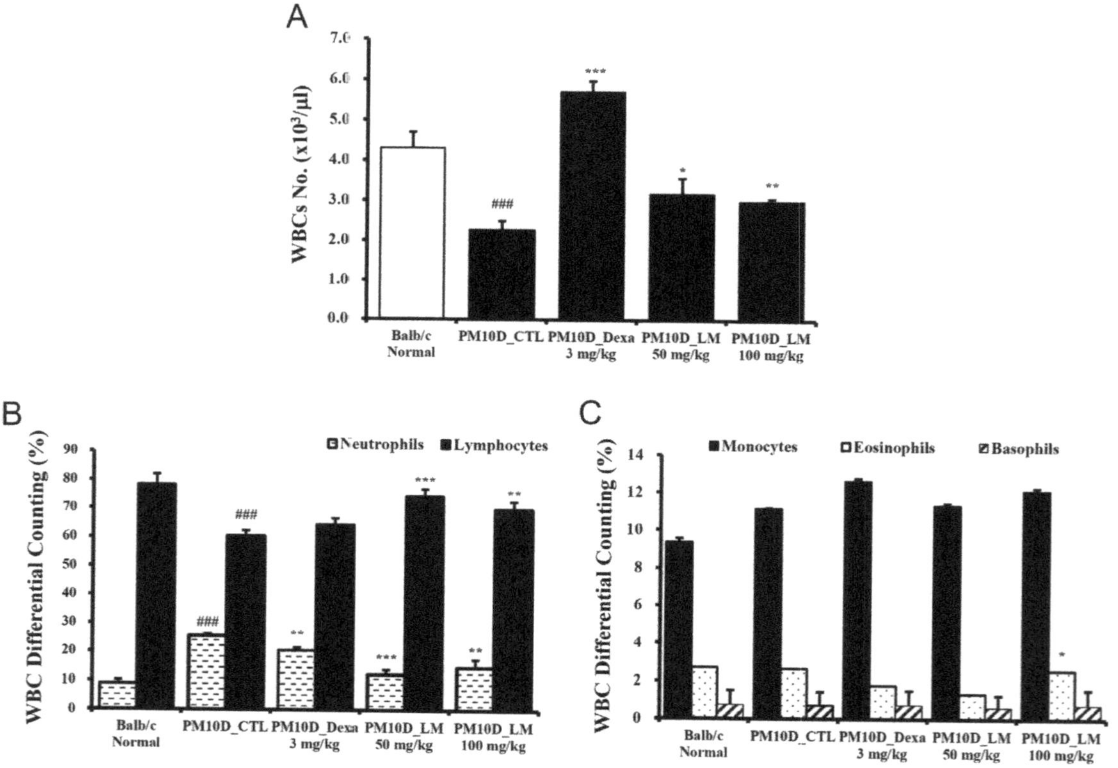

Figure 3. Effect of *Lysimachia mauritiana* extract on (**A**) the number of white blood cells (WBCs) and (**B**,**C**) WBC differential cell counting. N = 6/group. ### $p < 0.001$ vs. normal. * $p < 0.05$, ** $p < 0.01$ and *** $p < 0.001$ vs. particulate matter with a diameter less than 10 μm plus diesel exhaust particles (PM10D) control (CTL).

3.3. Effects of LM Extract on the Secretion of Inflammatory Mediators in BALF

The secretion of mediators containing cytokines and chemokines contributes to the pathology of airway inflammatory [16]. Figure 4A–E shows that IL-1α, IL-17, CXCL1, TNF-α, and MIP-2 levels in the BALF were elevated by PM10D exposure and then significantly inhibited by the administration of dexamethasone or LM extract. This effect was dose-dependent and the high dose of LM exerted almost the same effect as dexamethasone.

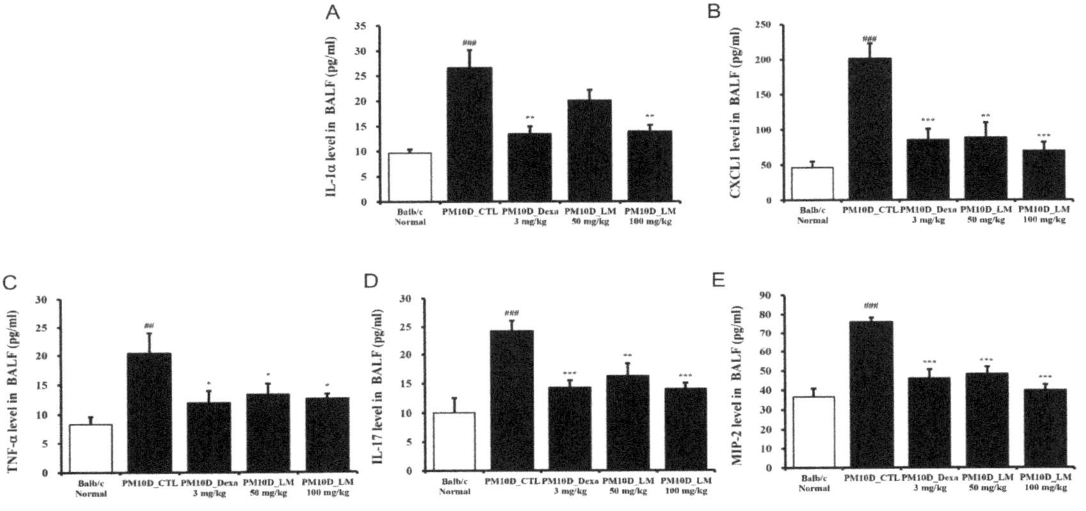

Figure 4. Effect of *Lysimachia mauritiana* extract on the release of cytokines and chemokines in bronchoalveolar lavage fluid (BALF) in a model of airway inflammation induced by particulate matter with a diameter less than 10 μm plus diesel exhaust particles (PM10D). BALF production of (**A**) IL-1α, (**B**) CXCL1, (**C**) TNF-α, (**D**) IL-17, and (**E**) MIP-2 (n = 6/group). ## $p < 0.01$ and ### $p < 0.001$ vs. normal. * $p < 0.05$, ** $p < 0.01$, and *** $p < 0.001$ vs. PM10D control (CTL).

3.4. Effect of LM Extract on Lung Histopathology

To investigate the activities of LM extract in the histopathological analysis of PM10D-induced airway inflammation, the lungs were stained using Masson's trichrome or H and E. Thickening of the airway wall, inflammatory cell infiltration around the airway, and collagen fibrosis were observed in the lung sections of the PM10D-treated group, and this airway inflammation was reduced in the mice treated with dexamethasone or LM extract (Figure 5A,B). These results indicate that LM extract prevented the histopathological changes in airway inflammation in the lungs of PM10D-treated mice.

3.5. Effects of LM Extract on the Expression of Inflammatory Mediators in the Lungs

To examine the effects of LM extract on airway inflammation, the mRNA expression levels of inflammation-related genes were investigated in the lung tissue. Figure 6 shows that mRNA expression of CXCL1, transient receptor potential (TRP) vanilloid 1 (TRPV1), TRP ankyrin 1 (TRPA1), MIP-2, TNF-α, and mucin 5AC (MUC5AC) was elevated in the lung tissues from the group treated only with PM10D compared with the standard (healthy normal control) group and was significantly suppressed by the administration of dexamethasone or LM extract. This effect on the mRNA expression was dose-dependent and the high dose of LM exerted almost the same effect as dexamethasone.

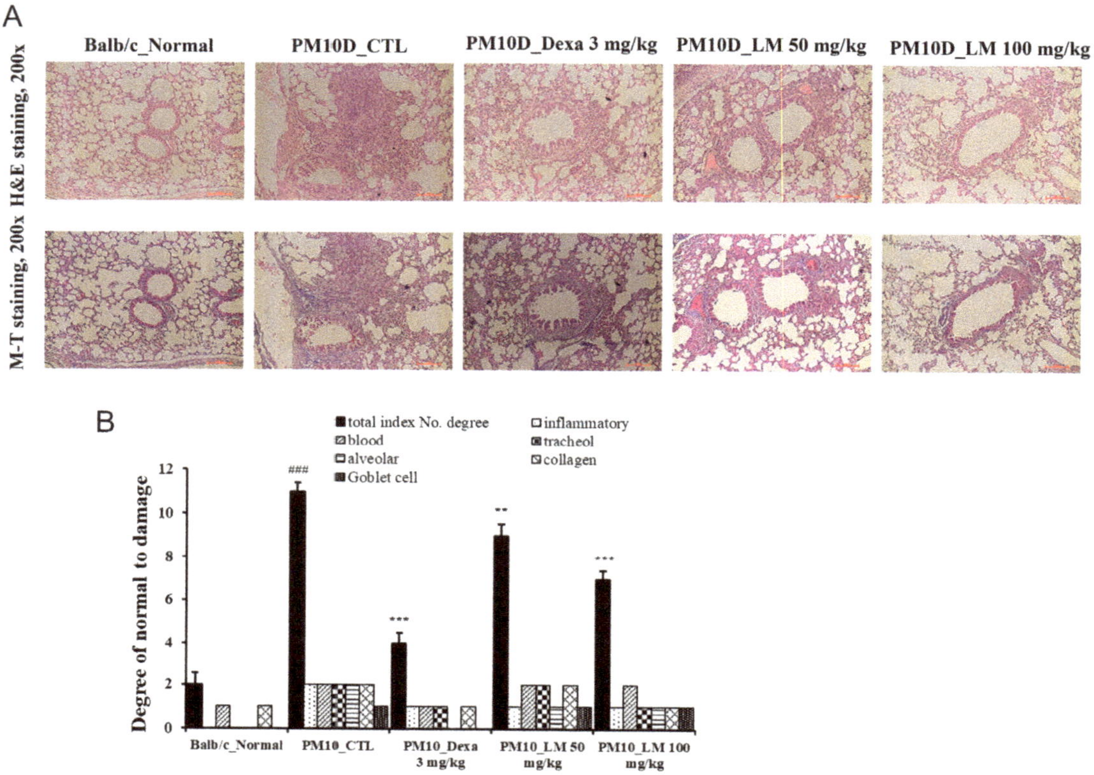

Figure 5. Effect of *Lysimachia mauritiana* extract on lung histopathology. (**A**) Hematoxylin and eosin (H and E) staining and Masson's trichrome (MT) staining of the lung tissue of mice with airway inflammation induced by particulate matter with a diameter less than 10 μm plus diesel exhaust particles (PM10D) (magnification: 200×) (n = 6). (**B**) Histopathological cell damage. ### $p < 0.001$ vs. normal., ** $p < 0.01$ and *** $p < 0.001$ vs. PM10D control (CTL).

3.6. Effects of LM Extract on Immune Cell Numbers in the BALF and Lungs

The effect of LM extract on the change in immune cell numbers was investigated through flow cytometry analysis of the BALF and lungs. The numbers of neutrophils in the BALF and lungs were elevated following exposure to PM10D and were reduced following the administration of LM extract (50 or 100 mg/kg) (Table 2). The absolute number of CD4+, CD8+, and CD62L−/CD44high+-activated T lymphocytes and Gr-1+SiglecF− cells in the BALF increased following PM10D exposure and decreased following the administration of dexamethasone or LM extract (50 or 100 mg/kg). In addition, the absolute numbers of CD62L−/CD44high+ T cells, Gr-1+SiglecF− neutrophils, CD21+/CD35+ B220+ B cells, and Gr-1+CD11b+ myeloid cells in the lungs were elevated by PM10D exposure and decreased following the administration of dexamethasone or LM extract (50 or 100 mg/kg). These results indicate that LM extract ameliorated the neutrophil-dependent airway inflammation caused by exposure to PM10D.

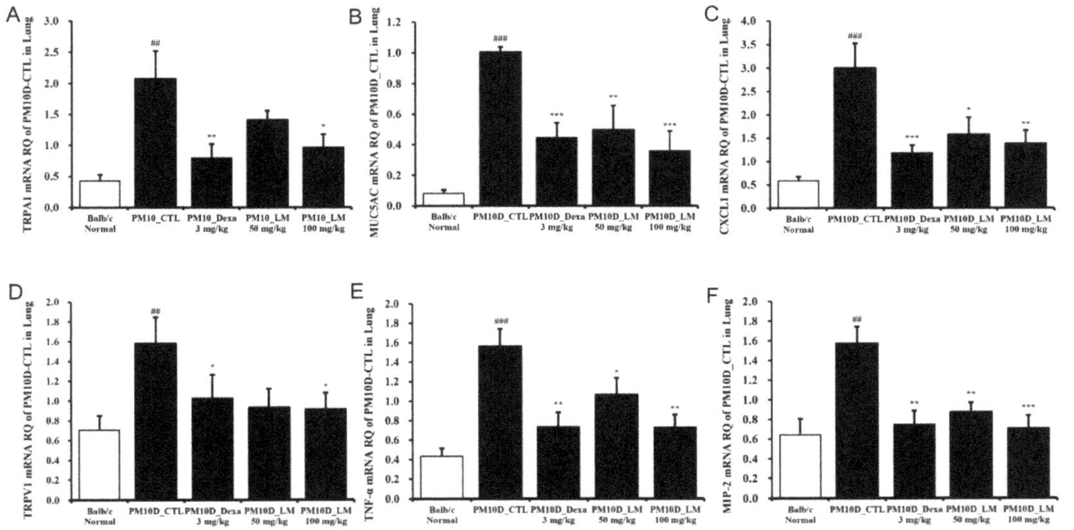

Figure 6. Effect of *Lysimachia mauritiana* extract on the mRNA expression of airway inflammation–related genes in the lung tissue of mice with airway inflammation induced by particulate matter with a diameter less than 10 μm plus diesel exhaust particles (PM10D). mRNA expression levels of (**A**) TRPA1, (**B**) MUC5AC, (**C**) CXCL1, (**D**) TRPV1, (**E**) TNF-α, and (**F**) MIP-2 (n = 6). ## $p < 0.01$ and ### $p < 0.001$ vs. normal. * $p < 0.05$, ** $p < 0.01$, and *** $p < 0.001$ vs. PM10D control (CTL).

Table 2. The effects of LM extract on airway immune cell numbers and neutrophilic airway inflammation in PM10D-induced inflammation model; fluorescence-activated cell sorting (FACS) analysis.

Cell Types	Absolute No. (Mean ± Standard Error of the Mean)				
	Balb/c Normal	PM10D-CTL	PM10D-Dexa 3 mg/kg	PM10D-LM 50 mg/kg	PM10D-LM 100 mg/kg
BALF					
Lymphocytes ($\times 10^4$ cells)	2.73 ± 0.68	7.45 ± 1.76 #	4.20 ± 1.02	4.46 ± 0.35	3.06 ± 0.26 *
Neutrophils ($\times 10^4$ cells)	5.41 ± 1.14	53.09 ± 6.44 ###	21.19 ± 5.56 **	26.32 ± 6.81 **	9.98 ± 2.49 ***
Eosinophils ($\times 10^4$ cells)	11.74 ± 3.89	48.90 ± 12.93 ##	44.74 ± 16.68	34.26 ± 10.56	27.26 ± 3.56
$CD4^+$ ($\times 10^4$ cells)	0.55 ± 0.25	31.56 ± 8.11 ##	10.51 ± 2.32 **	14.63 ± 3.60	6.85 ± 0.61 **
$CD8^+$ ($\times 10^4$ cells)	0.10 ± 0.06	17.01 ± 2.15 ###	3.98 ± 1.01 ***	6.92 ± 1.47 **	5.23 ± 2.68 **
$CD62L^-/CD44^{high+}$($\times 10^4$cells)	1.64 ± 0.39	89.75 ± 15.92 ###	55.28 ± 15.35	44.74 ± 11.58	25.01 ± 2.27 ***
$Gr\text{-}1^+SiglecF^-$ ($\times 10^4$ cells)	1.09 ± 0.53	53.18 ± 9.61 ###	14.35 ± 4.32 **	25.72 ± 6.35 *	6.91 ± 2.42 ***
Lung					
Lymphocytes ($\times 10^4$ cells)	14.46 ± 1.96	24.06 ± 4.26 #	33.31 ± 2.46	21.02 ± 4.11	21.75 ± 0.65
Neutrophils ($\times 10^4$ cells)	24.15 ± 5.70	81.34 ± 17.00 ##	50.86 ± 2.19	47.85 ± 6.31	42.20 ± 5.42 *
Eosinophils ($\times 10^4$ cells)	5.96 ± 0.73	12.20 ± 2.48 #	12.53 ± 0.55	9.37 ± 0.37	12.10 ± 0.99
$CD4^+$ ($\times 10^4$ cells)	15.94 ± 3.51	34.79 ± 5.47 ##	33.93 ± 1.28	31.43 ± 4.08	31.49 ± 2.09
$CD8^+$ ($\times 10^4$ cells)	6.68 ± 1.49	21.77 ± 4.24 ##	17.45 ± 0.79	13.71 ± 2.12	12.80 ± 1.41 *
$CD4^+CD69^+$ ($\times 10^4$ cells)	1.38 ± 0.44	4.06 ± 0.67 ##	2.41 ± 0.34 *	3.54 ± 0.47	2.56 ± 0.42
$CD62L^-/CD44^{high+}$($\times 10^4$ cells)	3.88 ± 0.76	17.88 ± 1.47 ###	9.00 ± 1.01 ***	11.62 ± 3.24	10.03 ± 2.06 **
$CD21^+/CD35^+B220^+$ ($\times 10^4$ cells)	4.33 ± 2.15	21.08 ± 4.84 ##	8.09 ± 2.14 *	9.99 ± 1.05 *	6.59 ± 0.16 **
$Gr\text{-}1^+SiglecF^-$ ($\times 10^4$ cells)	9.49 ± 2.76	41.83 ± 3.15 ###	19.26 ± 2.26 ***	25.51 ± 2.61 **	17.64 ± 3.23 ***
$Gr\text{-}1^+CD11b^+$ ($\times 10^4$ cells)	15.58 ± 3.13	56.92 ± 7.92 ###	28.78 ± 2.15 **	33.84 ± 5.44 *	25.32 ± 4.35 **

Abbreviations: CTL, control; Dexa, dexamethasone. The data are presented as means ± SEM (n = 8). # $p < 0.05$, ## $p < 0.01$, ### $p < 0.001$ versus the Normal group, and * $p < 0.05$, ** $p < 0.01$, *** $p < 0.001$ versus the CTL group, as determined by analyses of variance (ANOVA) followed by Duncan's multiple range tests.

3.7. Effects of LM Extract on the MAPK/NF-κB Pathway

To identify the potential pathways responsible for regulating the inhibitory effects of LM extract on the airway inflammatory responses in PM10D-induced mice, we analyzed the MAPK/NF-κB pathway in the lungs (Figure 7, Supplementary Figure S1). Dexamethasone as a positive control is a glucocorticoid that is available and is used for the treatment of various inflammatory conditions. The phosphorylation of p38, ERK, and JNK was elevated by PM10D exposure and suppressed to the normal (negative control) level by dexamethasone or LM extract (100 mg/kg) administration. The low dose of LM decreased the p-p38 level significantly, but this effect was less potent than that observed by the high dose. This effect on the phosphorylation of p38, ERK, and JNK was dose-dependent and the high dose of LM exerted almost the same effect as dexamethasone. NF-κB–p65 phosphorylation was also increased by PM10D exposure and decreased to the normal (negative control) level following the administration of dexamethasone or LM extract (50 and 100 mg/kg). The protective effects of LM were similar to those of dexamethasone. These results demonstrate that the inhibitory effects of LM extract on airway inflammation are due to the suppression of phosphorylation of p38, ERK, JNK, and NF-κB in the MAPK/NF-κB signaling pathway.

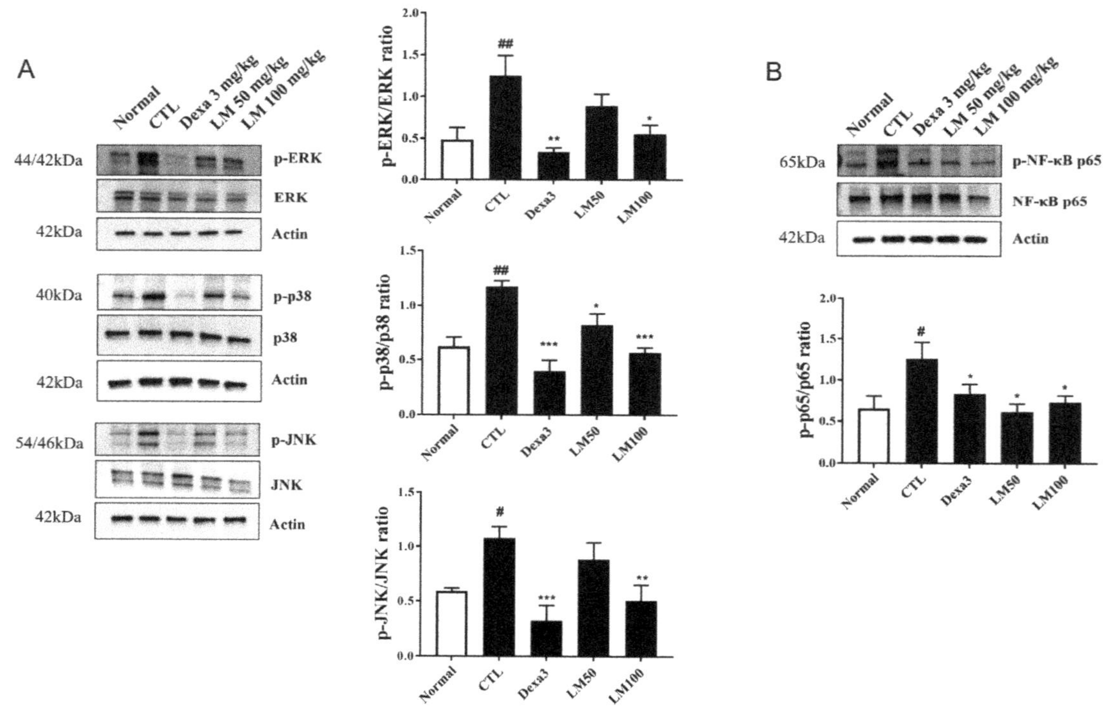

Figure 7. Effect of *Lysimachia mauritiana* extract on mitogen-activated protein kinase (MAPK)/nuclear factor-kappa B (NF-κB) signaling induced by particulate matter with a diameter less than 10 μm plus diesel exhaust particles (PM10D) in the lung tissue of mice with PM10D-induced airway inflammation. (**A**) Protein expression of phospho-ERK, ERK, phospho-p38, p38, phospho-JNK, JNK, phospho-p65, p65, and β-actin. (**B**) Quantitative analysis of each protein band using ImageJ (n = 3). # $p < 0.05$ and ## $p < 0.01$vs. normal. * $p < 0.05$, ** $p < 0.01$, and *** $p < 0.001$ vs. PM10D control (CTL).

3.8. Expectorant Effect of LM Extract According to Phenol Red Secretion

To evaluate the effect of LM extract on expectoration, the sputum excretion content in the trachea was measured using the phenol red secretion method in ICR mice. Since phenol red is a carcinogen that can cause toxicity, the ICR mouse model, a model commonly used in toxicity studies, was used. Oral administration of 200 mg of Levosol/kg (the positive control) and 100 mg of LM extract/kg significantly increased phenol red release compared with the control (1.37-fold and 1.57-fold, respectively) (Figure 8). These results illustrate the expectorant activity of LM extract.

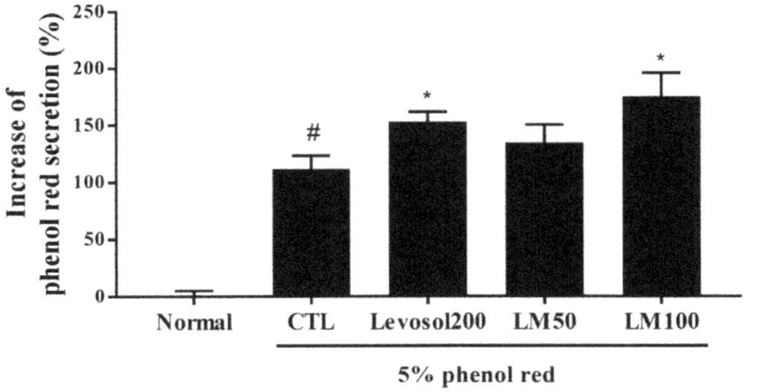

Figure 8. Effect of *Lysimachia mauritiana* extract on phenol red secretion in ICR mice. The amount of phenol red secretion in the airways was measured by injecting 5% phenol red into mice treated with Levosol (positive control) or LM extract for 3 days. N = 12/group. # $p < 0.05$ vs. normal, and * $p < 0.05$ vs. control.

4. Discussion

Airway inflammation, characterized by the mobilization and activation of immune cells (mainly neutrophils) and the immoderate production of molecular mediators, is considered a primary component of the pathogenesis of lung parenchymal destruction (emphysema) and airway remodeling (chronic bronchitis) in respiratory disorders such as chronic obstructive pulmonary disease (COPD) [17]. Neutrophils must be inhibited in inflamed airways to allow individuals to recover from lung damage in chronic respiratory disease [18].

Some pathological features similar to COPD were reproduced in PM10D-exposed experimental mice, including the agglutination and penetration of immune cells, the stenosis of the small airway, airway wall thickening, and pulmonary collagen fibrosis [19–21]. However, the histopathological changes in the lungs improved in the groups that received LM extract compared with the PM10D control group. The differential immune cell counts demonstrated that the BALF of normal mice had few neutrophils, eosinophils, and lymphocytes and that PM10D exposure obviously changed this cell composition. The numbers of eosinophils, lymphocytes, and, predominantly, neutrophils were increased in PM10D-exposed control mice. Furthermore, the infiltration and persistent recruitment of neutrophils were induced in the lung tissues, a typical feature of COPD. Compared with the PM10D controls, the elevated number of neutrophils and the increased expression of inflammatory cytokines (such as IL-1α, IL-17, MIP-2, CXCL1, and TNF-α) in the lungs and BALF were obviously lower in the LM groups, markedly reducing neutrophilic inflammation.

Previous studies have indicated that PM-induced respiratory inflammation mainly relates to small airway disease, lung parenchyma, and chronic bronchitis and is characterized by the recruitment and persistence of immune cells, predominantly neutrophils [22,23]. Neutrophils contribute to airway remodeling by producing proinflammatory cytokines containing TNF-α and IL-1 [24]. The functions of neutrophils and proinflammatory mediators in the pathophysiology of airway inflammatory disease are well known. TNF-α is a major neutrophil chemoattractant and multifunctional proinflammatory cytokine [25]. IL-1α stimulates the migration of neutrophils by inducing CXCL1, a key chemoattractant of neutrophils [26]. Studies have shown that IL-17(A) and TNF-α increase endothelial expression of the neutrophilic chemokines CXCL2 (MIP-2), CXCL1, and CXCL5 and enhance the influx of neutrophils to inflammation sites [27,28]. In this study, the increased expression levels of TRPA1, TRPV1, and MUC5AC in the lungs of PM10D-exposed control mice were inhibited by the administration of LM extract. The TRP receptor proteins (e.g., TRPV1 and TRPA1), which are irritant-sensing ion channels expressed in airway chemosensory nerves, are related to leukocyte infiltration in the airway, cytokine production, and cough response [29,30]. MUC5AC mucin is a main constituent of airway mucus, and mucus hypersecretion is a pathological feature of airway diseases [31]. Thus, the decrease in TRPA1, TRPV1, and MUC5AC in the lungs following the administration of LM extract should improve respiratory disease symptoms, such as cough and mucus production, in mice.

In the present study, we determined the mechanism responsible for these effects of LM. We investigated the activation of the MAPK/NF-κB signaling pathway in the lungs of PM10D-exposed mice and found that the increased ERK/p-38/JNK MAPK and NF-κB signals were suppressed by the administration of LM extract. These pathways are responsible for regulating the production of inflammatory mediators and the consequential neutrophilic infiltration and activation in chronic pulmonary disease [32]. Therefore, our results suggest that the reduction in neutrophilic airway inflammation following the administration of LM extract may be majorly attributed to the suppression of the MAPK/NF-κB signaling pathway.

According to the UPLC-QTof MS analysis, kaempferol 3-O-(2,6-di-O-α-rhamnopyranosyl)-β-galactopyranoside, also termed mauritianin, was the main flavonoid glycoside found in LM. From the whole plant of LM, mauritianin was isolated together with kaempferol-3-O-α-rhamnopyranosyl-(1–2)-β-galactopyranoside, kaempferol-3-O-robinobioside, and hyperin [7]. Mauritianin is a flavonoid that is rare in plants. As previously reported, mauritianin showed cytoprotective, antioxidant, neuroprotective, and antitumor-promoting activities [33–35]. However, mauritianin has not yet been reported to have effects against airway inflammation or related pulmonary diseases. Previous phytochemical investigations showed that *Lysimachia* species contain triterpenoid saponins and flavonoids [36]. Saponins in plants are important natural anti-inflammatory compounds that act on the activity of several proinflammatory cytokines in various inflammatory models [37]. These findings suggest that these compounds from LM could be potential anti-inflammatory agents for the protection of respiratory diseases. To our knowledge, this is the first study to demonstrate that LM exhibits an anti-inflammatory effect against inflammation-induced respiratory disease. Further investigation into the effects of other compounds with mauritianin from LM on airway inflammation is therefore required.

5. Conclusions

LM extract ameliorated neutrophilic airway inflammation via the suppression of the MAPK/NF-κB signaling pathway in mice with PM10D-induced respiratory inflammation. The results of our study suggest that LM may be an effective candidate for the prevention/treatment of respiratory disease.

Supplementary Materials: The following supporting information can be downloaded at: https://www.mdpi.com/article/10.3390/nu16213732/s1, Figure S1: Original Western blot result of lung tissue.

Author Contributions: Conceptualization, Y.-Y.S. and D.-S.K.; methodology, Y.-Y.S. and S.-H.K.; validation, H.J.Y.; investigation, Y.-Y.S., S.-H.K., W.-K.Y. and M.-S.K.; resources, D.-S.K.; data curation, Y.-Y.S.; writing—original draft preparation, Y.-Y.S.; writing—review and editing, Y.-Y.S.; visualization, S.-H.K.; supervision, Y.-Y.S.; funding acquisition, Y.-Y.S. and D.-S.K. All authors have read and agreed to the published version of the manuscript.

Funding: This research was funded by the KIOM of the Republic of Korea (grant numbers KSN1824311 and KSN23214313).

Institutional Review Board Statement: The animal study protocol was approved by the Committee for Animal Welfare of Daejeon University (protocol code DJUARB2022-041, data of approval 2

September 2022) and by the Animal Ethics Committee of the Korea Institute of Oriental Medicine (protocol code 23-054, data of approval 25 May 2023) for studies involving animals.

Informed Consent Statement: Not applicable.

Data Availability Statement: The data used to support the findings of this study are included within this article.

Conflicts of Interest: The authors declare no conflicts of interest.

References

1. Shah, A.S.; Langrish, J.P.; Nair, H.; McAllister, D.A.; Hunter, A.L.; Donaldson, K.; Newby, D.E.; Mills, N.L. Global association of air pollution and heart failure: A systematic review and meta-analysis. *Lancet* **2013**, *382*, 1039–1048. [CrossRef] [PubMed]
2. Kim, K.H.; Kabir, E.; Kabir, S. A review on the human health impact of airborne particulate matter. *Environ. Int.* **2015**, *74*, 136–143. [CrossRef]
3. Park, E.; Kim, B.Y.; Lee, S.; Son, K.H.; Bang, J.; Hong, S.H.; Lee, J.W.; Uhm, K.O.; Kwak, H.J.; Lim, H.J. Diesel exhaust particle exposure exacerbates ciliary and epithelial barrier dysfunction in the multiciliated bronchial epithelium models. *Ecotoxicol. Environ. Saf.* **2024**, *273*, 116090. [CrossRef] [PubMed]
4. Saba, E.; Lee, Y.S.; Yang, W.K.; Lee, Y.Y.; Kim, M.; Woo, S.M.; Kim, K.; Kwon, Y.S.; Kim, T.H.; Kwak, D.; et al. Effects of a herbal formulation, KGC3P, and its individual component, nepetin, on coal fly dust-induced airway inflammation. *Sci. Rep.* **2020**, *10*, 14036. [CrossRef] [PubMed]
5. Lee, Y.; Yun, N.; Kang, J.S.; Choi, S.; Paik, J.H. The complete chloroplast genome of the medicinal plant *Lysimachia mauritiana* (Lamarck, 1792). *Mitochondrial DNA B Resour.* **2022**, *7*, 554–555. [CrossRef]
6. Roh, S.S.; Seo, B.I.; Park, J.H. A herbological study on the native plants of Dokdo island. *Korea J. Herbol.* **2012**, *27*, 17–24. [CrossRef]
7. Yasukawa, K.; Takido, M. A flavonol glycoside from *Lysimachia mauritiana*. *Phytochemistry* **1987**, *26*, 1224–1226. [CrossRef]
8. Bae, S.; Song, Y.J. Inhibition of varicella-zoster virus replication by an ethanol extract of *Lysimachia mauritiana*. *Mol. Med. Rep.* **2017**, *15*, 3847–3851. [CrossRef]
9. Jin, S.E.; Kim, J.E.; Kim, S.Y.; Park, B.J.; Song, A.J. An ethanol extract of *Lysimachia mauritiana* exhibits inhibitory activity against hepatitis E virus genotype 3 replication. *J. Microbiol.* **2017**, *55*, 984–988. [CrossRef]
10. Pal, D. *Anti-Viral Metabolites from Medicinal Plants (Reference Series in Phytochemistry)*, 1st ed.; Springer International Publishing AG: New York, NY, USA, 2023; p. 666.
11. Jwon, H.S. An amazing herbal medicine with the efficacy of oriental medicine. In *Iksaeng Yaksul Daejeon*, 1st ed.; Academic Editing Center: Seoul, Republic of Korea, 2012; p. 97.
12. Herbal Medicine Research Society. *Herbal Medicine Encyclopedia*; Baekman Munhwasa: Seoul, Republic of Korea, 2020.
13. Sung, Y.Y.; Kim, M.; Yuk, H.J.; Kim, S.H.; Yang, W.K.; Park, G.D.; Kim, K.S.; Ham, W.J.; Kim, D.S. *Siraitia grosvenorii* extract attenuates airway inflammation in a mouse model of respiratory disease induced by particulate matter 10 plus diesel exhaust particle. *Nutrients* **2023**, *15*, 4140. [CrossRef]
14. Kim, M.S.; Kim, D.S.; Yuk, H.J.; Kim, S.H.; Yang, W.K.; Park, G.D.; Kim, K.S.; Ham, W.J.; Sung, Y.Y. *Siraitia grosvenorii* extract attenuates airway inflammation in a murine model of chronic obstructive pulmonary disease induced by cigarette smoke and lipopolysaccharide. *Nutrients* **2023**, *15*, 468. [CrossRef] [PubMed]
15. Jasper, A.E.; McIver, W.J.; Sapey, E.; Walton, G.M. Understanding the role of neutrophils in chronic inflammatory airway disease. *F1000Research* **2019**, *8*, F1000 Faculty Rev-557. [CrossRef]
16. Gandhi, V.D.; Vliagoftis, H. Secretion of inflammatory mediators containing cytokines and chemokines contribute to the pathology of airway inflammatory response. *Front. Immunol.* **2015**, *6*, 147.
17. Wei, K.; Zhang, X.; Yang, J.; Chen, J. Tobacco introduced *Perilla frutescens* and *Ocimum basilicum* genes attenuates neutrophilic inflammation in lung tissues of COPD rats. *Ecotoxicol. Environ. Saf.* **2024**, *271*, 115956. [CrossRef]
18. Keir, H.R.; Chalmers, J.D. Neutrophil extracellular traps in chronic lung disease: Implications for pathogenesis and therapy. *Eur. Respir. Rev.* **2022**, *31*, 210241. [CrossRef]
19. Lee, Y.S.; Yang, W.K.; Park, Y.R.; Park, Y.C.; Park, I.J.; Lee, G.J.; Kang, H.S.; Kim, B.K.; Kim, S.H. *Opuntia ficus-indica* alleviates particulate matter 10 plus diesel exhaust particles (PM10D)-induced airway inflammation by suppressing the expression of inflammatory cytokines and chemokines. *Plants* **2022**, *11*, 520. [CrossRef]
20. Lee, Y.S.; Park, G.S.; Ko, S.H.; Yang, W.K.; Seo, H.J.; Kim, S.H.; Jeong, N.; Kang, J. *Lactobacillus paracasei* ATG-E1 improves particulate matter 10 plus diesel exhaust particles (PM10D)-induced airway inflammation by regulating immune responses. *Front. Microbiol.* **2023**, *14*, 1145546. [CrossRef] [PubMed]
21. Jung, S.H.; Chung, K.S.; Na, C.S.; Ahn, H.S.; Shin, Y.K.; Lee, K.T. Ethanol extracts from the aerial parts of *Inula japonica* and *Potentilla chinensis* alleviate airway inflammation in mice that inhaled particulate matter 10 and diesel particulate matter. *Nutrients* **2023**, *15*, 4599. [CrossRef]
22. Ling, S.H.; Eeden, S.F.V. Particulate matter air pollution exposure: Role in the development and exacerbation of chronic obstructive pulmonary disease. *Int. J. Chron. Obstruct. Pulmon. Dis.* **2009**, *4*, 233–243. [CrossRef]

23. Parris, B.A.; O'Farrell, H.E.; Fong, K.M.; Yang, L.A. Chronic obstructive pulmonary disease (COPD) lung cancer: Common pathways for pathogenesis. *J. Thorac. Dis.* **2019**, *11*, S2155–S2172. [CrossRef]
24. Herrero-Cervera, A.; Soehnlein, O.; Kenne, E. Neutrophils in chronic inflammatory diseases. *Cell. Mol. Immunol.* **2022**, *19*, 177–191. [CrossRef] [PubMed]
25. Thomas, P. Tumour necrosis factor-a: The role of this multifunctional cytokine in asthma. *Immunol. Cell. Biol.* **2001**, *79*, 132–140. [CrossRef] [PubMed]
26. Lee, P.Y.; Kumagai, Y.; Xu, Y.; Li, Y.; Barker, T.; Liu, C.; Sobel, E.S.; Takeuchi, O.; Akira, S.; Satoh, M.; et al. IL-1α modulates neutrophil recruitment in chronic inflammation induced by hydrocarbon oil. *J. Immunol.* **2011**, *186*, 1747–1754. [CrossRef]
27. Griffin, G.K.; Newton, G.; Tarrio, M.L.; Bu, D.X.; Maganto-Garcia, E.; Azcutia, V.; Alcaide, P.; Grabie, N.; Luscinskas, F.W.; Croce, K.J.; et al. IL-17 and TNFα sustain neutrophil recruitment during inflammation through synergistic effects on endothelial activation. *J. Immunol.* **2012**, *188*, 6287–6299. [CrossRef]
28. Liu, Y.W.; Li, S.; Dai, S.S. Neutrophils in traumatic brain injury (TBI): Friend or foe? *J. Neuroinflamm.* **2018**, *15*, 146. [CrossRef] [PubMed]
29. Caceres, A.I.; Brackmann, M.; Elia, M.D.; Bessac, B.F.; del Camino, D.; D'Amours, M.; Witek, J.S.; Fanger, J.S.; Chong, J.A.; Hayward, N.J.; et al. A sensory neuronal ion channel essential for airway inflammation and hyperreactivity in asthma. *Proc. Natl. Acad. Sci. USA* **2009**, *106*, 9099–9104. [CrossRef]
30. Mukhopadhyay, I.; Kulkarni, A.; Khairatkar-Joshi, N. Blocking TRPA1 in respiratory disorders: Does it hold a promise? *Pharmaceuticals* **2016**, *9*, 70. [CrossRef]
31. Ou-Yang, H.F.; Wu, C.G.; Qu, S.Y.; Li, Z.K. Notch signaling downregulates MUC5AC expression in airway epithelial cells through Hes1-dependent mechanisms. *Respiration* **2013**, *86*, 341–346. [CrossRef]
32. Kojima, K.; Asai, K.; Kubo, H.; Sugitani, A.; Kyomoto, Y.; Okamoto, A.; Yamada, K.; Ijiri, N.; Watanabe, T.; Hirata, K.; et al. Isoflavone aglycones attenuate cigarette smoke-induced emphysema via suppression of neutrophilic inflammation in a COPD murine model. *Nutrients* **2019**, *11*, 2023. [CrossRef]
33. Krasteva, I.; Bratkov, V.; Bucar, F.; Kunert, O.; Kollroser, M.; Kondeva-Burdina, M.; Ionkova, I. Flavoalkaloids and Flavonoids from Astragalus monspessulanus. *J. Nat. Prod.* **2015**, *78*, 2565–2571. [CrossRef]
34. Yasukawa, K.; Takido, M.; Takeuchi, M.; Sato, Y.; Nitta, K.; Nakagawa, S. Inhibitory effects of flavonol glycosides on 12-O-tetradecanoylphorbol-13-acetate-induced tumor promotion. *Chem. Pharm. Bull.* **1990**, *38*, 774–776. [CrossRef] [PubMed]
35. Kicel, A.; Wolbiś, M. Study on the phenolic constituents of the flowers and leaves of *Trifolium repens* L. *Nat. Prod. Res.* **2012**, *26*, 2050–2054. [CrossRef] [PubMed]
36. Podolak, I.; Koczurkiewicz, P.; Galanty, A.; Michalik, M. Cytotoxic triterpene saponins from the underground parts of six *Lysimachia* L. species. *Biochem. Syst. Ecol.* **2013**, *47*, 116–120. [CrossRef]
37. Passos, F.R.S.; Araújo-Filho, H.G.; Monteiro, B.S.; Shanmugam, S.; Araújo, A.A.S.; Almeida, J.R.G.D.S.; Thangaraj, P.; Júnior, L.J.Q.; Quintans, J.S.S. Anti-inflammatory and modulatory effects of steroidal saponins and sapogenins on cytokines: A review of pre-clinical research. *Phytomedicine* **2022**, *96*, 153842. [CrossRef]

nutrients

MDPI

Article

Network Pharmacology Combined with Experimental Validation to Investigate the Mechanism of the Anti-Hyperuricemia Action of *Portulaca oleracea* Extract

Yiming Zhang [1,†], Shengying Zhu [1,†], Yueming Gu [1], Yanjing Feng [1] and Bo Gao [1,2,*]

[1] School of Life Sciences, Jilin University, Changchun 130012, China; yimingz21@mails.jlu.edu.cn (Y.Z.); zhusy22@mails.jlu.edu.cn (S.Z.); guym22@mails.jlu.edu.cn (Y.G.); fengyj23@mails.jlu.edu.cn (Y.F.)

[2] Key Laboratory for Molecular Enzymology and Engineering, Jilin University, Ministry of Education, Changchun 130012, China

[*] Correspondence: gaobo@jlu.edu.cn; Tel.: +86-131-3443-5290

[†] These authors contributed equally to this work.

Abstract: Background/Objectives: Hyperuricemia (HUA) is a common metabolic disease caused by purine metabolic disorders in the body. *Portulaca oleracea* L. (PO) is an edible wild vegetable. Methods: In this study, the regulatory effect of PO on HUA and its potential mechanism were initially elucidated through network pharmacology and experimental validation. Results: The results showed that PO from Sichuan province was superior to the plant collected from other habitats in inhibiting xanthine oxidase (XOD) activity. Berberine and stachydrine were isolated and identified from PO for the first time by UPLC-Q-Exactive Orbitrap MS. The potential molecular targets and related signaling pathways were predicted by network pharmacology and molecular docking techniques. Molecular docking showed that berberine had strong docking activity with XOD, and the results of in vitro experiments verified this prediction. Through experimental analysis of HUA mice, we found that PO can reduce the production of uric acid (UA) in the organism by inhibiting XOD activity. On the other hand, PO can reduce the body 's reabsorption of urate and aid in its excretion out of the body by inhibiting the urate transporter proteins (GLUT9, URAT1) and promoting the high expression of urate excretory protein (ABCG2). The results of H/E staining showed that, compared with the positive drug (allopurinol and benzbromarone) group, there was no obvious renal injury in the middle- and high-dose groups of PO extract. Conclusions: In summary, our findings reveal the potential of wild plant PO as a functional food for the treatment of hyperuricemia.

Keywords: hyperuricemia; *Portulaca oleracea*; xanthine oxidase; ABCG2; berberine

1. Introduction

With the improvement of modern living standards, people's dietary patterns have begun to develop towards high purines, and the number of patients with hyperuricemia (HUA) has, accordingly, also increased [1,2]. Many studies have shown that HUA is due to the disorder of the purine metabolism or the obstruction of UA excretion in the body, which eventually leads to a high concentration of UA in serum, which then evolves into a metabolic disease that endangers human health [3,4].

Uric acid (UA) is the end-product of a purine metabolism series in the body [5]. UA homeostasis is maintained by multiple organs in the body. After UA is formed, about 1/3 of it is excreted through the gastrointestinal tract and 2/3 is excreted through the kidney tissue [6]. Eventually, the remainder is reabsorbed into the bloodstream [7]. Researchers have found that with an increase of UA levels, urate crystals gradually formed in the tubules and interstitia of the kidneys, ultimately leading to pathological damage to kidney tissue [8,9]. Excessive accumulation of urate may trigger diseases such as gout, which seriously affects the daily lives of patients [10].

The main factor contributing to the cause of HUA is a dysfunction of urate transport in the kidneys or a blockage of the transport pathway. In renal tissues, urate transporter proteins include URAT1 (SLC22A12), OAT4 (SLC22A11), OAT10 (SLC22A13), and GLUT9 (SLC2A9). Excretory proteins include ABCG2, ABCC4, and NPT1 (SLC17A1). OAT1 (SLC22A6), OAT2 (SLC22A7), and OAT3 (SLC22A8) proteins, on the outside of the cellular basement membrane, are similarly involved in urate transport [11–15]. In addition, XOD, as a key enzyme in UA production, is often considered an important target in HUA studies [16]. Allopurinol, benzbromarone, and febuxostat, which are widely used in clinical practice, have been associated with serious adverse effects [17–20]. In contrast, natural drug preparations often have the advantages of multi-target regulation and low levels of side-effects, and have shown great potential in the field of HUA treatment in recent years [21–23].

Portulaca oleracea L. (PO) is an annual herb of Caryophyllaceae and Portulacaceae, with fleshy, branched, and light-red stems. It is distributed all over the world, mainly in temperate and tropical regions, and is distributed throughout many provinces in China. It is an edible wild plant [24]. People in many countries, such as Spain, Greece, Italy, Turkey, the United States, and China, cook it as a traditional dish. It is one of the famous medicinal and edible wild plants in China, one which is called the "longevity vegetable" in traditional folklore [25–28]. PO is rich in a variety of bioactive substances, including polysaccharides, alkaloids, unsaturated fatty acids, flavonoids, terpenoids, proteins, vitamins, and minerals [29,30]. In ancient Chinese traditional prescriptions, it has the functions of detoxification, detumescence, anti-inflammation, diuresis, and so on. In folk medicine, it is used to treat bloody diarrhea [28,31]. In recent years, studies have found that the extracts of PO have a wide range of pharmacological activities, including anti-inflammatory [32], anti-diabetic [33], anti-bacterial [34], anti-ulcer [35], anti-oxidation, and immunomodulatory effects [36]. However, there have not yet been any clinical reports demonstrating its efficacy in lowering UA.

Within the realm of traditional Chinese medicine, considerable emphasis is placed on authentic medicinal materials, denoting those cultivated in specific regions and possessing superior therapeutic efficacy and a more stable quality compared with the same herbs from other origins. Consequently, we meticulously chose four emblematic regions across China, varying in both longitude and latitude, specifically, Sichuan, Henan, Guangdong, and Jilin, to meticulously analyze and juxtapose the inhibitory prowess of PO against XOD, whilst theoretically forecasting PO's plausible targets in HUA treatment through the application of LC-MS technology, network pharmacology, and molecular docking. Finally, the pertinent mechanism was further elucidated by in vivo experiments.

2. Materials and Methods

2.1. Materials

The aerial parts of PO were harvested from four distinct locations: Mianyang City, Sichuan Province (104°44′ E, 31°53′ N); Luoyang City, Henan Province (112°4′ E, 34°20′ N); Guangzhou City, Guangdong Province (113°15′ E, 23°06′ N); and Changchun City, Jilin Province (125°42′ E, 31°53′ N). These specimens were meticulously identified by Professor Shuwen Guan of the College of Life Sciences, Jilin University.

XOD and xanthine (XA) were purchased from Shanghai Yuanye Bio-Technology Co., Ltd. (Shanghai, China). Methanol and formic acid were purchased from ThermoFisher, Waltham, MA, USA. Berberine (HPLC $\geq$ 98%) and stachydrine (HPLC $\geq$ 98%) were purchased from Aladdin Reagent Co., Ltd. (Shanghai, China). Yeast extract was purchased from Beijing Oberstar Biotechnology Co., Ltd. (Beijing, China). Allopurinol was purchased from Jiangsu World Trade Tianjie Pharmaceutical Co., Ltd. (Yancheng, China). Benzbromarone was purchased from Herman Pharma Kft. (Hungary, Germany). UA, XOD, blood urea nitrogen (BUN), and serum creatinine (SCr) kits were purchased from Nanjing Jiancheng Bioengineering Institute (Nanjing, China). The following primary antibodies were purchased from Proteintech Group, Inc. (Wuhan, China): ABCG2 (27286-1-AP,

1:1000), GLUT9 (26486-1-AP, 1:600), and URAT1 (14937-1-AP, 1:1500). The β-actin (GB15003, 1:2000) and horseradish peroxidase (HRP)-labeled anti-rabbit IgG (GB23303, 1:5000) were purchased from Wuhan Servicebio Technology Co., Ltd. (Wuhan, China).

2.2. Preparation of PO Extract

The aerial parts of freshly picked PO were dried and crushed, and then passed through a 60-mesh sieve. PO powder was mixed with distilled water at a ratio of 1:12 (w/v) and extracted at 60 °C for 3 h. During the extraction, PO water extract and water-extract residue were obtained by ultrasonic-assisted extraction and vacuum filtration. Then, ethanol was used to extract the water extraction-filter residue under the same conditions to obtain the ethanol extract. The water extract and the ethanol extract were then mixed and, following this, concentrated using a vacuum rotary evaporator, and the PO extract was obtained after vacuum drying. Subsequently, the extract was resuspended in ultrapure water for subsequent experiments.

2.3. XOD Inhibition-Ability Experiment

Based on the formation of UA catalyzed by XOD, a stable enzymatic reaction system was established [37]. Firstly, 0.08 U/mL XOD was added to the system containing substrate (1.5 mm xanthine, XA) and inhibitor (sample concentrations were 1000, 500, 400, 250, 200, and 100 μg/mL, respectively), and then the catalytic reaction was carried out at 37 °C for 30 min. Subsequently, the absorbance was measured by a spectrophotometer at 295 nm, and the XOD inhibition rate was calculated according to the following formula:

$$\text{XOD Inhibition rate } (\%) = \frac{(\text{A} - \text{B}) - (\text{C} - \text{D})}{\text{A} - \text{B}} \times 100\%$$

A: OD295 nm solution containing XA and XOD.
B: OD295 nm solution containing only XA.
C: OD295 nm solution containing inhibitors, XA, and XOD.
D: OD295 nm solution containing inhibitors and XA.

2.4. Compositional Analysis

PO extracts were identified by UPLC-Q-Exactive Orbitrap MS [38]. A sample of 0.15 g was weighed, and 1000 μL 80% methanol and grinding beads were added. Grinding proceeded for 5 min, and then the mixture was vortexed for 10 min. During the centrifugation at 4 °C for 10 min, the centrifugal force was 20,000× g. The supernatant was then filtered and injected for analysis.

An Ultimate AQ-C18 chromatographic column (150 × 2.1 mm, 1.8 μm, Welch Technology (SHANGHAI) Co., Ltd., Shanghai, China) was used in this study. The mobile phase A was composed of 0.1% (v/v) formic acid and water. The B phase was methanol. Gradient elution was performed under the following conditions: 98% A phase (0–1 min), 98–80% A phase (1–5 min), 80–50% A phase (5–10 min), 50–20% A phase (10–15 min), 20–5% A phase (15–20 min), 5% A phase (20–27 min), 5–98% A phase (27–28 min), and 98% A phase (28–30 min). The fixed flow rate was 0.30 mL/min, the temperature of the automatic sampler was 10.0 °C, the column temperature was 35 °C, and the injection volume was 5.00 μL. The mass spectrometer was equipped with a Q Exactive ESI source with a scan range of m/z 150–2000. The detection method selected was data-dependent tandem mass spectrometry (dd-MS2) for full-mass scanning. The resolution of the full-mass scanning was 70,000, and the resolution for the dd-MS2 was 17,500. The voltage of the ion jet needle was 3.2 kV (positive). The capillary temperature was 300 °C. The collision gas was high-purity argon (purity ≥ 99.999%). The sheath gas was nitrogen (purity ≥ 99.999%) 40 Arb; the auxiliary gas was nitrogen (purity ≥ 99.999%), 15 Arb; and the heater temperature was 350 °C. The data acquisition time was 30.0 min.

The analysis of berberine and stachydrine in the PO was based on the methods of Ren et al. [39] and Yan et al. [40]. Berberine (HPLC ≥ 98%) and stachydrine (HPLC ≥ 98%)

were dissolved in methanol and treated with ultrasound for 5 min to prepare a standard stock solution, with a concentration of 5 μg/mL, for subsequent analysis.

2.5. Identification of Candidate Targets of PO with Effects on HUA

The PO potential targets were predicted by the TCMSP database [41] (https://tcmsp-e.com/index.php/, accessed on 12 March 2024), Targetnet database [42], and SwissTargetPrediction [43] (http://www.swisstargetprediction.ch/, accessed on 12 March 2024). The above collected targets were merged and de-weighted using the UniProt database [44] (http://www.uniprot.org, accessed on 12 March 2024) and further standardized into official gene names for subsequent analysis. Employing "hyperuricemia" as the search term, disease-associated targets were explored within the CTD [45] (http://ctdbase.org/, accessed on 12 March 2024), OMIM [46] (https://omim.org/, accessed on 12 March 2024), and DisGeNET databases [47] (https://www.disgenet.org/, accessed on 12 March 2024), with the results subsequently being merged and de-duplicated to procure hyperuricemia-associated targets. Finally, the Venny2.1.0 online utility (https://bioinfogp.cnb.csic.es/tools/venny, accessed on 12 March 2024) was employed for visual examination of the intersecting elements between the disease-associated and PO targets. The members of the intersecting target ensemble were regarded as putative therapeutic targets for both PO and HUA.

2.6. Analysis of Protein—Protein Interaction Network

The collected intersecting targets were imported into the String database [48] (https://cn.string-db.org/, accessed on 12 March 2024), the free genes were removed, and confidence levels were selected to obtain a PPI network graph for PO treatment of HUA, in which the nodes represent the potential targets and the connecting lines represent their interactions. The nodes were saved and imported into Cytoscape 3.7.1 software [49] for visualization and analysis, and the importance of the nodes in the network was evaluated by using the degree value after the topological network analysis; the larger the value of the degree was, the greater was the relevance and the more effective the effect of the node in the network.

2.7. Construction of Gene Enrichment Analysis

The bioinformatics analysis platform DAVID database [50] (https://david.ncifcrf.gov/, accessed on 13 March 2024) was used to perform GO annotation of biological processes, cellular components, and molecular functions, in addition to KEGG pathway enrichment analysis of the above PO and HUA intersection targets. The obtained results were arranged in descending order according to their −lg(P) values, and the results were visualized and analyzed using the microbiology platform (https://www.bioinformatics.com.cn/login/, accessed on 13 March 2024) in order to explore the relevant mechanism of action of PO in treating HUA.

2.8. Molecular Docking Validation

The 3D structural information associated with the berberine molecule was downloaded using the PubChem database [51] (pubchem.ncbi.nlm.nih.gov/, accessed on 13 March 2024), and the XOD protein and its ligand complexes were obtained from the PDB protein structure database (htps://www.rcsb.org/, accessed on 13 March 2024); water molecules and ligands of target proteins were removed using PyMOL 2.5.7 software, the 3D structure of SDF was converted to PDB format, and the receptor and ligand were pre-processed using AutbDock Tools and then saved in PDBQT format for use. Finally, molecular docking of the ligand and receptor was performed using AutoDock 4.2.6 software [52]. It is generally accepted that when the docking score is less than −7.0, it indicates significant binding activity between the active ingredient and the target; less than −5.0 indicates good binding activity between the two; less than −4.25 indicates the presence of some binding activity [53].

2.9. Establishment of HUA Mouse Model

All experimental procedures involving animals adhered strictly to the guiding principles for animal care and use outlined by the Animal Experiment Ethics Committee of Jilin University (Changchun, China), in accordance with the regulations stipulated by the Committee for Animal Use and Care and the principles established in the Helsinki Declaration. SPF-grade male C57BL/6J mice, aged 4–6 weeks, weighing 20 ± 2 g, were purchased from Liaoning Changsheng Biotechnology Co., Ltd. (Shenyang, China), under license number SCXK (Liao) 2020-0001. The experimental animals were not genetically modified during the experiment. The mice were accommodated in the Jilin University Experimental Animal Platform, where they had unrestricted access to sterile water and food. The animals were maintained under controlled conditions of (22 ± 2) °C and 60% humidity, and subjected to a 12 h light/dark cycle. After 1 week of adaptive feeding, the mice were randomly divided into groups. The change in body weight of each mouse was recorded for subsequent equivalent dose conversion based on body weight.

Referring to the method of Dai et al. [54], the HUA mouse model was induced using gastric gavage with yeast paste. Except for the control group ($n = 8$), the mice received daily gastric gavage of yeast paste at a dosage of 20 g/kg. After 14 days of pretreatment, the mice were randomly divided into six groups as follows: the model group; the allopurinol group (7.6 mg/kg); the benzbromarone group (7.6 mg/kg); and low-, medium-, and high-dose PO groups (0.5, 1, and 2 g/kg, LPO, MPO, HPO, respectively) (n = 8 per group). Following this, daily gastric gavage with yeast paste was performed every morning to sustain clinical manifestations of HUA, followed by daily drug administration for 7 consecutive days in the afternoon. On the final day of treatment, mice were euthanized with carbon dioxide 2 h after administration. Blood samples were collected and centrifuged at 3000 rpm, 4 °C for 15 min to separate serum. The levels of UA, XOD, creatinine (SCr), and urea nitrogen (BUN) in serum were detected by detection kit. Following extraction, mice liver and kidney tissues were rinsed with physiological saline, air-dried, and weighed post-absorption of moisture; the left kidney tissues were fixed in 4% paraformaldehyde for histopathological examination, and the right kidney tissues were stored at −80 °C for subsequent analysis.

2.10. Western Blot Analysis

Kidney tissues were subjected to lysis utilizing RIPA buffer supplemented with protease inhibitors. Protein concentration was quantified employing the bicinchoninic acid (BCA) protein assay kit. Subsequently, proteins were fractionated via sodium dodecyl sulfate-polyacrylamide gel electrophoresis (SDS-PAGE) and subsequently transferred onto polyvinylidene difluoride (PVDF) membranes. Following blocking with 5% non-fat milk for 2 h, the membranes were then incubated overnight at 4 °C with antibodies targeting ABCG2, GLUT9, and URAT1. Subsequent to this, the membranes were exposed to secondary antibodies for a duration of 1.5 h. Lastly, the membranes underwent washing and imaging utilizing an enhanced chemiluminescence (ECL) detection kit. Band intensities were quantified utilizing Image J software (version 1.54).

2.11. H/E Staining and IHC Analysis

The kidney tissues, fixed and embedded, underwent precision slicing into 4 μm sections. Following meticulous deparaffinization employing a gradient of xylene and ethanol, the sections underwent staining with hematoxylin/eosin (H/E).

Upon deparaffinization, endogenous peroxidase activity was effectively inhibited using 3% hydrogen peroxide, and subsequent blocking of the sections was achieved with 3% BSA. Subsequently, the sections were incubated overnight at 4 °C with primary antibodies targeting ABCG2, GLUT9, and URAT1. Following this, the sections were subjected to a 1 h incubation at room temperature with secondary antibodies, followed by detection utilizing DAB chromogen and subsequent counterstaining with hematoxylin.

2.12. Statistical Analysis

The values are expressed as the mean ± SEM/SD in multigroup animal experiments. One-way ANOVA was used to analyze the significance of differences, and a value of $p < 0.05$ was considered statistically significant; highly significant differences were indicated at $p < 0.01$. All statistical analyses were performed using GraphPad Prism 8 software. IHC and Western Blot analyses were performed by Image J, and subsequently employed for densitometric analysis.

3. Results

3.1. In Vitro XOD Inhibition Experiment

Figure 1 demonstrates the inhibition effect of PO on XOD for the Sichuan, Henan, Guangdong, and Jilin samples; the degree of inhibition of XOD by PO extracts from different geographical regions and different concentrations was calculated based on the absorbance (OD) at 295 nm of the reaction systems of each group. The corresponding IC50 inhibition curves were plotted using GraphPad Prism 8. According to the enzyme inhibition rate curves, it can be seen that the PO extracts showed concentration dependence, and the best inhibition of XOD was achieved by the PO from Sichuan, with an IC50 value of 160 μg/mL; we therefore chose the PO from Sichuan for the subsequent experiments.

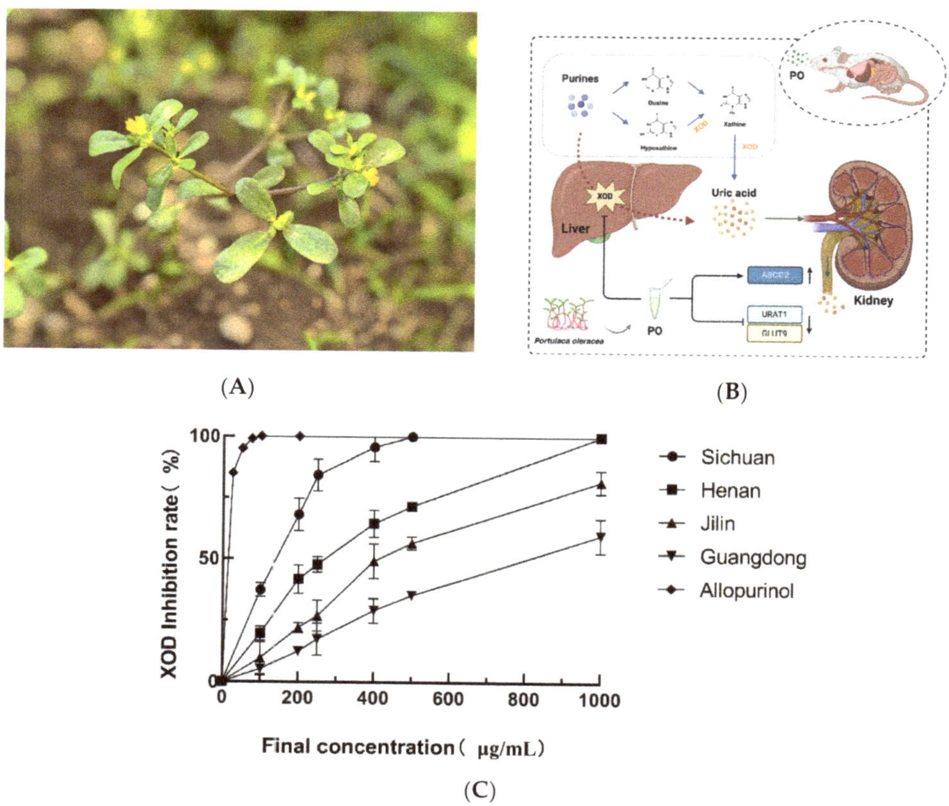

Figure 1. (**A**) Photograph of the aerial parts of *Portulaca Oleracea*. (**B**) Mechanism map of purine metabolism and uric acid excretion pathway (Created in bioRender). (**C**) Inhibitory effect of PO extracts from different producing areas on XOD, in vitro.

3.2. Analysis of PO Components from Sichuan

UPLC-Q-Orbitrap MS was used to characterize the major components in the PO extract in both positive and negative ion modes. The total ion chromatogram of PO is shown in Figure 2A. The compounds with the best matching score for mzCloud (above 90) in the possible molecular formula deduced from the high-resolution mass spectrometry information were selected and analyzed, in combination with data from the literature. Trigonelline, betaine, stachydrine, berberine, salsolinol, baicalin, tangeritin, nobiletin, curcumin, scopoletin, vanillin, lupeol, cafestol, oleanolic acid, salsolinol, and other components were screened. Among them, stachydrine and berberine were, for the first time, detected in PO, in the sample produced in Sichuan. Berberine has broad-spectrum antibacterial activity and can potentially be used as a drug for the treatment of various diseases [55]. Stachydrine is a multifunctional bioactive substance with great potential in the treatment of many diseases [56].

In order to verify the presence of stachydrine and berberine in PO samples more accurately, they were compared with the corresponding standards using the LC-MS technique. In Figure 2B,C, the retention times of the samples showed RT1 = 2.36 min and RT2 = 3.41 min, values which were consistent with the retention times of the standards, which were Rt = 2.37 and 3.41 min, respectively. Furthermore, in the MS2 spectra shown in Figure 2D,E, target compound 1 was found to produce ions at m/z 144.10 [M + H], m/z 84.24, m/z 58.33 and m/z 42.48, yielding fragment ions in agreement with the stachydrine standard comparison. Similarly, target compound 2 produced fragment ions at m/z 336.12 [M + H], m/z 320.17, and m/z 292.10, in agreement with the berberine standards. Eventually, the two compounds were identified as stachydrine and berberine.

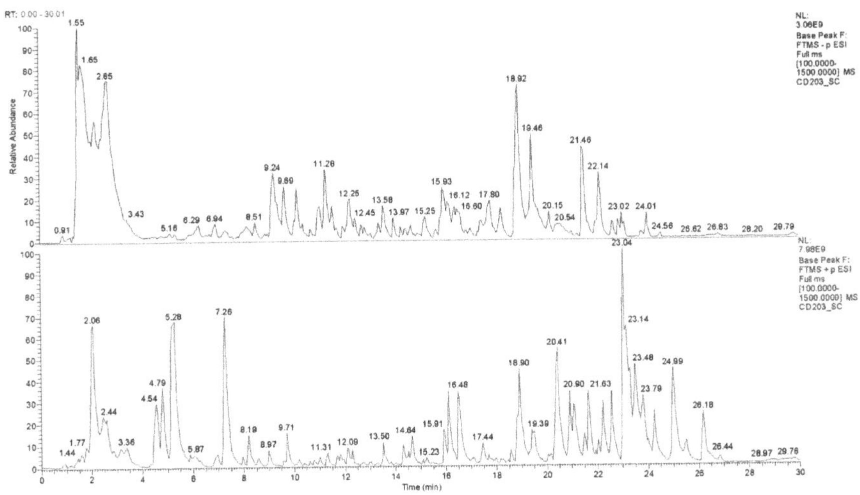

(A)

Figure 2. *Cont.*

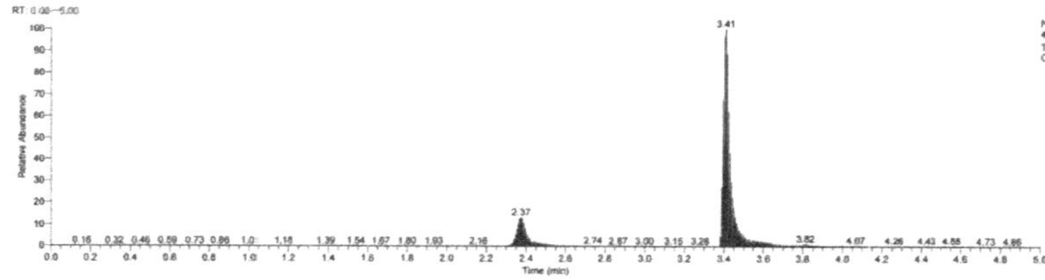

(B)

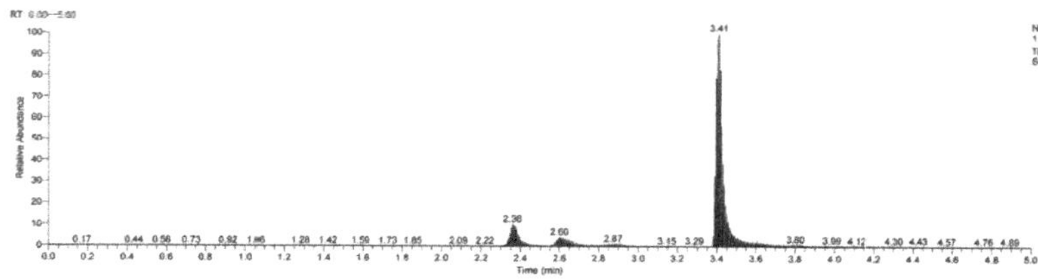

(C)

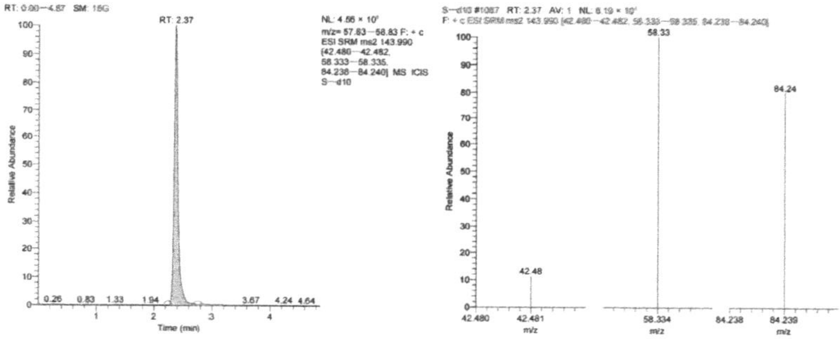

(D)

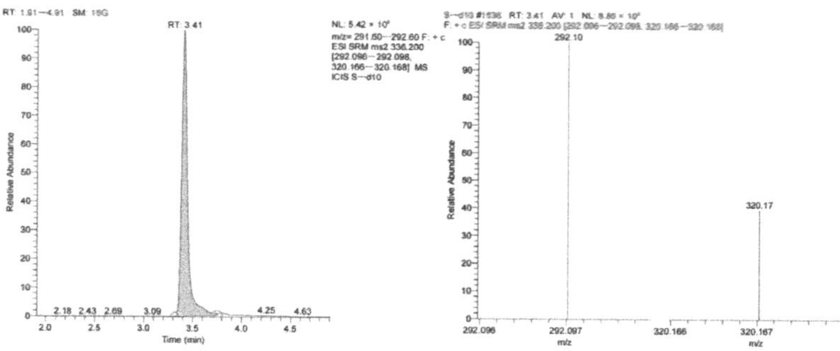

(E)

Figure 2. PO component analysis by UPLC-Q-Orbitrap MS. (**A**) Total ion chromatogram (TIC). (**B**) LC-MS chromatograms of the stachydrine (RT: 2.37) and berberine (RT: 3.41) standards. (**C**) LC-MS chromatograms of the stachydrine (RT: 2.36) and berberine (RT: 3.41) in the sample. (**D**) LC-MS chromatograms of the stachydrine ion channel (**left**) and MS2 spectra (**right**) for the separated sample. (**E**) Ion channel chromatogram (**left**) and MS2 spectra (**right**) of berberine in the separated sample.

3.3. Construction of the Component–Target–Disease Network and Analysis of the PPI Network

A total of 82 cross-targets were screened by the Venn intersection of PO component-related targets and HUA disease-related targets which had been identified as potential therapeutic targets for HUA (Figure 3A). The interactions between target proteins are shown in Figure 3B. The PPI network contained 82 nodes and 712 edges. After processing, a total of 15 key targets were obtained: ABCG2, PPARG, HMGCR, CASP3, PARP1, MCL1, BCL2, ESR1, TNF, ACE, SIRT1, ICAM1, REN, PTGS2, GCG. Through the analysis of these key targets, it was found that the XDH (XOD), ABCG2 protein and its associated SLC22A12 (URAT1) protein were closely related to urate transport, anion transport, small molecule transport, and purine-containing compound metabolism, which are common targets in HUA research. Therefore, we selected proteins such as ABCG2 and URAT1 for further study.

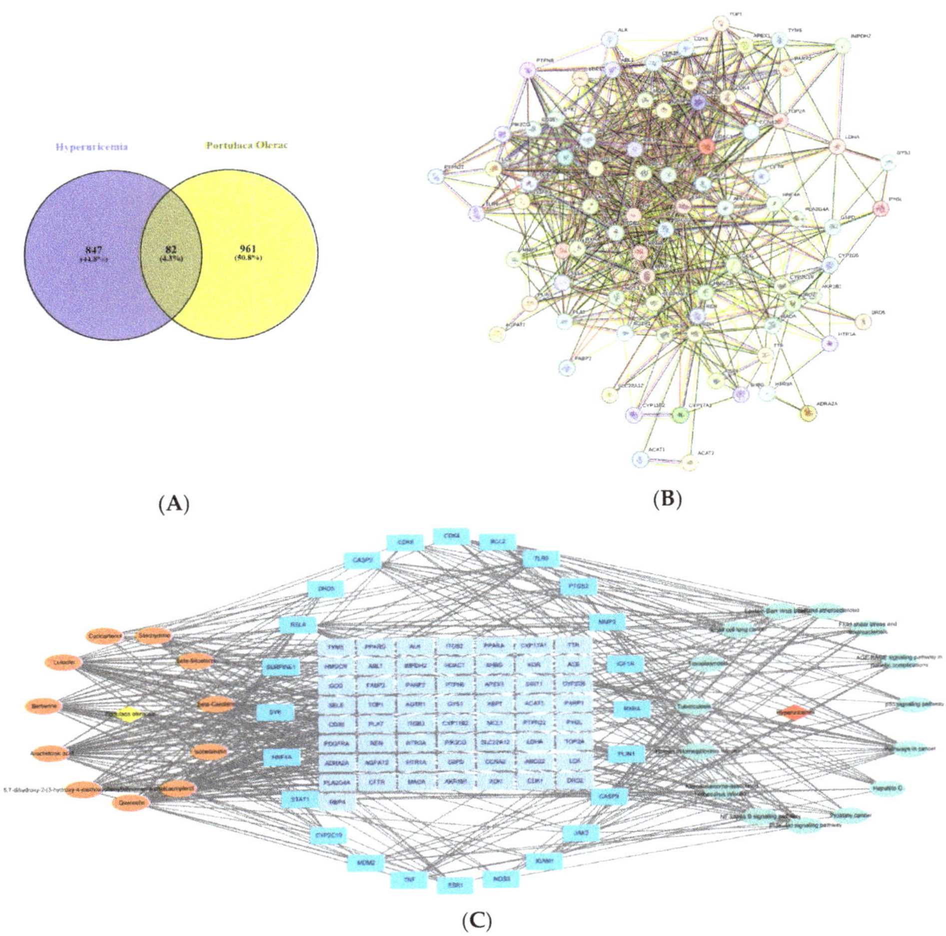

Figure 3. PPI network of PO active-compound targets. (**A**) Venn diagram of active compounds in PO and intersection targets in HUA. (**B**) Potential-target PPI network diagram. (**C**) Component–target–pathway network diagram for PO in the treatment of HUA.

The intricate network depicting the components, targets, and pathways influenced by PO in addressing HUA is visually represented in Figure 3C. The left side, depicted in orange, signifies the active constituents present in PO, while the right side, in green, delineates the pertinent signaling pathways identified through KEGG enrichment analysis. The intersecting targets of these components and pathways are depicted in blue. Subsequent topological analysis, facilitated by plugins, unveiled potential biological impacts of PO on HUA, targeting key elements like RELA, CASP9, BCL2, CASP3, CDK4, and TNF. These interactions are implicated in pivotal signaling cascades, encompassing the cancer, PI3K-Akt, p53, and NF-κB pathways, among others.

3.4. Enrichment Analysis of Related Pathways and the Biological Process

The comprehensive GO analysis resulted in the identification of a remarkable 1124 entries related to biological processes (BP), encompassing a diverse array of phenomena ranging from rhythmic processes to intricate hormonal regulatory mechanisms and responsive reactions to organic substances, among others (as illustrated in Figure 4A). Moreover, the analysis unveiled 46 distinct entries associated with cellular components (CC), spanning crucial entities like the cytoplasm, receptors, and extracellular regions. Additionally, it elucidated 97 entries pertaining to molecular functions (MF), exemplified by crucial interactions such as protein kinase binding, chromatin binding, and oxidoreductase activity, among others.

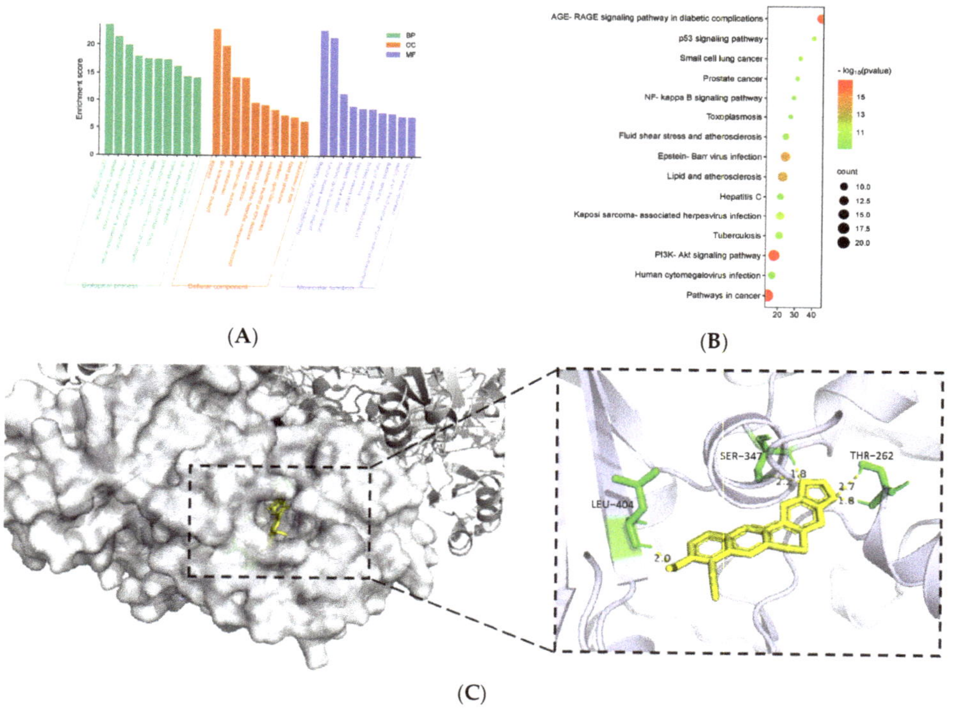

Figure 4. (**A**) GO function annotation. (**B**) KEGG pathway enrichment analysis. (**C**) Visualization of berberine and XOD molecular docking results. The white structure represents the ABCG2 protein, the yellow structure represents the active compound, and the green structure represents the binding site between the two. The value represents the binding affinity, and the unit is kcal/mol.

Subsequent enrichment analysis of KEGG pathways unveiled their intricate association with various critical signaling cascades, notably encompassing cancer-related pathways, the AGE-RAGE signaling pathway implicated in diabetic complications, the pivotal PI3K-Akt signaling cascade, the regulatory p53 signaling pathway, and the intricate NF-κB signaling pathway, among others (as depicted in Figure 4B).

3.5. Molecular Docking and Residue Interaction

With the aid of PyMOL software, the binding pocket of the berberine–XOD complex was visualized (Figure 4C), having a binding energy of approximately -10.00 kJ-mol^{-1}, in which amino acid residues located within approximately 4.0 Å (Å) of the berberine have been highlighted. After careful screening, we have targeted a series of key active site residues, including THR262, SER347, and LEU404, which are uniquely located and surrounded near the active center of molybdenum chalcogenide, and the results indicate that berberine has strong docking activity with XOD. The binding energy of stachydrine with XOD was about -3.51 kJ-mol^{-1}, which is a weak binding ability. Therefore, according to the experimental steps described in Section 2.3, the IC50 value of berberine was about 74 μg/mL, demonstrating a good inhibitory effect on XOD in vitro (Figure S1).

3.6. In Vivo Studies on the Reduction of Uric Acid

UA levels in serum samples from each group of mice were measured using the colorimetric method to compare the changes in serum-UA levels in mice after drug administration. After 14 days of modeling, compared with the control group, the serum UA in the model group was significantly increased ($^{###}$ $p < 0.001$), indicating that the model construction method used was effective and successful. The serum-UA levels of mice in different treatment groups showed a decreasing trend after gavage administration, among which the positive control group and the HPO group showed excellent UA-lowering efficacy (*** $p < 0.001$); no statistically significant difference was observed in the comparison between the groups (Figure 5A).

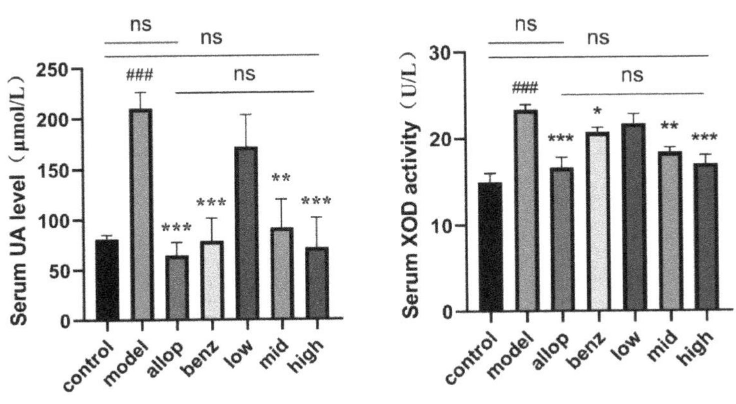

Figure 5. Serum levels of UA and XOD in mice after intragastric administration. (**A**) Serum uric acid level in mice after intragastric administration. (**B**) The level of XOD in serum of mice after intragastric administration. $^{###}$ $p < 0.001$ compared with the control group. * $p < 0.05$, ** $p < 0.01$, and *** $p < 0.001$, compared with the model group. ns (no significance).

Since the level of XOD activity is proportional to the rate of UA production, we measured the XOD activity in the serums of mice to reflect the level of XOD inhibition of the drug. The results of the XOD activity assay showed that the treatment of yeast-paste gavage modeling resulted in a significant effect on the XOD activity of the mice in each group (### $p < 0.001$); this is because, after the mice received yeast paste gastric gavage, the purine-like substances in the body accumulated in large quantities, which led to the elevation of XOD activity in the body and the production of large quantities of UA. The XOD-inhibitor allopurinol group and the HPO group showed significantly inhibited levels of XOD activity and lowered serum-UA levels, and there were no statistically significant differences compared with the control group (Figure 5B).

3.7. Renal Protection Properties of PO

The centrifuged serums were immediately, and following the operating instructions in the biochemical kit, tested for the determination of SCr levels, as shown in Figure 6A; the SCr values in the model group of mice showed a significantly higher trend compared with the normal group (### $p < 0.001$), and after the administration of the drug, the SCr levels in the allopurinol group, the benzbromarone group, the MPO group, and the HPO group were significantly decreased (* $p < 0.05$, ** $p < 0.01$, *** $p < 0.001$), and there was no significant difference in SCr value between the HPO group and the control group. BUN levels were measured by the 96-well plate colorimetric method (Figure 6B), and from the results returned by the biochemical assay kit, it could be seen that the BUN levels of mice in the model group were significantly higher than those in the control group (### $p < 0.001$), while after the administration of the drug, the BUN levels of the mice in all the groups appeared to be reduced to varying degrees; the dose-dependencies between the various administration groups of PO are presented, and the BUN levels of the HPO group can be seen to be significantly lower than those of the model group (*** $p < 0.001$).

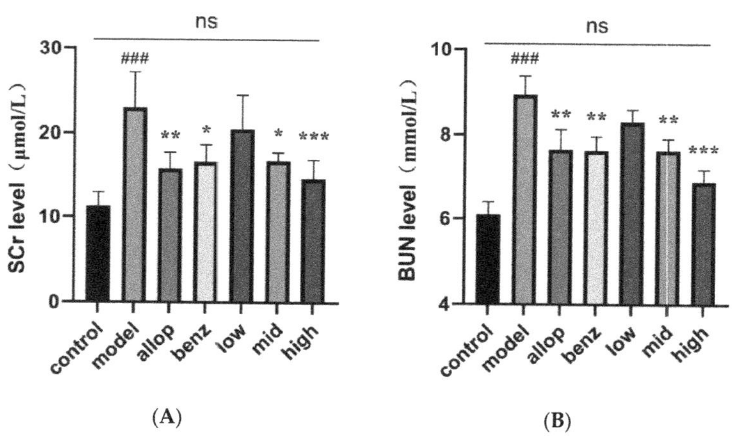

Figure 6. Serum levels of SCr and BUN in mice after intragastric administration. (**A**) The level of SCr in serum of mice after intragastric administration. (**B**) The level of BUN in serum of mice after intragastric administration. ### $p < 0.001$ compared with the control group. * $p < 0.05$, ** $p < 0.01$, and *** $p < 0.001$, compared with the model group. ns (no significance).

3.8. Effects of PO on Renal Histopathology

Illustrated in Figure 7, the histological analysis of renal tissues from individual mouse cohorts subsequent to H/E staining illuminated that within the control cohort, renal tubules manifested an exemplary preservation of morphology, which was characterized by proximal epithelial cells presenting a plump appearance and the renal interstitia being densely populated. Nonetheless, subsequent to gastric gavage with yeast paste to instigate the experimental model, the experimental cohort displayed conspicuous eosinophilia alongside pronounced tubular vacuolization. Analogous eosinophilic modifications, coupled with a degree of tubular vacuolization, were discernible within the allopurinol cohort, the benzbromarone cohort, and the LPO cohort, coinciding with a concurrent relaxation of tissue architecture. Conversely, there was an absence of noteworthy morphological aberrations concerning tubular cell integrity and tissue structure within the MPO and HPO cohorts when juxtaposed with the pristine control cohort.

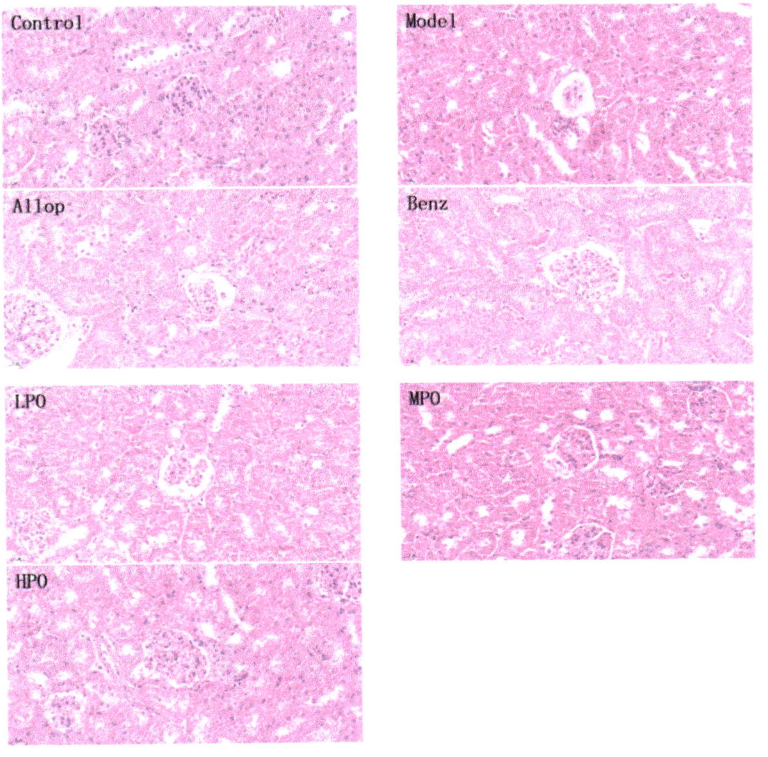

Figure 7. H/E-stained pathological sections of mouse kidney tissue (400×).

3.9. Western Blot Analysis of Kidney Tissues

The expression level of urate transporters in the kidney tissue for each group of mice was obtained by Western Blot, as shown in Figure 8A. The relative content of the protein sample can be obtained by comparing the gray value of the protein index with the gray value of the internal reference band. By analyzing these data, the expression level of urate transporter in the kidney tissue of HUA mice was explored. Compared with the normal group, the expression of ABCG2 protein in the model group was significantly decreased ($^{##}$ $p < 0.01$), while the expression intensity of ABCG2 protein in the PO group was dose-dependent, and there was no significant difference in the expression level between the high-dose group and the normal group, indicating that PO can increase the excretion of UA in mice by promoting the expression of ABCG2 protein (Figure 8B). Compared with the model group, GLUT9 protein levels were significantly down-regulated in the allopurinol group, benzbromarone group, MPO group, and HPO group (** $p < 0.01$) (Figure 8C). Compared with the control group, the expression of URAT1 protein in the model group was significantly up-regulated ($^{##}$ $p < 0.01$), while benzbromarone, as an inhibitor of URAT1 protein, significantly down-regulated its expression level. In addition, the PO administration group showed a dose-dependent downward trend, and there was no statistical difference in the expression level of URAT1 protein between the HPO group and the control group (Figure 8D).

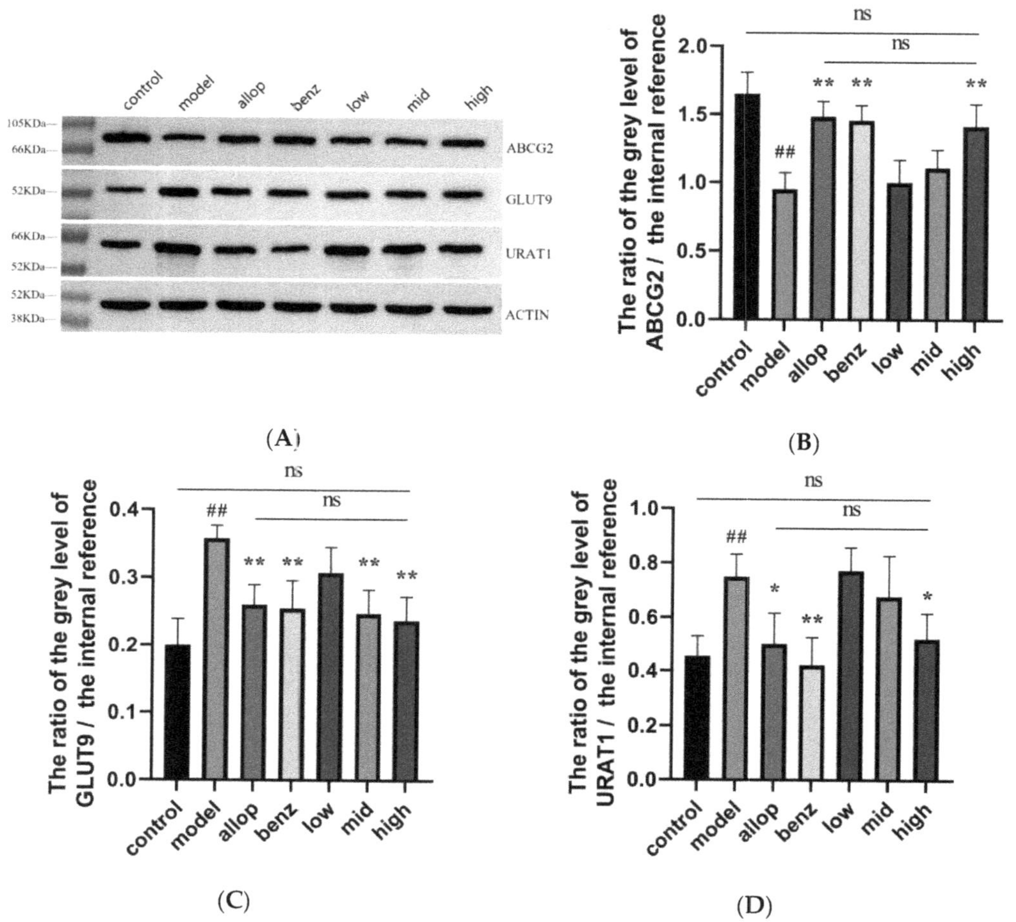

Figure 8. (**A**) Western Blot analysis of kidney tissues after drug administration in each group of mice. (**B**) ABCG2 protein expression level. (**C**) GLUT9 protein expression level. (**D**) URAT1 protein expression level. ## $p < 0.01$ compared with the control group. * $p < 0.05$ and ** $p < 0.01$, compared with the model. ns (no significance).

3.10. Effects of PO on Urate Transport Proteins

IHC analysis was performed on the kidney tissue sections of mice in each experimental group. The brown specific staining area observed by the microscope indicated the positive reaction of antigen–antibody binding, while the light yellow area represented the background color. According to the staining area and depth, the intensity of antigen–antibody binding can be intuitively reflected.

As shown in Figure 9A–C, the renal cortex region showed different degrees of positive reaction. URAT1 protein was widely expressed in renal tubular cells, and the expression levels of the benzbromarone group and HPO group were significantly lower than that of the model group. The ABCG2 protein was widely expressed in the cytoplasm of the renal tubular epithelial cells in each group. Compared with the model group, the control group and the HPO group had stronger positive localization.

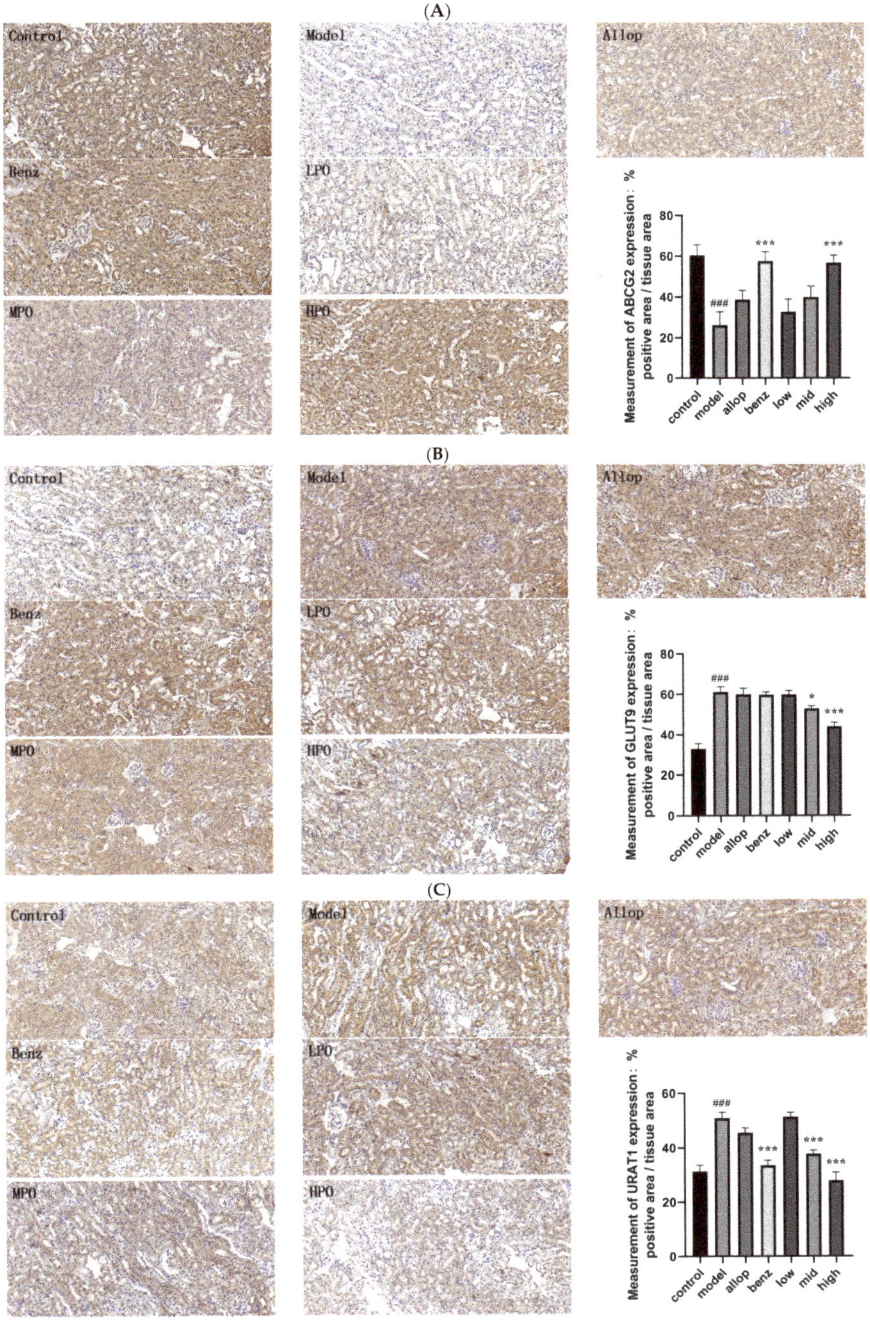

Figure 9. IHC analysis of renal tissues after drug administration in each group of mice (200×). (**A**) ABCG2 protein IHC expression level. (**B**) GLUT9 protein IHC expression level. (**C**) URAT1 protein IHC expression level. ### $p < 0.001$ vs. control. * $p < 0.05$ and *** $p < 0.001$, vs. model. Positive area values were analyzed by Image.

IHC results showed that the ABCG2 protein was widely distributed in the kidney of PO-treated mice, covering the renal cortex and renal tubular cells, and was more dense than that of the HUA model mice in the control group. This indicates that the ABCG2 protein can maintain the homeostasis of UA in the body by promoting UA excretion. In the IHC test results of the HPO group, the expression intensity levels of the URAT1 and GLUT9 proteins were the same as those shown in the Western Blot results, further confirming that the HPO group indeed exerted a significant regulatory effect on the urate transporters.

4. Discussion

Currently, allopurinol, benzbromarone, febuxostat, and other drugs are extensively utilized in the clinical management of HUA [19,57]. Nevertheless, due to varying degrees of adverse reactions associated with these agents, there is a growing interest in natural remedies with diminished side effects [58,59]. Studies have found that many plants that people eat daily have been found to have uric acid-lowering effects [60]. In addition, some traditional Chinese herbal medicines have been shown to have some effect in alleviating hyperuricemia, especially in the protection of liver and kidney function [61]. Among them, many plant-based active ingredients such as flavonoids, phenolic acids, saponins, etc., have been shown to reduce uric acid levels in a variety of ways without obvious side effects [62,63]. In summary, plant-derived functional foods and their active ingredients have shown potential in the treatment of hyperuricemia. These findings provide a treatment plan with small side effects, good therapeutic effects, and easier acceptance for people, and one which may become a safe and effective natural alternative therapy for hyperuricemia.

Studies have shown that the same plant in different habitats may have different pharmacological effects, and the theory of dao-di herbs is also mentioned in the field of traditional Chinese medicine [64,65]. In order to further study the active substances and pharmacological effects of PO, we meticulously procured fresh PO samples from four provinces in China with great climate differences, including Sichuan, Henan, Guangdong, and Jilin, for subsequent extraction and purification. Employing LC-MS technology alongside the XOD enzymatic reaction system enabled thorough identification and comparative analysis. Notably, findings revealed a marginally superior XOD inhibition efficacy in Sichuan specimens compared to samples of the plant collected from other habitats. Studies have reported that different conditions of cultivation and crop management lead to changes in PO's active ingredients [27,66]. At the same time, our findings also reveal that different geographical and climatic conditions may be one of the reasons for the changes in bioactive substances in PO, which also confirms the dao-di herbs theory in the field of traditional Chinese medicine.

Furthermore, subsequent to the analysis of Liquid Chromatography-Mass Spectrometry (LC-MS) identification outcomes and the review of pertinent literature, berberine and stachydrine were discerned within Sichuan-derived PO. Subsequently, we verified the presence of these two components in PO by standard control. This is the first time that berberine and stachydrine were identified from PO. Many studies have shown that berberine [55,67–69] and stachydrine [56,70–72] have a variety of physiological activities, which lays a theoretical foundation for further study of the effective components of PO and the related mechanism of network pharmacology. At the same time, the results of molecular docking showed that berberine had strong docking activity with XOD, and the studies reported in [73,74] also showed that berberine had the effect of reducing uric acid. Therefore, we speculated that berberine was one of the active substances of PO in the reduction of uric acid.

With the development of modern society, people's eating habits have gradually shown a trend of high levels of purine [75]. Studies have shown that the risk of hyperuricemia is positively correlated with red meat, seafood, alcohol, and fructose intake [76]. In order to more accurately replicate the physiological conversion of exogenous purines into UA within the human body, we employed the technique of gavaging yeast paste to establish an experimental model of HUA mice [54]. In addition, we selected the XOD inhibitor allopurinol and the uric acid-promoting drug benzbromarone as two positive drug groups to better study the uric acid-lowering mechanism of PO. By assessing serum biochemical indices in the murine bloodstream, we observed a gradual normalization of serum-UA levels in mice administered medium (1 g/kg) and high (2 g/kg) doses of PO after one week (** $p < 0.01$), with no statistical variance compared to either the allopurinol or benzbromarone groups. Furthermore, compared with the model group, the content levels of SCr and BUN also decreased significantly (** $p < 0.01$), and the BUN level in the HPO group was more similar to that in the control group, which indicated that PO had weaker hepatorenal toxicity than did allopurinol or benzbromarone. Studies have shown that elevated serum-UA levels are a risk factor for decreased renal function, and elevated UA levels can lead to a series of immune and inflammatory responses [77,78]. Our in vivo results showed that PO extract effectively inhibited XOD activity, and potential renal tissue damage caused by elevated UA levels was effectively alleviated in mice.

At present, XOD inhibitors and uric acid excretory drugs are often used in clinical treatment of gout patients, but these drugs can also cause certain forms of damage to the kidney [79,80]. Allopurinol can inhibit XOD activity and prevent the conversion of hypoxanthine and xanthine to UA [81]. Benzbromarone can promote UA excretion by inhibiting URAT1 transporters [82]. In vivo experiments and serum XOD activity analysis showed that the XOD activity of the HPO group (** $p < 0.01$) was significantly reduced, and there was no significant difference from the allopurinol group, indicating that the HPO group had good XOD inhibition performance. Through histological examination utilizing H/E staining of murine renal tissues, the model group exhibited notable pathological alterations, including eosinophilic degeneration resultant from urate accumulation and pronounced dilatation of renal tubules. Conversely, the MPO and HPO groups displayed no discernible morphological aberrations within renal tubular cells or tissue architecture, which indicated that the PO extract had no obvious nephrotoxicity. The above results show that PO extract is safer than allopurinol and benzbromarone and has better clinical application value.

Studies have shown that various urate transporters in the kidney are involved in the regulation of serum-UA levels [83]. Investigation into hyperuricemia-induced renal tissue in mice revealed that PO exerts efficacious synergistic regulation over UA excretion protein ABCG2 and urate transporters URAT1 and GLUT9, thereby preserving murine UA homeostasis. Consequently, we posit that PO has the dual capacity to attenuate UA synthesis by suppressing XOD activity and to diminish UA reabsorption while facilitating its excretion by modulating the overexpression of urate transporters and bolstering UA excretion proteins. In general, PO effectively reduces serum-UA levels through the synergistic effects of various components, targets, and pathways, thereby maintaining UA homeostasis.

5. Conclusions

In this study, we first screened the PO from Sichuan, determining that it demonstrated the best in vitro XOD inhibitory activity among the plant samples from the four habitats, and berberine and stachydrine were isolated and identified from this PO for the first time. This finding reveals that different geographical and climatic conditions may be one of the reasons for the changes of bioactive substances in PO. Then ABCG2, URAT1, and other proteins were screened out as research targets by network pharmacology. Molecular docking prediction and in vitro verification showed that berberine had strong docking activity with XOD. Finally, in vivo results showed that PO could inhibit excessive uric acid production and promote uric acid excretion by inhibiting XOD activity, inhibiting the expression of uric acid transporters (GLUT9, URAT1) and promoting the expression of uric acid excretion protein (ABCG2), and thereby effectively reducing serum-UA levels in mouse models. In addition, compared with positive drugs, PO extracts showed less nephrotoxicity and increased safety. In summary, our study showed the potential of purslane to reduce uric acid, and provided a theoretical basis for the development of the edible wild plant purslane.

6. Patents

An extraction method of effective components of purslane and its application in reducing uric acid. Bo Gao; Yiming Zhang; Fei Ye; Ming Kang; Zhenlong Ge; Shengying Zhu; Yanjing Feng; Hao Chang. ZL 2024 1 0543667.X.

Supplementary Materials: The following supporting information can be downloaded at: https://www.mdpi.com/article/10.3390/nu16203549/s1, Figure S1: Berberine in vitro XOD inhibition-ability experiment.

Author Contributions: Y.Z. and S.Z.: Writing—original draft, Data curation, Investigation, Visualization. S.Z. and Y.F.: Writing—review and editing. Y.Z. and B.G.: Conceptualization, Methodology. Y.Z., S.Z. and Y.G.: Investigation. Y.Z. and Y.G.: Formal analysis. B.G.: Resources, Supervision, Funding acquisition, Project administration. All authors have read and agreed to the published version of the manuscript.

Funding: This research was funded by Jilin province school co-construction plan special, grant number SXGJSF2017-1-1(06).

Institutional Review Board Statement: The animal study protocol was approved by the Animal Experiment Ethics Committee of Jilin University (protocol code: 2023029; approval date: 29 March 2023).

Informed Consent Statement: Not applicable.

Data Availability Statement: Data are contained within the article and Supplementary Materials.

Conflicts of Interest: The authors declare no conflicts of interest.

References

1. Dehlin, M.; Jacobsson, L.; Roddy, E. Global epidemiology of gout: Prevalence, incidence, treatment patterns and risk factors. *Nat. Rev. Rheumatol.* **2020**, *16*, 380–390. [CrossRef] [PubMed]
2. He, Q.; Mok, T.N.; Sin, T.H.; Yin, J.; Li, S.; Yin, Y.; Ming, W.K.; Feng, B. Global, Regional, and National Prevalence of Gout From 1990 to 2019: Age-Period-Cohort Analysis with Future Burden Prediction. *JMIR Public Health Surveill* **2023**, *9*, e45943. [CrossRef] [PubMed]
3. Yanai, H.; Adachi, H.; Hakoshima, M.; Katsuyama, H. Molecular Biological and Clinical Understanding of the Pathophysiology and Treatments of Hyperuricemia and Its Association with Metabolic Syndrome, Cardiovascular Diseases and Chronic Kidney Disease. *Int. J. Mol. Sci.* **2021**, *22*, 9221. [CrossRef]
4. Crawley, W.T.; Jungels, C.G.; Stenmark, K.R.; Fini, M.A. U-shaped association of uric acid to overall-cause mortality and its impact on clinical management of hyperuricemia. *Redox Biol.* **2022**, *51*, 102271. [CrossRef] [PubMed]
5. Cicero, A.F.G.; Fogacci, F.; Kuwabara, M.; Borghi, C. Therapeutic Strategies for the Treatment of Chronic Hyperuricemia: An Evidence-Based Update. *Medicina* **2021**, *57*, 58. [CrossRef]
6. Kielstein, J.T.; Pontremoli, R.; Burnier, M. Management of Hyperuricemia in Patients with Chronic Kidney Disease: A Focus on Renal Protection. *Curr. Hypertens. Rep.* **2020**, *22*, 102. [CrossRef]
7. Maiuolo, J.; Oppedisano, F.; Gratteri, S.; Muscoli, C.; Mollace, V. Regulation of uric acid metabolism and excretion. *Int. J. Cardiol.* **2016**, *213*, 8–14. [CrossRef]
8. Su, H.Y.; Yang, C.; Liang, D.; Liu, H.F. Research Advances in the Mechanisms of Hyperuricemia-Induced Renal Injury. *BioMed Res. Int.* **2020**, *2020*, 5817348. [CrossRef]
9. Sivera, F.; Andres, M.; Dalbeth, N. A glance into the future of gout. *Ther. Adv. Musculoskelet. Dis.* **2022**, *14*, 1759720x221114098. [CrossRef]
10. Wen, S.; Arakawa, H.; Tamai, I. Uric acid in health and disease: From physiological functions to pathogenic mechanisms. *Pharmacol. Ther.* **2024**, *256*, 108615. [CrossRef]
11. Engelhart, D.C.; Granados, J.C.; Shi, D.; Saier, M.H., Jr.; Baker, M.E.; Abagyan, R.; Nigam, S.K. Systems Biology Analysis Reveals Eight SLC22 Transporter Subgroups, Including OATs, OCTs, and OCTNs. *Int. J. Mol. Sci.* **2020**, *21*, 1791. [CrossRef] [PubMed]
12. Enomoto, A.; Kimura, H.; Chairoungdua, A.; Shigeta, Y.; Jutabha, P.; Cha, S.H.; Hosoyamada, M.; Takeda, M.; Sekine, T.; Igarashi, T.; et al. Molecular identification of a renal urate anion exchanger that regulates blood urate levels. *Nature* **2002**, *417*, 447–452. [CrossRef] [PubMed]

13. Ekaratanawong, S.; Anzai, N.; Jutabha, P.; Miyazaki, H.; Noshiro, R.; Takeda, M.; Kanai, Y.; Sophasan, S.; Endou, H. Human Organic Anion Transporter 4 Is a Renal Apical Organic Anion/Dicarboxylate Exchanger in the Proximal Tubules. *J. Pharmacol. Sci.* **2004**, *94*, 297–304. [CrossRef] [PubMed]
14. Vitart, V.; Rudan, I.; Hayward, C.; Gray, N.K.; Floyd, J.; Palmer, C.N.; Knott, S.A.; Kolcic, I.; Polasek, O.; Graessler, J.; et al. SLC2A9 is a newly identified urate transporter influencing serum urate concentration, urate excretion and gout. *Nat. Genet.* **2008**, *40*, 437–442. [CrossRef]
15. Eraly, S.A.; Vallon, V.; Rieg, T.; Gangoiti, J.A.; Wikoff, W.R.; Siuzdak, G.; Barshop, B.A.; Nigam, S.K. Multiple organic anion transporters contribute to net renal excretion of uric acid. *Physiol. Genom.* **2008**, *33*, 180–192. [CrossRef]
16. Ojha, R.; Singh, J.; Ojha, A.; Singh, H.; Sharma, S.; Nepali, K. An updated patent review: Xanthine oxidase inhibitors for the treatment of hyperuricemia and gout (2011–2015). *Expert Opin. Ther. Pat.* **2017**, *27*, 311–345. [CrossRef] [PubMed]
17. Terkeltaub, R. Emerging Urate-Lowering Drugs and Pharmacologic Treatment Strategies for Gout: A Narrative Review. *Drugs* **2023**, *83*, 1501–1521. [CrossRef]
18. Stamp, L.K.; Chapman, P.T. Allopurinol hypersensitivity: Pathogenesis and prevention. *Best Pr. Res. Clin. Rheumatol.* **2020**, *34*, 101501. [CrossRef]
19. Chou, H.W.; Chiu, H.T.; Tsai, C.W.; Ting, I.W.; Yeh, H.C.; Huang, H.C.; Kuo, C.C. Comparative effectiveness of allopurinol, febuxostat and benzbromarone on renal function in chronic kidney disease patients with hyperuricemia: A 13-year inception cohort study. *Nephrol. Dial. Transpl.* **2018**, *33*, 1620–1627. [CrossRef]
20. Liu, N.; Xu, H.; Sun, Q.; Yu, X.; Chen, W.; Wei, H.; Jiang, J.; Xu, Y.; Lu, W. The Role of Oxidative Stress in Hyperuricemia and Xanthine Oxidoreductase (XOR) Inhibitors. *Oxid. Med. Cell Longev.* **2021**, *2021*, 470380. [CrossRef]
21. Xiang, L.; Huang, Y.; Li, R.; Tao, Y.; Wu, T.; Pan, S.; Xu, X. Artemisia selengensis Turcz. leaves extract ameliorates hyperuricemia in mice by inhibiting hepatic xanthine oxidase activity, modulating renal uric acid transporters, and improving metabolic disorders. *Food Biosci.* **2023**, *56*, 102639. [CrossRef]
22. Song, D.; Zhao, H.; Wang, L.; Wang, F.; Fang, L.; Zhao, X. Ethanol extract of Sophora japonica flower bud, an effective potential dietary supplement for the treatment of hyperuricemia. *Food Biosci.* **2023**, *52*, 102457. [CrossRef]
23. Mehmood, A.; Zhao, L.; Ishaq, M.; Xin, W.; Zhao, L.; Wang, C.; Hossen, I.; Zhang, H.; Lian, Y.; Xu, M. Anti-hyperuricemic potential of stevia (*Stevia rebaudiana* Bertoni) residue extract in hyperuricemic mice. *Food Funct.* **2020**, *11*, 6387–6406. [CrossRef] [PubMed]
24. Carrascosa, A.; Pascual, J.A.; Ros, M.; Petropoulos, S.A.; Alguacil, M.d.M. Agronomical Practices and Management for Commercial Cultivation of *Portulaca oleracea* as a Crop: A Review. *Plants* **2023**, *12*, 1246. [CrossRef]
25. Hou, Y.; Jiang, J.G. Origin and concept of medicine food homology and its application in modern functional foods. *Food Funct.* **2013**, *4*, 1727–1741. [CrossRef]
26. Lu, Q.; Li, R.; Yang, Y.; Zhang, Y.; Zhao, Q.; Li, J. Ingredients with anti-inflammatory effect from medicine food homology plants. *Food Chem.* **2022**, *368*, 130610. [CrossRef]
27. Montoya-García, C.O.; García-Mateos, R.; Becerra-Martínez, E.; Toledo-Aguilar, R.; Volke-Haller, V.H.; Jesús Magdaleno-Villar, J. Bioactive compounds of purslane (*Portulaca oleracea* L.) according to the production system: A review. *Sci. Hortic.* **2023**, *308*, 111584. [CrossRef]
28. Chen, C.-J.; Wang, W.-Y.; Wang, X.-L.; Dong, L.-W.; Yue, Y.-T.; Xin, H.-L.; Ling, C.-Q.; Li, M. Anti-hypoxic activity of the ethanol extract from *Portulaca oleracea* in mice. *J. Ethnopharmacol.* **2009**, *124*, 246–250. [CrossRef]
29. Srivastava, R.; Srivastava, V.; Singh, A. Multipurpose Benefits of an Underexplored Species Purslane (*Portulaca oleracea* L.): A Critical Review. *Environ. Manag.* **2023**, *72*, 309–320. [CrossRef]
30. Kumar, A.; Sreedharan, S.; Kashyap, A.K.; Singh, P.; Ramchiary, N. A review on bioactive phytochemicals and ethnopharmacological potential of purslane (*Portulaca oleracea* L.). *Heliyon* **2022**, *8*, e08669. [CrossRef]
31. Jin, R.; Lin, Z.J.; Xue, C.M.; Zhang, B. An improved association-mining research for exploring Chinese herbal property theory: Based on data of the Shennong's Classic of Materia Medica. *J. Integr. Med.* **2013**, *11*, 352–365. [CrossRef] [PubMed]
32. Liu, F.X.; Cui, X.Y.; Duan, Y.; Guo, S.N.; Liu, J.P.; Ying, X.X. A new alkaloid from *Portulaca oleracea* L. and its anti-inflammatory activity. *Nat. Prod. Res.* **2022**, *36*, 4709–4713. [CrossRef] [PubMed]
33. Bao, M.; Hou, K.; Xin, C.; Zeng, D.; Cheng, C.; Zhao, H.; Wang, Z.; Wang, L. Portulaca oleracea L. Extract Alleviated Type 2 Diabetes Via Modulating the Gut Microbiota and Serum Branched-Chain Amino Acid Metabolism. *Mol. Nutr. Food Res.* **2022**, *66*, e2101030. [CrossRef] [PubMed]
34. Tleubayeva, M.I.; Datkhayev, U.M.; Alimzhanova, M.; Ishmuratova, M.Y.; Korotetskaya, N.V.; Abdullabekova, R.M.; Flisyuk, E.V.; Gemejiyeva, N.G. Component Composition and Antimicrobial Activity of CO2 Extract of *Portulaca oleracea*, Growing in the Territory of Kazakhstan. *Sci. World J.* **2021**, *2021*, 5434525. [CrossRef] [PubMed]
35. Karimi, G.; Hosseinzadeh, H.; Ettehad, N. Evaluation of the gastric antiulcerogenic effects of *Portulaca oleracea* L. extracts in mice. *Phytother. Res.* **2004**, *18*, 484–487. [CrossRef]
36. Ghorani, V.; Saadat, S.; Khazdair, M.R.; Gholamnezhad, Z.; El-Seedi, H.; Boskabady, M.H. Phytochemical Characteristics and Anti-Inflammatory, Immunoregulatory, and Antioxidant Effects of *Portulaca oleracea* L.: A Comprehensive Review. *Evid. Based Complement. Altern. Med.* **2023**, *2023*, 2075444. [CrossRef]
37. Dai, H.; Lv, S.; Fu, X.; Li, W. Identification of Scopoletin and Chlorogenic Acid as Potential Active Components in Sunflower Calathide Enzymatically Hydrolyzed Extract towards Hyperuricemia. *Appl. Sci.* **2021**, *11*, 10306. [CrossRef]

38. Voynikov, Y.; Nedialkov, P.; Gevrenova, R.; Zheleva-Dimitrova, D.; Balabanova, V.; Dimitrov, I. UHPLC-Orbitrap-MS Tentative Identification of 51 Oleraceins (Cyclo-Dopa Amides) in *Portulaca oleracea* L. Cluster Analysis and MS(2) Filtering by Mass Difference. *Plants* **2021**, *10*, 1921. [CrossRef]
39. Ren, L.; Xue, X.; Zhang, F.; Xu, Q.; Liang, X. High performance liquid chromatography-mass spectrometry analysis of protoberberine alkaloids in medicine herbs. *J. Sep. Sci.* **2007**, *30*, 833–842. [CrossRef]
40. Yan, S.; Wang, X.; Zhao, H.; Lu, H.; Tian, W.; Wu, L.; Xue, X. Metabolomics-based screening and chemically identifying abundant stachydrine as quality characteristic of rare Leucosceptrum canum Smith honey. *J. Food Compos. Anal.* **2022**, *114*, 104759. [CrossRef]
41. Ru, J.; Li, P.; Wang, J.; Zhou, W.; Li, B.; Huang, C.; Li, P.; Guo, Z.; Tao, W.; Yang, Y.; et al. TCMSP: A database of systems pharmacology for drug discovery from herbal medicines. *J. Cheminform.* **2014**, *6*, 13. [CrossRef] [PubMed]
42. Yao, Z.J.; Dong, J.; Che, Y.J.; Zhu, M.F.; Wen, M.; Wang, N.N.; Wang, S.; Lu, A.P.; Cao, D.S. TargetNet: A web service for predicting potential drug-target interaction profiling via multi-target SAR models. *J. Comput. Aided. Mol. Des.* **2016**, *30*, 413–424. [CrossRef] [PubMed]
43. Daina, A.; Michielin, O.; Zoete, V. SwissTargetPrediction: Updated data and new features for efficient prediction of protein targets of small molecules. *Nucleic Acids Res.* **2019**, *47*, W357–W364. [CrossRef]
44. UniProt: A worldwide hub of protein knowledge. *Nucleic Acids Res.* **2019**, *47*, D506–D515. [CrossRef]
45. Davis, A.P.; Grondin, C.J.; Johnson, R.J.; Sciaky, D.; Wiegers, J.; Wiegers, T.C.; Mattingly, C.J. Comparative Toxicogenomics Database (CTD): Update 2021. *Nucleic Acids Res.* **2021**, *49*, D1138–D1143. [CrossRef]
46. Amberger, J.S.; Bocchini, C.A.; Schiettecatte, F.; Scott, A.F.; Hamosh, A. OMIM.org: Online Mendelian Inheritance in Man (OMIM®), an online catalog of human genes and genetic disorders. *Nucleic Acids Res.* **2015**, *43*, D789–D798. [CrossRef]
47. Piñero, J.; Ramírez-Anguita, J.M.; Saüch-Pitarch, J.; Ronzano, F.; Centeno, E.; Sanz, F.; Furlong, L.I. The DisGeNET knowledge platform for disease genomics: 2019 update. *Nucleic Acids Res.* **2020**, *48*, D845–D855. [CrossRef] [PubMed]
48. Szklarczyk, D.; Morris, J.H.; Cook, H.; Kuhn, M.; Wyder, S.; Simonovic, M.; Santos, A.; Doncheva, N.T.; Roth, A.; Bork, P.; et al. The STRING database in 2017: Quality-controlled protein-protein association networks, made broadly accessible. *Nucleic Acids Res.* **2017**, *45*, D362–D368. [CrossRef]
49. Otasek, D.; Morris, J.H.; Bouças, J.; Pico, A.R.; Demchak, B. Cytoscape Automation: Empowering workflow-based network analysis. *Genome Biol.* **2019**, *20*, 185. [CrossRef]
50. Huang, D.W.; Sherman, B.T.; Lempicki, R.A. Systematic and integrative analysis of large gene lists using DAVID bioinformatics resources. *Nat. Protoc.* **2009**, *4*, 44–57. [CrossRef]
51. Kim, S.; Thiessen, P.A.; Bolton, E.E.; Chen, J.; Fu, G.; Gindulyte, A.; Han, L.; He, J.; He, S.; Shoemaker, B.A.; et al. PubChem Substance and Compound databases. *Nucleic Acids Res.* **2016**, *44*, D1202–D1213. [CrossRef] [PubMed]
52. Trott, O.; Olson, A.J. AutoDock Vina: Improving the speed and accuracy of docking with a new scoring function, efficient optimization, and multithreading. *J. Comput. Chem.* **2010**, *31*, 455–461. [CrossRef] [PubMed]
53. Tang, Z.; Li, L.; Xia, Z. Exploring Anti-Nonalcoholic Fatty Liver Disease Mechanism of Gardeniae Fructus by Network Pharmacology, Molecular Docking, and Experiment Validation. *ACS Omega* **2022**, *7*, 25521–25531. [CrossRef] [PubMed]
54. Dai, H.; Lv, S.; Qiao, Z.; Wang, K.; Zhou, X.; Bao, C.; Zhang, S.; Fu, X.; Li, W. The Active Components of Sunflower (*Helianthus annuus* L.) Calathide and the Effects on Urate Nephropathy Based on COX-2/PGE2 Signaling Pathway and the Urate Transporter URAT1, ABCG2, and GLUT9. *Front. Nutr.* **2021**, *8*, 769555. [CrossRef]
55. Gasmi, A.; Asghar, F.; Zafar, S.; Oliinyk, P.; Khavrona, O.; Lysiuk, R.; Peana, M.; Piscopo, S.; Antonyak, H.; Pen, J.J.; et al. Berberine: Pharmacological Features in Health, Disease and Aging. *Curr. Med. Chem.* **2024**, *31*, 1214–1234. [CrossRef]
56. He, Z.; Li, P.; Liu, P.; Xu, P. Exploring stachydrine: From natural occurrence to biological activities and metabolic pathways. *Front. Plant Sci.* **2024**, *15*, 1442879. [CrossRef]
57. Ramirez-Sandoval, J.C.; Madero, M. Treatment of Hyperuricemia in Chronic Kidney Disease. *Contrib. Nephrol.* **2018**, *192*, 135–146.
58. Wang, X.; Dong, L.; Dong, Y.; Bao, Z.; Lin, S. Corn Silk Flavonoids Ameliorate Hyperuricemia via PI3K/AKT/NF-κB Pathway. *J. Agric. Food Chem.* **2023**, *71*, 9429–9440. [CrossRef] [PubMed]
59. Wu, D.; Chen, R.; Li, Q.; Lai, X.; Sun, L.; Zhang, Z.; Wen, S.; Sun, S.; Cao, F. Tea (*Camellia sinensis*) Ameliorates Hyperuricemia via Uric Acid Metabolic Pathways and Gut Microbiota. *Nutrients* **2022**, *14*, 2666. [CrossRef]
60. Cheng-Yuan, W.; Jian-Gang, D. Research progress on the prevention and treatment of hyperuricemia by medicinal and edible plants and its bioactive components. *Front. Nutr.* **2023**, *10*, 1186161. [CrossRef]
61. Xu, L.; Lu, L.L.; Gao, J.D. Traditional Chinese Herbal Medicine Plays a Role in the Liver, Kidney, and Intestine to Ameliorate Hyperuricemia according to Experimental Studies. *Evid. Based Complement. Altern. Med.* **2021**, *2021*, 4618352. [CrossRef] [PubMed]
62. Mehmood, A.; Zhao, L.; Wang, C.; Nadeem, M.; Raza, A.; Ali, N.; Shah, A.A. Management of hyperuricemia through dietary polyphenols as a natural medicament: A comprehensive review. *Crit. Rev. Food Sci. Nutr.* **2019**, *59*, 1433–1455. [CrossRef] [PubMed]
63. Jiang, L.L.; Gong, X.; Ji, M.Y.; Wang, C.C.; Wang, J.H.; Li, M.H. Bioactive Compounds from Plant-Based Functional Foods: A Promising Choice for the Prevention and Management of Hyperuricemia. *Foods* **2020**, *9*, 973. [CrossRef] [PubMed]

64. Huang, Y.; Wang, L.; Xie, J.; Chen, H.; Ou, G.; Zeng, L.; Li, Y.; Li, W.; Fan, H.; Zheng, J. Exploring the chemical composition, medicinal benefits, and antioxidant activity of Plumula nelumbinis essential oil from different habitats in China. *Saudi Pharm. J.* **2023**, *31*, 101829. [CrossRef] [PubMed]
65. Luo, H.; Zhao, Y.; Hua, H.; Zhang, Y.; Zhang, X.; Fang, Q.; Li, Q.; Zhang, Y.; Tan, P.; Yang, A.; et al. Research progress on quality assurance of genuine Chinese medicinal in Sichuan. *Chin. Med.* **2021**, *16*, 19. [CrossRef]
66. Petropoulos, S.; Karkanis, A.; Martins, N.; Ferreira, I.C.F.R. Phytochemical composition and bioactive compounds of common purslane (*Portulaca oleracea* L.) as affected by crop management practices. *Trends Food Sci. Technol.* **2016**, *55*, 1–10. [CrossRef]
67. Song, D.; Hao, J.; Fan, D. Biological properties and clinical applications of berberine. *Front. Med.* **2020**, *14*, 564–582. [CrossRef]
68. Xu, X.; Yi, H.; Wu, J.; Kuang, T.; Zhang, J.; Li, Q.; Du, H.; Xu, T.; Jiang, G.; Fan, G. Therapeutic effect of berberine on metabolic diseases: Both pharmacological data and clinical evidence. *Biomed. Pharmacother.* **2021**, *133*, 110984. [CrossRef]
69. Shou, J.W.; Shaw, P.C. Therapeutic Efficacies of Berberine against Neurological Disorders: An Update of Pharmacological Effects and Mechanisms. *Cells* **2022**, *11*, 796. [CrossRef]
70. Cheng, F.; Zhou, Y.; Wang, M.; Guo, C.; Cao, Z.; Zhang, R.; Peng, C. A review of pharmacological and pharmacokinetic properties of stachydrine. *Pharmacol. Res.* **2020**, *155*, 104755. [CrossRef]
71. Liao, L.; Tang, Y.; Li, B.; Tang, J.; Xu, H.; Zhao, K.; Zhang, X. Stachydrine, a potential drug for the treatment of cardiovascular system and central nervous system diseases. *Biomed. Pharmacother.* **2023**, *161*, 114489. [CrossRef] [PubMed]
72. Sun, Y.; Xia, X.; Yuan, G.; Zhang, T.; Deng, B.; Feng, X.; Wang, Q. Stachydrine, a Bioactive Equilibrist for Synephrine, Identified from Four Citrus Chinese Herbs. *Molecules* **2023**, *28*, 3813. [CrossRef] [PubMed]
73. Li, Q.; Huang, Z.; Liu, D.; Zheng, J.; Xie, J.; Chen, J.; Zeng, H.; Su, Z.; Li, Y. Effect of Berberine on Hyperuricemia and Kidney Injury: A Network Pharmacology Analysis and Experimental Validation in a Mouse Model. *Drug Des. Devel. Ther.* **2021**, *15*, 3241–3254. [CrossRef]
74. Chen, Q.; Li, D.; Wu, F.; He, X.; Zhou, Y.; Sun, C.; Wang, H.; Liu, Y. Berberine Regulates the Metabolism of Uric Acid and Modulates Intestinal Flora in Hyperuricemia Rats Model. *Comb. Chem. High Throughput Screen* **2023**, *26*, 2057–2066. [CrossRef] [PubMed]
75. Aihemaitijiang, S.; Zhang, Y.; Zhang, L.; Yang, J.; Ye, C.; Halimulati, M.; Zhang, W.; Zhang, Z. The Association between Purine-Rich Food Intake and Hyperuricemia: A Cross-Sectional Study in Chinese Adult Residents. *Nutrients* **2020**, *12*, 3835. [CrossRef]
76. Li, R.; Yu, K.; Li, C. Dietary factors and risk of gout and hyperuricemia: A meta-analysis and systematic review. *Asia Pac. J. Clin. Nutr.* **2018**, *27*, 1344–1356.
77. Jung, S.W.; Kim, S.-M.; Kim, Y.G.; Lee, S.-H.; Moon, J.-Y. Uric acid and inflammation in kidney disease. *Am. J. Physiol.-Ren. Physiol.* **2020**, *318*, F1327–F1340. [CrossRef]
78. Shahin, L.; Patel, K.M.; Heydari, M.K.; Kesselman, M.M. Hyperuricemia and Cardiovascular Risk. *Cureus* **2021**, *13*, e14855. [CrossRef]
79. Hansildaar, R.; Vedder, D.; Baniaamam, M.; Tausche, A.K.; Gerritsen, M.; Nurmohamed, M.T. Cardiovascular risk in inflammatory arthritis: Rheumatoid arthritis and gout. *Lancet Rheumatol.* **2021**, 3, e58–e70. [CrossRef]
80. Ye, X.; Wu, J.; Tang, K.; Li, W.; Xiong, C.; Zhuo, L. Benzbromarone as a possible cause of acute kidney injury in patients with urolithiasis: Two case reports. *Medicine* **2019**, *98*, e15214. [CrossRef]
81. Sekine, M.; Okamoto, K.; Pai, E.F.; Nagata, K.; Ichida, K.; Hille, R.; Nishino, T. Allopurinol and oxypurinol differ in their strength and mechanisms of inhibition of xanthine oxidoreductase. *J. Biol. Chem.* **2023**, *299*, 105189. [CrossRef] [PubMed]
82. Li, X.; Yan, Z.; Tian, J.; Zhang, X.; Han, H.; Ye, F. Urate Transporter URAT1 in Hyperuricemia: New Insights from Hyperuricemic Models. *Ann. Clin. Lab. Sci.* **2019**, *49*, 756–762. [PubMed]
83. Chung, S.; Kim, G.H. Urate Transporters in the Kidney: What Clinicians Need to Know. *Electrolyte Blood Press.* **2021**, *19*, 1–9. [CrossRef] [PubMed]

nutrients

MDPI

Article

The Protective Effects of an Aged Black Garlic Water Extract on the Prostate

Maria Loreta Libero [1,2,3,†], Antonio J. Montero-Hidalgo [2,3,4,5,†], Lucia Recinella [1,*], Raúl M. Luque [2,3,4,5,*], Daniele Generali [6,7], Alessandra Acquaviva [1], Giustino Orlando [1], Claudio Ferrante [1], Luigi Menghini [1], Simonetta Cristina Di Simone [1], Nilofar Nilofar [1], Annalisa Chiavaroli [1], Luigi Brunetti [1] and Sheila Leone [1]

1 Department of Pharmacy, "G. d'Annunzio" University, 66013 Chieti, Italy; maria.libero@unich.it (M.L.L.); alessandra.acquaviva@unich.it (A.A.); giustino.orlando@unich.it (G.O.); claudio.ferrante@unich.it (C.F.); luigi.menghini@unich.it (L.M.); simonetta.disimone@unich.it (S.C.D.S.); nilofar.nilofar@unich.it (N.N.); annalisa.chiavaroli@unich.it (A.C.); luigi.brunetti@unich.it (L.B.); sheila.leone@unich.it (S.L.)

2 Department of Cell Biology, Physiology and Immunology, University of Cordoba, 14014 Cordoba, Spain; b42mohia@uco.es

3 Maimonides Biomedical Research Institute of Cordoba (IMIBIC), 14004 Cordoba, Spain

4 Reina Sofia University Hospital (HURS), 14004 Cordoba, Spain

5 Centro de Investigación Biomédica en Red de Fisiopatología de la Obesidad y Nutrición (CIBERobn), 14004 Cordoba, Spain

6 Department of Medical, Surgical and Health Sciences, University of Trieste, 34149 Trieste, Italy; dgenerali@units.it

7 Department of Advanced Translational Microbiology, Institute for Maternal and Child Health-IRCCS "Burlo Garofolo", 34137 Trieste, Italy

* Correspondence: lucia.recinella@unich.it (L.R.); raul.luque@uco.es (R.M.L.); Tel.: +39-0871-3554754 (L.R.); +34-957-213740 (R.M.L.)

† These authors contributed equally to this work.

Abstract: Chronic inflammation is a recognized risk factor for various cancers, including prostate cancer (PCa). We aim to explore the potential protective effects of aged black garlic extract (ABGE) against inflammation-induced prostate damage and its impact on prostate cancer cell lines. We used an ex vivo model of inflammation induced by Escherichia coli lipopolysaccharide (LPS) on C57BL/6 male mouse prostate specimens to investigate the anti-inflammatory properties of ABGE. The gene expression levels of pro-inflammatory biomarkers (*COX-2*, *NF-κB*, and *TNF-α*, *IL-6*) were measured. Additionally, we evaluated ABGE's therapeutic effects on the prostate cancer cell lines through in vitro functional assays, including colony formation, tumorsphere formation, migration assays, and phosphorylation arrays to assess the signaling pathways (MAPK, AKT, JAK/STAT, and TGF-β). ABGE demonstrated significant anti-inflammatory and antioxidant effects in preclinical models, partly attributed to its polyphenolic content, notably catechin and gallic acid. In the ex vivo model, ABGE reduced the gene expression levels of *COX-2*, *NF-κB*, *TNF-α*, and *IL-6*. The in vitro studies showed that ABGE inhibited cell proliferation, colony and tumorsphere formation, and cell migration in the prostate cancer cells, suggesting its potential as a therapeutic agent. ABGE exhibits promising anti-inflammatory and anti-cancer properties, supporting further investigation into ABGE as a potential agent for managing inflammation and prostate cancer.

Keywords: ABGE; prostate; inflammation; cancer

1. Introduction

Prostatitis is a prostate gland inflammation, which encompasses a range of disorders, such as acute and chronic bacterial prostatitis. These conditions can be caused by bacterial infections, immune responses, or non-infectious factors such as trauma or stress [1].

In particular, acute prostatic inflammation in mice induced an epithelial transformation, named proliferative inflammatory atrophy, which could promote prostatic intraepithelial neoplasia [1].

In this context, chronic inflammation is often linked with the process of carcinogenesis and is recognized as both a hallmark and a potential risk factor for various cancers [2]. Specifically, for prostate cancer (PCa), chronic inflammation is suggested as a bridge between environmental factors and tumor development [3–5].

Numerous studies have explored the relationship between prostate gland abnormalities and the inflammatory process, showing a strong prevalence of mild chronic inflammation in PCa [6].

Chronic inflammation can create a microenvironment conducive to carcinogenesis by producing pro-inflammatory cytokines, reactive oxygen species, and DNA damage [7].

In line with this, NLRP3 inflammasome is critically involved in PCa aggressiveness [8].

Altogether, the presented evidence indicates the proficient pro-oncogenic role of certain inflammatory processes in PCa [9,10].

Various biomarkers, such as tumor necrosis factor (TNF)-α, nuclear factor (NF)-kB, interleukin (IL)-6, and cyclooxygenase (COX)-2, play a critical role in inflammatory responses. In particular, Baud and their collaborators (2001) reported that TNF-α is a potent pro-inflammatory cytokine whose involvement in inflammation, cell proliferation, differentiation, and apoptosis is well known. Increased serum levels of pro-inflammatory markers such as TNF-α are related to accelerated progression and a poor prognosis in PCa [11,12].

Furthermore, NF-κB is essential for regulating both the innate and adaptive immune responses, particularly in inflammation. Besides its role in the survival and activation of immune cells, NF-κB stimulates the release of pro-inflammatory genes, including cytokines and chemokines, and regulates inflammasome activity. Moreover, the dysregulation of NF-κB contributes to various inflammatory diseases, including rheumatic diseases and asthma [13,14]. Interestingly, a wide body of evidence suggested that NF-κB activation, as well as various signals linked to inflammation, are well known to be involved in the modulation of PCa malignancy [15]. In particular, NF-κB activation exerts modulatory effects on the expression of the cytokines and factors involved in cancer development and progression, including IL-6 [15]. Moreover, the activation of IL-6 signaling was found to induce growth, proliferative activity, and the migration of PCa cells [16].

COX-2 is also critically involved in carcinogenesis in various tissues, including breasts and lungs, as well as the prostate [17].

Various studies suggested the potential activity of a number of herbal extracts commonly used in traditional medicine as well as natural compounds exhibiting an innovative action mode as a possible remedy for PCa [18,19].

In this context, aged black garlic (ABG) has garnered attention for its bioactive compound profile and biological activities [20].

ABG is produced by fermenting fresh garlic at controlled high humidity (80–90%) and temperature (60–90 °C) conditions over several weeks. As previously reported [20], the temperature and humidity conditions of the thermal treatment chosen during ABG production are strongly involved in the quality of ABG.

This process alters garlic's organoleptic properties, making it sweeter and less pungent, and increases the concentration of bioactive compounds, such as S-allylcysteine, polyphenols, and flavonoids [21]. These compounds were found to be able to exert various beneficial effects, including the suppression of cell proliferative activity, as well as the stimulation of apoptosis and the modulation of the cell cycle, all of which are relevant in cancer prevention and treatment [22,23].

Interestingly, in the previous studies of ours, a water extract of ABG (ABGE) showed anti-inflammatory and antioxidant effects in preclinical models [24,25]. In particular, the protective effects induced by ABGE were suggested to be partly related to the polyphenolic content in the same extract, notably catechin and gallic acid [24,25]. We previously performed the quantification of polyphenolic content in the extract using high-performance liquid chromatography coupled with a photo diode array detector (HPLC-DAD) analytical method. In particular, various compounds were identified in ABGE, with gallic acid and catechin being the more representative phytochemicals [26].

This research aims to explore the potential benefits of ABGE on inflammation and prostate cancer. Building on these findings, we sought to explore the potential protective effects of ABGE against inflammation-induced prostate damage using an ex vivo experimental model, as well as its impact on prostate cancer cell lines through in vitro studies. We investigated the anti-inflammatory properties of ABGE using a well-established ex vivo model of inflammation composed of mouse prostate specimens exposed to *Escherichia coli* lipopolysaccharide (LPS) [26,27]. In this setting, we examined the gene expression levels of the key pro-inflammatory biomarkers, including *COX-2*, *NF-κB*, *TNF-α*, and *IL-6*. Furthermore, we assessed the potential therapeutic effects of ABGE on the prostate cancer cell lines using in vitro experimental models through functional parameters (colony formation, tumorsphere formation, and a migration assay) and molecular studies to evaluate the potential involvement of different signaling pathways, such as mitogen-activated protein kinase (MAPK), protein kinase B (AKT), Janus kinases/the signal transducer and activator of transcription proteins (JAK/STAT), and transforming growth factor (TGF-β).

2. Materials and Methods

2.1. Extraction and Sample Preparation of ABGE

Dried ABG cloves were provided by il Grappolo S.r.l. (Soliera, Modena, Italy). The preparation of ABGE followed the method described in the previous studies [24,28,29].

A detailed protocol is included in the Supplementary Materials.

2.2. Ex Vivo Studies

Adult C57BL/6 male mice (3 months old, weight 20–25 g, n = 25) were housed and maintained as described in the Supplementary Materials Section. The housing conditions and experimentation procedures were strictly in agreement with the European Community ethical regulations (EU Directive no. 26/2014) for the care of animals for scientific research. In agreement with the recognized principles of "Replacement, Refinement and Reduction in Animals in Research", prostate specimens were obtained as residual materials from the vehicle-treated mice randomized in our previous experiments, approved by the local ethical committee ('G. d'Annunzio' University, Chieti, Italy) and the Italian Health Ministry (Project no. 885/2018-PR).

Mouse sacrifice was performed by CO_2 inhalation (100% CO_2 at a flow rate of 20% of the chamber volume per min). After collection, the isolated prostate specimens were maintained in a humidified incubator with 5% CO_2 at 37 °C for 4 h, as previously described [26,30] and reported in the Supplementary Materials Section.

Total RNA was extracted from the prostate specimens using TRI reagent (Sigma-Aldrich, St. Louis, MO, USA) following the manufacturer's protocol. The gene expression of COX-2, NF-kB, TNF-α, and iNOS was quantified by real-time PCR with TaqMan probe-based chemistry, as previously described [27,31,32]. The detailed protocol can be found in the Supplementary Materials Section.

2.3. Cell Culture

Cell lines from control prostate (PNT-2), androgen-dependent PCa (LNCaP), and androgen-independent PCa (PC-3) (American Type Culture Collection, Manassas, VA, USA) were maintained in a humidified incubator with 5% CO_2 at 37 °C following the manufacturer's guidelines as previously outlined [33,34] (Supplementary Materials Section).

2.4. Cell Proliferation

Cell proliferation was evaluated using resazurin reagent (Canvax Biotech, Cordoba, Spain) [33]. Cell proliferation was measured at the start and after 24, 48, and 72 h of treatment (Supplementary Materials Section).

2.5. Clonogenic Assay

A clonogenic assay was performed on the LNCaP and PC-3 PCa cells treated with 1000 μg/mL of ABGE and incubated for 10 days. The results were expressed as a percentage of the number of colonies relative to the control [34] (Supplementary Materials Section).

2.6. Tumorsphere Formation

The tumorsphere formation assay was conducted as previously described on LNCaP and PC-3 [35,36]. A minimum of three experiments with two replicates for each condition were performed. The results are expressed as a percentage of tumorsphere area relative to the control [35] (Supplementary Materials Section).

2.7. Cell Migration Assay

Cell migration was assessed using a wound healing assay as previously detailed [33,35,36]. The results are presented as the percentage of the migration rate relative to the control. A minimum of three experiments with three replicates for each condition were performed. This experiment was conducted using PC-3 cell lines, but not LNCaP cells due to their lower migration capacity (Supplementary Materials Section).

2.8. Phosphorylation Array

Protein extracts from the LNCaP cells were collected in lysis buffer from 6-well plates after 24 h of treatment with 1000 μg/mL ABGE. The determination of protein content was conducted using a Pierce BCA Protein assay (ThermoFisher Scientific, Madrid, Spain) and adjusted with assay buffer. The data were normalized following the manufacturer's instructions. In brief, the membranes designed for the semi-quantitative detection of 55 phosphorylated human proteins, which are part of the MAPK, AKT, JAK/STAT, and TGF-β signaling pathways, were incubated with blocking buffer for 30 min at 25 °C. The array spots' densitometric analysis was performed using ImageJ software (version number 1.54j), with positive control spots used for normalization. The results are expressed as the log2 Fold Change in each protein signal relative to the control signal, with a log2 Fold Change of 0.2 set as the threshold [37] (Supplementary Materials Section).

2.9. Statistical Analysis

To calculate sample size, we performed power analysis by using G*Power 3.1.9.4 software (effect size = 0.6, $\alpha = 0.05$, power = 0.85) [38]. As for the ex vivo evaluations, the experimental procedures were performed by a researcher blinded to the treatment. All experiments were conducted at least three times independently ($n \geq 3$). The results from ex vivo and in vitro studies are expressed as means ± SEM. Statistical differences between the two groups were evaluated using either an unpaired parametric *t*-test or a nonparametric Mann–Whitney U test, depending on normality as determined by a Kolmogorov–Smirnov test. For comparisons involving more than two groups, a One-Way ANOVA was employed. Statistical significance was set at $p < 0.05$. All statistical analyses were performed using GraphPad Prism 9 (GraphPad Software, La Jolla, CA, USA).

3. Results and Discussion

In the present study, we aimed to study the potential effects of ABGE on proliferation, colony formation, tumor spheroid formation, cell migration, and the phosphorylation array in three prostate cell lines: PNT-2, LNCaP, and PC-3.

3.1. Ex Vivo Studies

Considering the critical role of chronic inflammation in PCa, we first investigated the potential beneficial activities exerted by ABGE (10–1000 μg/mL) as a validated experimental model of inflammation [24,39]. We studied the effects of ABGE on the gene expression of pro-inflammatory mediators, including *COX-2*, *NF-kB*, *TNF-α*, and *IL-6*, on isolated LPS-stimulated prostate specimens by RT-PCR. In this context, we found that

ABGE (10–1000 μg/mL) was able to inhibit gene expression of all the markers investigated, with 1000 μg/mL being the most effective dose (Figure 1a–d).

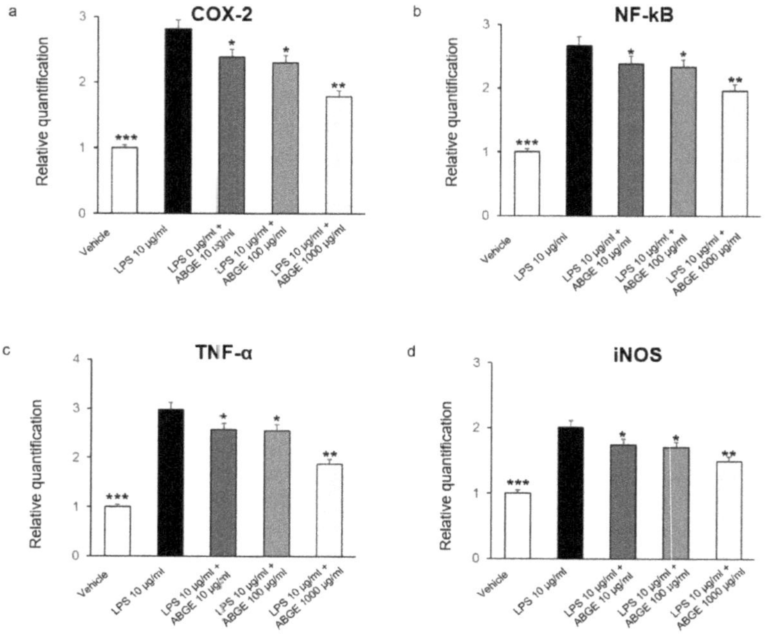

Figure 1. Effects of aged black garlic water extract (ABGE) (10–1000 μg/mL) on LPS-induced *cyclooxygenase (COX)-2* (**a**), *nuclear factor kappa (NF-κ) B* (**b**), *tumor necrosis factor (TNF)-α* (**c**), and *interleukin (IL)-6* (**d**) gene expression (RQ, relative quantification) in mouse prostate specimens. Data shown are means ± SEM of two independent experiments with triplicate determinations. ANOVA, * $p < 0.05$, ** $p < 0.005$; and *** $p < 0.001$ vs. LPS.

Various pro-inflammatory markers were shown to be implicated in prostatic inflammation. In this context, different phytochemicals, such as catechins, were found to modulate a number of inflammation targets, including TNF-α, COX-2, and interleukins. In the previous studies, we demonstrated that ABGE induced protective activities on colon and heart tissues treated ex vivo with LPS, which have been hypothesized to be related, at least partially, to its polyphenolic composition, with particular regards to gallic acid and catechin [24,25]. Accordingly, BenSaad et al. (2017) found that gallic acid suppressed the LPS-induced production of prostaglandin E2 and IL-6 in RAW264.7 cells [40].

Furthermore, we previously found that ABGE (1 g kg^{-1}) exerted protective effects in rats in vivo [25] in a dose which could be translated to 1 g day in humans.

3.2. Cell Proliferation in Basal Conditions

Cell proliferation was measured after 24, 48, and 72 h of the treatment with ABGE (10, 100, 500, and 1000 μg/mL) in basal conditions. The non-tumor prostate cell line PNT-2 was used as the control cell line. In the control prostate line PNT-2, ABGE (10–1000 μg/mL) did not affect cell proliferation more compared to that of the control group at any concentration at the different times. In agreement, we previously reported that ABGE did not modify the viability of cardiomyoblast (H9c2) cells or the human fibroblast HFF-1 cell line [24,25] (Figure 2a).

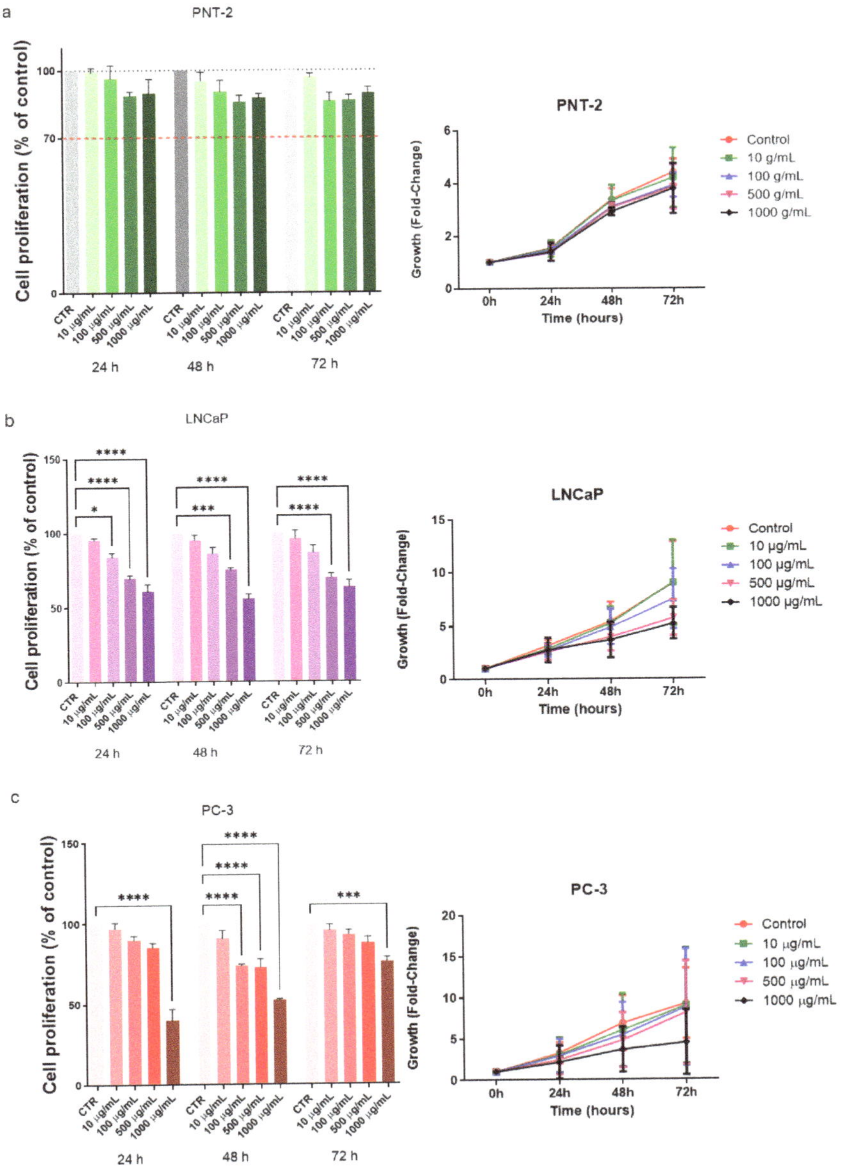

Figure 2. Effects of aged black garlic water extract (ABGE) on cell proliferation of control prostate (PNT-2) (**a**), androgen-dependent (LNCaP) (**b**), and androgen-independent (PC-3) (**c**) prostate cancer (PCa) cells. Cell proliferation and growth were evaluated by resazurin reagent after incubation for 24, 48, and 72 h of PNT-2, LNCaP, and PC-3 cell lines with ABGE at different concentrations (10, 100, 500, and 1000 µg/mL) or vehicle. Data shown are means ± SEM of 3 independent experiments with 3 replicates of each condition. ANOVA, * $p < 0.05$, *** $p = 0.001$, **** $p < 0.0001$ vs. vehicle.

The LNCaP cell line is derived from lymph node metastasis specimens of individuals with prostate cancer [41].

It retains the characteristics of prostate cancer tumor cytology as well as its early differentiation function, which represents the early androgen-dependent notable features of prostate cancer.

On the other hand, ABGE (10–1000 μg/mL) was able to significantly suppress LNCaP cell proliferation. Interestingly, the inhibitory effect on cell proliferation was dose-dependent, with a greater reduction at higher concentrations and longer exposure times (Figure 2b). Figure 2b shows inhibitory effects in cell proliferation after just 24 h, starting at a concentration of 100 μg/mL. The inhibition induced by the extract is also confirmed following 48 and 72 h of treatment at 500 and 1000 μg/mL concentrations.

The PC-3 cell line was isolated from human prostate cancer bone metastases with a low differentiation degree [42] and represents an androgen-independent prostate cancer cell with moderate metastatic potential in the absence of endogenous androgen receptors.

Similarly, the PC-3 cell line showed a significant reduction in cell proliferation following the treatment with ABGE (10–1000 μg/mL) compared to that of the control, with a greater decrease at higher concentrations (Figure 2c), thus confirming its antiproliferative activity also against androgen-independent cancer cells. After 48 h, we showed a significant decrease in cell proliferation starting from 100 μg/mL.

The mechanism underlying the inhibition of cell proliferation induced by ABGE is not yet clear. Dong and their collaborators (2014) demonstrated that an alcohol extract of ABG inhibited the growth of HT129 colon cancer cells probably by the inhibition of the PI3K/Akt pathway [22].

Additionally, Wang and their collaborators (2012) have demonstrated that aged black garlic water extract can inhibit the growth of gastric cancer cells in both in vitro and in vivo [23].

Moreover, an aged black garlic water extract showed dose-dependent apoptosis in human gastric cancer cell lines [23]. Notably, the extract in the prostate did not induce apoptosis in the LNCaP cells (Figure S1, Supplementary Materials).

Meanwhile, in vivo study highlighted the anti-cancer properties of the extract, including the inhibition of tumor growth in mice with tumors. The researchers proposed that the anti-cancer effects of the aged black garlic extract might be due to its antioxidant and immunomodulatory characteristics [23].

Multiple studies have indicated that black garlic possesses anti-tumor properties by inhibiting cell proliferation in both colon and gastric cancers. Jikihara et al. (2014) have performed an experiment using aged garlic extract on F344 rats and DLD-1 human colon cancer cells. The findings revealed antiproliferative effects in both adenoma and adenocarcinoma lesions [43].

3.3. Colony Formation

The analysis of the colony-forming ability of the LNCaP and PC-3 cell lines was performed after the treatment with ABGE (1000 μg/mL) or the vehicle. The highest concentration was chosen because it proved to be the most effective, while remaining biocompatible. In the LNCaP cell line (Figure 3a), the treatment with 1000 μg/mL of ABGE significantly reduced number of colonies formed compared to that of the control, suggesting that ABGE is effective in decreasing the long-term proliferative capacity of androgen-dependent cancer cells. Similarly, in the PC-3 cell line, the treatment with ABGE (1000 μg/mL) (Figure 3b) led to more inhibitory effects in colony formation compared to those of the control, further supporting the potential activity of the extract as an anti-tumor agent. These effects might be due to the presence of polyphenolic compounds in ABGE. In agreement, Jang et al. (2020) demonstrated that gallic acid can inhibit colony formation in various cancer cell lines [40].

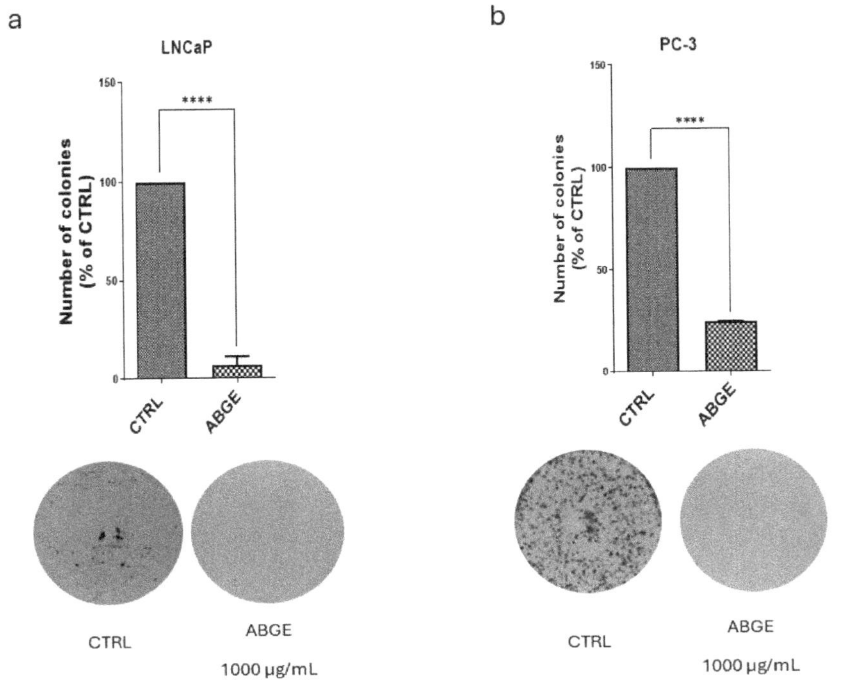

Figure 3. Effects of aged black garlic water extract (ABGE) on colony formation of LNCaP (**a**) and PC-3 (**b**) cell lines in response to ABGE at 1000 µg/mL or vehicle. Data shown are means ± SEM of 3 independent experiments with 3 replicates of each condition. ANOVA, **** $p < 0.0001$ vs. vehicle.

3.4. Tumor Spheroid Formation

Tumor spheroid formation was assessed by measuring the number of spheroids after the treatment with ABGE (1000 µg/mL) or the vehicle in the LNCaP and PC-3 cell lines. In the LNCaP cells (Figure 4a), the treatment with ABGE (1000 µg/mL) did not significantly affect the number of spheroids, which remained unchanged compared to that of the vehicle. However, our present findings also showed that in the PC-3 cells (Figure 4b), ABGE (1000 µg/mL) significantly reduced the number of spheroids compared to that of the control, suggesting that ABGE impedes the proliferation of cancer cells.

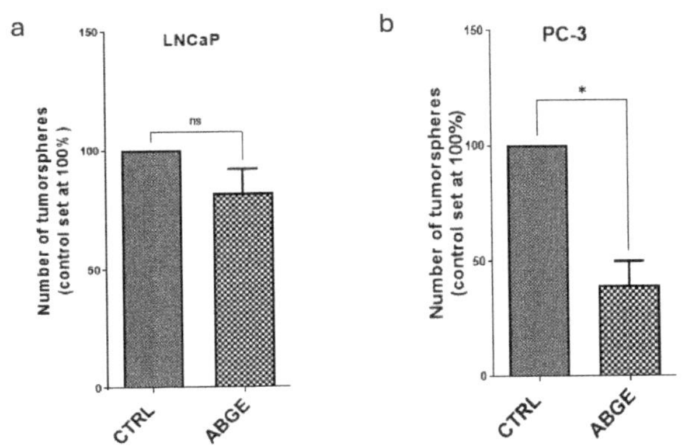

Figure 4. *Cont.*

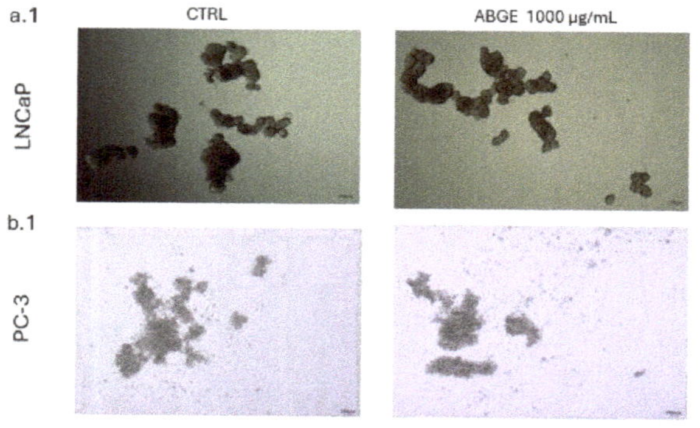

Figure 4. Effects of aged black garlic water extract (ABGE) on tumor spheroid formation of LNCaP (**a**,**a.1**) and PC-3 (**b**,**b.1**) cell line with ABGE at 1000 µg/mL or vehicle. Data shown are means ± SEM of 3 independent experiments with 3 replicates of each condition. ANOVA, * $p < 0.05$ vs. vehicle.

3.5. Migration Assay

The cell migration assay was conducted only on the PC-3 cell line because the morphology of LNCaP cells does not allow for accurate migration assessment. The treatment with 1000 µg/mL of ABGE more significantly reduced the cell migration rate compared to that of the control after 24 h of incubation. The reduction in cell migration in PC-3 (Figure 5) suggests that ABGE may also limit the capacity of cancer cells to spread. In agreement, recently, ABG (dissolved in 0.9% normal saline) extract was found able to impede cell migration in breast cancer cells [44].

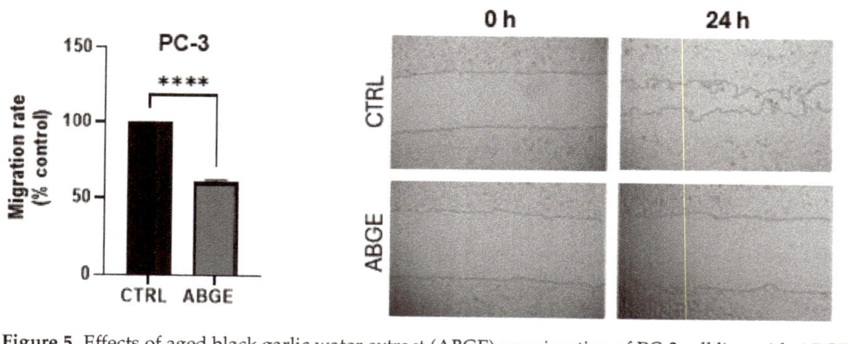

Figure 5. Effects of aged black garlic water extract (ABGE) on migration of PC-3 cell line with ABGE at 1000 µg/mL or vehicle for 24 h. Data shown are means ± SEM of 3 independent experiments with 3 replicates of each condition. ANOVA, **** $p < 0.0001$ vs. vehicle.

3.6. Cell Proliferation after LPS Pre-Treatment

Considering the previously found effects of ABGE into a pro-inflammatory cell context [18], we then decided to evaluate its potential interaction with LPS. We studied the effects of ABGE (10–1000 µg/mL) on LPS-treated cell proliferation in the PC-3 line (Figure 6), which was chosen for its higher aggressiveness compared to that of the LNCaP cell line, as supported by previous studies [45]. In this context, Xu and their collaborators (2021) showed that LPS combined with ATP significantly increased the proliferation and migration of PC-3 cells, reducing apoptosis. This effect was related to the stimulation of the NLRP3/caspase-1 inflammasome, hypothesizing that inflammation plays a crucial role in prostate cancer progression [8]. Interestingly, our data indicate that the LPS pre-treatment may sensitize the PCa cells to ABGE (Figure 6).

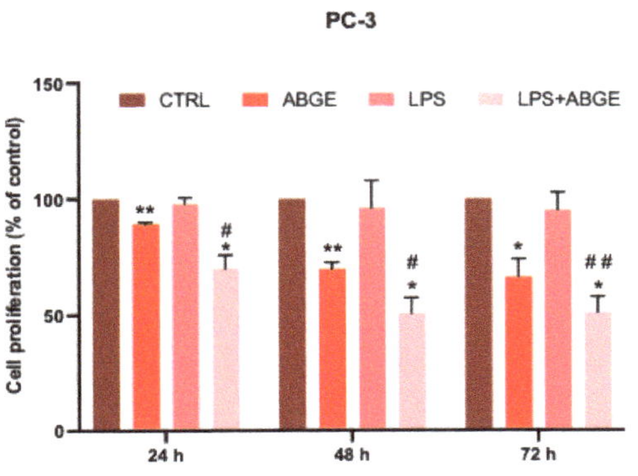

Figure 6. Effects of aged black garlic water extract (ABGE) in combination to LPS on cell proliferation of androgen-independent PC-3 cells. Cell proliferation was evaluated by resazurin reagent after incubation for 24, 48, and 72 h of PC-3 cell line with ABGE at 1000 μg/mL or vehicle. Data shown are means ± SEM of 3 independent experiments with 3 replicates of each condition. ANOVA, * $p < 0.05$, ** $p < 0.005$ vs. vehicle. ANOVA, # $p < 0.05$, ## $p < 0.005$ vs. ABGE.

Gallic acid and catechin, which are the main components of ABGE, as previously shown [24,25], are well known to suppress, proliferate, and stimulate the apoptosis of PCa cells [39,40].

Moreover, a previous study showed that gallic acid decreased the viability of PCa cell lines, but not normal cells' viability [46]. In agreement, we could suggest the potential involvement of polyphenolic compounds, with particular regards to gallic acid and catechin, due to the beneficial effects induced by ABGE on PCa proliferation.

3.7. Phosphorylation Array

A wide body of evidence shows that the MAPK, AKT, JAK/STAT, and TGF-β pathways play a key role in cell proliferation, survival, apoptosis, and growth [23,39–41]. In our study, we analyzed the phosphorylation of the key proteins that participate in these signaling pathways in response to the treatment with ABGE (1000 μg/mL) or the vehicle using a phosphorylation array.

Specifically, the MAPK signaling pathway showed significant modulation in response to the treatment with ABGE (Figure 7). Proteins such as ERK1/2 and JNK showed reduced phosphorylation, suggesting that ABGE (1000 μg/mL) could inhibit these signaling pathways. In this context, the MAPK signaling pathway is critically related to cell proliferation and survival [47]. Furthermore, the reduced phosphorylation of ERK1/2 (T202/Y204) and JNK (T183/Y185) suggests reduced cell proliferation and the potential inhibition of the apoptotic response [48].

p53 is involved in regulation of cell growth, DNA repair, survival, cycle, autophagy, senescence, and apoptosis [49,50].

After the injection of knockdown of ribosomal S6 protein kinases (RSK) 1 and RSK2 in mouse femurs, there was a reduction in osteolytic lesions in the PC3 cells compared to those in the control cells [51].

In our present study, we found that ABGE increased the quantity of LPS-treated p53, while decreased the RSK2 phosphorylation levels (Figure 7), which could be related to the anti-cancer properties of the extract.

The role of AKT signaling pathway in cell survival and growth is also well known [23]. ABGE (1000 μg/mL) showed variable effects on the phosphorylation of both the AKT and downstream proteins (Figure 8).

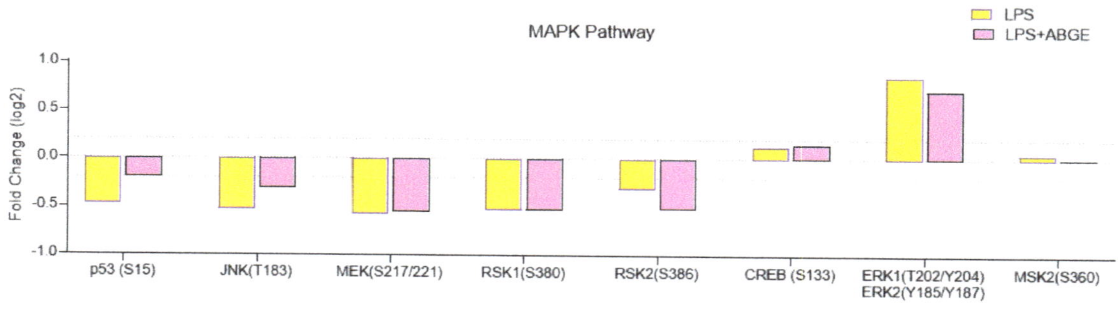

Figure 7. The MAPK signaling pathway in the phosphoprotein array in response to 24 h treatment of 1000 μg/mL ABGE. The log2 Fold Change in the phosphorylation protein level in comparison with that for the control condition (threshold: log2 Fold Change = 0.2).

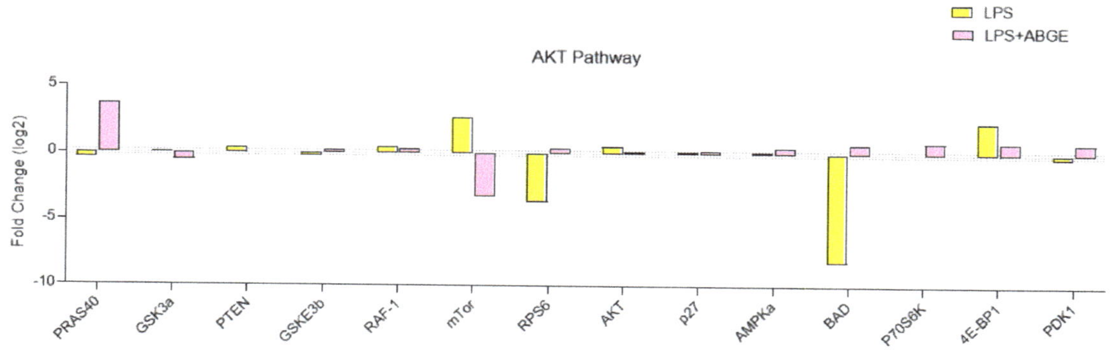

Figure 8. The AKT signaling pathway in the phosphoprotein array in response to 24 h treatment of 1000 μg/mL ABGE. The log2 Fold Change in the phosphorylation protein level in comparison with that for the control condition (threshold: log2 Fold Change = 0.2).

The reduced phosphorylation of mTOR suggests decreased protein synthesis and cell growth [52]. mTOR activation has been shown to induce the phosphorylation of many substrates, such as eukaryotic translation initiation factor 4E (eIF4E)-binding proteins (4E-BP1), and mTOR kinase inhibitors have been reported to block p4E-BP1 [53].

Our findings show that ABGE reduced the LPS-treated mTOR and 4E-BP1 phosphorylation levels. In agreement, considering that high levels of 4E-BP1 have been measured in prostate cancer cells, we can speculate that mTOR and 4E-BP1 could be involved, at least in part, in the beneficial effects induced by ABGE [54].

Moreover, ABGE also lowers the LPS-treated levels of glycogen synthase kinase (GSK)-3, phosphatase, tensin-homolog in chromosome 10 (PTEN), and serine/threonine kinase Raf-1 (RAF-1), which are involved in cancer development and progression [55–57].

On the other hand, ABGE increased the LPS-treated levels of p27 and AMP-activated protein kinase (AMPK), which possess a well-known suppressor role in carcinogenesis [58,59].

The JAK/STAT signaling pathway plays a key role in numerous essential biological processes, such as differentiation, cell proliferation, immune regulation, and apoptosis [48]. The inactivation of Src induced a reduction in the migration and growth in PCa cell lines [60,61].

In addition, the reduced phosphorylation of STAT1, STAT2, STAT3, and STAT5 (Figure 9) indicates a potential decrease in proliferative signaling and cancer development [62–65].

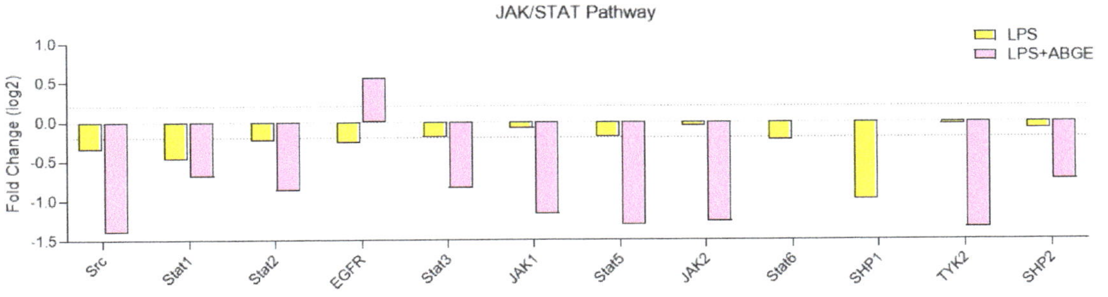

Figure 9. The JAK/STAT signaling pathway in the phosphoprotein array in response to 24 h treatment of 1000 μg/mL ABGE. The log2 Fold Change in the phosphorylation protein level in comparison with that for the control condition (threshold: log2 Fold Change = 0.2).

Moreover, the decreased phosphorylation of JAK1 and JAK2 suggests decreased signal transduction promoting prostate cancer cell proliferation and survival [66,67].

In agreement, TYK2 signaling promotes the invasiveness of prostate cancer cells [68].

Accordingly, the involvement of SHP2 in several cancer-related processes has been reported [69].

Actually, our findings, showing that ABGE decreased the LPS-treated Src, STAT1, STAT2, STAT3, STAT5, JAK1, JAK 2, TYK2, and SHP2 phosphorylation levels, could suggest the potential protective role of the extract in PC-3 cells.

Regarding the TGF-β pathway (Figure 10) involved in cell growth regulation and tumor progression [49], we showed that ABGE (1000 μg/mL) decreased the phosphorylation of SMAD1, suggesting reduced TGF-β signaling, which may be associated with reduced cell invasiveness [70].

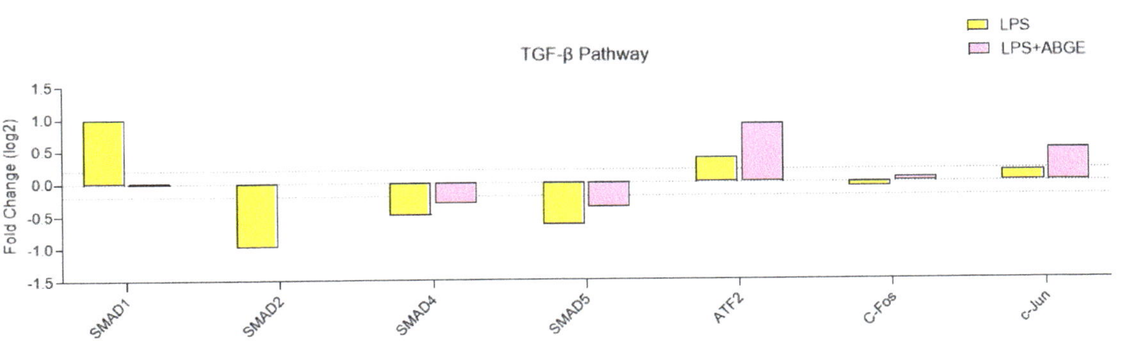

Figure 10. The TGF-β pathway in the phosphoprotein array in response to 24 h treatment of 1000 μg/mL ABGE. The log2 Fold Change in the phosphorylation protein level in comparison with that for the control condition (threshold: log2 Fold Change = 0.2).

The previous studies reported a correlation between SMAD2 and SMAD4, which are involved in the inhibition of cell growth [71].

ATF2 has been found as a tumor promoter in various human cancers, such as prostate cancer [72].

Furthermore, c-Jun or c-Fos overexpression has been directly related with PCa cell line invasiveness, and the phosphorylated c-Jun levels are high in PCa [73].

In our study, we showed that ABGE decreased the quantity of LPS-treated SMAD1, while it increased the SMAD2, SMAD4, AFT2, c-Jun, and c-Fos phosphorylation levels, further confirming the potential protective role of the extract.

In the literature, there are not many studies about the effects of ABGE on the prostate; thus, its mechanisms are not particularly well known.

4. Conclusions

In conclusion, our results showed the potential anti-inflammatory and anti-proliferative effects of ABGE on prostate cancer. In this context, ABGE reduced the gene expression of the different biomarkers involved in inflammatory response, such as *COX-2*, *TNF-α*, *IL-6*, and *NF-kB*, also modulating relevant signaling pathways, including AKT, MAPK, TGF-β, and JAK/STAT. Furthermore, we performed different in vitro assays, where ABGE had beneficial effects on both the prostate cancer lines. Therefore, our results suggest that ABGE might be potentially used as a diet supplement for health promotion and a source of bio-organic compounds with antitumor properties in PCa.

A limitation of our study is that we have not evaluated specific targeting, as well as the signaling pathways modulating the potential anti-inflammatory and anti-cancer effects of the extract. However, further studies are needed in the future to accurately evaluate the in vivo activity of ABGE in reducing inflammation and cancer, as well as its potential negative effects on the body.

Supplementary Materials: The following supporting information can be downloaded at: https://www.mdpi.com/article/10.3390/nu16173025/s1. Figure S1: Apoptosis induction in response to ABGE (1000 μg/mL) in LNCaP cells. Annexin V positive cells were considered as apoptotic. Annexin positivity was determined by flow cytometry (LSRFortessa SORP) with FITC Annexin V Apoptosis Detection Kit I (BD Pharmingen, San Jose, CA, USA; #556547) at 10 μg/mL in PBS. References [24,27–29,31–38] are cited in the supplementary materials.

Author Contributions: Conceptualization, M.L.L., L.R., R.M.L. and S.L.; methodology, M.L.L., A.J.M.-H., L.R., R.M.L., L.B. and S.L.; software, G.O., C.F. and L.M.; validation, G.O., C.F. and L.M.; formal analysis, M.L.L., A.J.M.-H.. D.G., A.A., G.O., C.F., L.M., S.C.D.S., N.N. and A.C.; investigation, M.L.L., A.J.M.-H., D.G., A.A., G.O., C.F., L.M., S.C.D.S., N.N. and A.C.; resources, M.L.L., A.J.M.-H., L.R., R.M.L., L.B. and S.L.; data curation, M.L.L., A.J.M.-H., L.R., R.M.L. and S.L.; writing—original draft preparation, M.L.L., L.R., L.B. and S.L.; writing—review and editing, M.L.L., A.J.M.-H., L.R., R.M.L. and S.L.; visualization, M.L.L., A.J.M.-H., L.R., R.M.L. and S.L.; supervision, L.R., R.M.L. and S.L.; project administration, L.R., R.M.L., L.B. and S.L.; funding acquisition, L.R., A.J.M.-H., R.M.L., L.B. and S.L. All authors have read and agreed to the published version of the manuscript.

Funding: This research was funded by il Grappolo S.r.l. 2021 (Soliera, Modena, Italy) (Grant 2021) (Principal Investigators: Luigi Brunetti, Sheila Leone, and Lucia Recinella), by MEDnoTE S.r.l. 2024 (Grant 2024) (Principal Investigator: Sheila Leone, Coordinators: Luigi Brunetti, Lucia Recinella and Maria Loreta Libero), and by the Spanish Ministry of Science, Innovation, and Universities (Research-Grant: PID2022-1381850B-I00; Predoctoral contracts: FPU18/02485).

Institutional Review Board Statement: The housing conditions and experimentation procedures were strictly in agreement with the European Community ethical regulations (EU Directive no. 26/2014) on the care of animals for scientific research. In agreement with the recognized principles of "Replacement, Refinement and Reduction in Animals in Research", the prostate specimens were obtained as residual materials from the vehicle-treated mice randomized in our previous experiments, approved on 23 November 2018 by the local ethical committee ('G. d'Annunzio' University, Chieti, Italy) and the Italian Health Ministry (Project no. 885/2018-PR).

Informed Consent Statement: Not applicable.

Data Availability Statement: The original contributions presented in the study are included in the article and Supplementary Materials, further inquiries can be directed to the corresponding authors request.

Conflicts of Interest: The authors declare that this study received funding from Grappolo S.r.l. and MEDnoTE S.r.l. The funders were not involved in the study design, collection, analysis, interpretation of data, the writing of this article or the decision to submit it for publication.

References

1. de Bono, J.S.; Guo, C.; Gurel, B.; De Marzo, A.M.; Sfanos, K.S.; Mani, R.S.; Gil, J.; Drake, C.G.; Alimonti, A. Prostate Carcinogenesis: Inflammatory Storms. *Nat. Rev. Cancer* **2020**, *20*, 455–469. [CrossRef] [PubMed]
2. Mantovani, A.; Allavena, P.; Sica, A.; Balkwill, F. Cancer-Related Inflammation. *Nature* **2008**, *454*, 436–444. [CrossRef] [PubMed]
3. Pérez-Gómez, J.M.; Montero-Hidalgo, A.J.; Fuentes-Fayos, A.C.; Sarmento-Cabral, A.; Guzmán-Ruiz, R.; Malagón, M.M.; Herrera-Martínez, A.D.; Gahete, M.D.; Luque, R.M. Exploring the Role of the Inflammasomes on Prostate Cancer: Interplay with Obesity. *Rev. Endocr. Metab. Disord.* **2023**, *24*, 1165–1187. [CrossRef]
4. Zhou, M.; Liang, J.; Hui, J.; Xu, J. Inflammation-Related Indicators Have a Potential to Increase Overall Quality of the Prostate Cancer Management: A Narrative Review. *Transl. Androl. Urol.* **2023**, *12*, 809–822. [CrossRef]
5. Oseni, S.O.; Naar, C.; Pavlović, M.; Asghar, W.; Hartmann, J.X.; Fields, G.B.; Esiobu, N.; Kumi-Diaka, J. The Molecular Basis and Clinical Consequences of Chronic Inflammation in Prostatic Diseases: Prostatitis, Benign Prostatic Hyperplasia, and Prostate Cancer. *Cancers* **2023**, *15*, 3110. [CrossRef]
6. Sessa, F.; Nicoletti, R.; De Nunzio, C.; Porreca, A.; Magrini, S.M.; Mirone, V.; Tubaro, A.; Serni, S.; Gontero, P.; Noale, M.; et al. Inflammation and Prostate Cancer: Pathological Analysis from Pros-IT CNR 2. *Cancers* **2023**, *15*, 630. [CrossRef] [PubMed]
7. Zhao, H.; Wu, L.; Yan, G.; Chen, Y.; Zhou, M.; Wu, Y.; Li, Y. Inflammation and Tumor Progression: Signaling Pathways and Targeted Intervention. *Signal Transduct. Target. Ther.* **2021**, *6*, 263. [CrossRef]
8. Xu, Z.; Wang, H.; Qin, Z.; Zhao, F.; Zhou, L.; Xu, L.; Jia, R. NLRP3 Inflammasome Promoted the Malignant Progression of Prostate Cancer via the Activation of Caspase-1. *Cell Death Discov.* **2021**, *7*, 399. [CrossRef]
9. Hou, J.; Karin, M.; Sun, B. Targeting Cancer-Promoting Inflammation—Have Anti-Inflammatory Therapies Come of Age? *Nat. Rev. Clin. Oncol.* **2021**, *18*, 261–279. [CrossRef]
10. Koliaraki, V.; Prados, A.; Armaka, M.; Kollias, G. The Mesenchymal Context in Inflammation, Immunity and Cancer. *Nat. Immunol.* **2020**, *21*, 974–982. [CrossRef]
11. Baud, V.; Karin, M. Signal Transduction by Tumor Necrosis Factor and Its Relatives. *Trends Cell Biol.* **2001**, *11*, 372–377. [CrossRef]
12. Sharma, J.; Gray, K.P.; Harshman, L.C.; Evan, C.; Nakabayashi, M.; Fichorova, R.; Rider, J.; Mucci, L.; Kantoff, P.W.; Sweeney, C.J. Elevated IL-8, TNF-α, and MCP-1 in Men with Metastatic Prostate Cancer Starting Androgen-Deprivation Therapy (ADT) Are Associated with Shorter Time to Castration-Resistance and Overall Survival. *Prostate* **2014**, *74*, 820–828. [CrossRef] [PubMed]
13. Liu, T.; Zhang, L.; Joo, D.; Sun, S.-C. NF-κB Signaling in Inflammation. *Signal Transduct. Target. Ther.* **2017**, *2*, 17023. [CrossRef] [PubMed]
14. Pai, S.; Thomas, R. Immune Deficiency or Hyperactivity-Nf-Kb Illuminates Autoimmunity. *J. Autoimmun.* **2008**, *31*, 245–251. [CrossRef]
15. Staal, J.; Beyaert, R. Inflammation and NF-κB Signaling in Prostate Cancer: Mechanisms and Clinical Implications. *Cells* **2018**, *7*, 122. [CrossRef]
16. Liu, X.-H.; Kirschenbaum, A.; Lu, M.; Yao, S.; Klausner, A.; Preston, C.; Holland, J.F.; Levine, A.C. Prostaglandin E(2) Stimulates Prostatic Intraepithelial Neoplasia Cell Growth through Activation of the Interleukin-6/GP130/STAT-3 Signaling Pathway. *Biochem. Biophys. Res. Commun.* **2002**, *290*, 249–255. [CrossRef]
17. Zha, S.; Gage, W.R.; Sauvageot, J.; Saria, E.A.; Putzi, M.J.; Ewing, C.M.; Faith, D.A.; Nelson, W.G.; De Marzo, A.M.; Isaacs, W.B. Cyclooxygenase-2 Is up-Regulated in Proliferative Inflammatory Atrophy of the Prostate, but Not in Prostate Carcinoma. *Cancer Res.* **2001**, *61*, 8617–8623.
18. Cragg, G.M.; Newman, D.J. Natural Products: A Continuing Source of Novel Drug Leads. *Biochim. Biophys. Acta* **2013**, *1830*, 3670–3695. [CrossRef]
19. Seca, A.M.L.; Pinto, D.C.G.A. Plant Secondary Metabolites as Anticancer Agents: Successes in Clinical Trials and Therapeutic Application. *Int. J. Mol. Sci.* **2018**, *19*, 263. [CrossRef] [PubMed]
20. Ahmed, T.; Wang, C.-K. Black Garlic and Its Bioactive Compounds on Human Health Diseases: A Review. *Molecules* **2021**, *26*, 5028. [CrossRef]
21. Ma, L.; Zhao, C.; Chen, J.; Zheng, J. Effects of Anaerobic Fermentation on Black Garlic Extract by Lactobacillus: Changes in Flavor and Functional Components. *Front. Nutr.* **2021**, *8*, 645416. [CrossRef]
22. Dong, M.; Yang, G.; Liu, H.; Liu, X.; Lin, S.; Sun, D.; Wang, Y. Aged Black Garlic Extract Inhibits HT29 Colon Cancer Cell Growth via the PI3K/Akt Signaling Pathway. *Biomed. Rep.* **2014**, *2*, 250–254. [CrossRef]
23. Wang, X.; Jiao, F.; Wang, Q.-W.; Wang, J.; Yang, K.; Hu, R.-R.; Liu, H.-C.; Wang, H.-Y.; Wang, Y.-S. Aged Black Garlic Extract Induces Inhibition of Gastric Cancer Cell Growth in Vitro and in Vivo. *Mol. Med. Rep.* **2012**, *5*, 66–72. [CrossRef] [PubMed]
24. Recinella, L.; Libero, M.L.; Citi, V.; Chiavaroli, A.; Martelli, A.; Foligni, R.; Mannozzi, C.; Acquaviva, A.; Di Simone, S.; Calderone, V.; et al. Anti-Inflammatory and Vasorelaxant Effects Induced by an Aqueous Aged Black Garlic Extract Supplemented with Vitamins D, C, and B12 on Cardiovascular System. *Foods* **2023**, *12*, 1558. [CrossRef]
25. Libero, M.L.; Lucarini, E.; Recinella, L.; Ciampi, C.; Veschi, S.; Piro, A.; Chiavaroli, A.; Acquaviva, A.; Nilofar, N.; Orlando, G.; et al. Anti-Inflammatory and Anti-Hyperalgesic Effects Induced by an Aqueous Aged Black Garlic Extract in Rodent Models of Ulcerative Colitis and Colitis-Associated Visceral Pain. *Phytother. Res.* **2024**, *38*, 4177–4188. [CrossRef] [PubMed]
26. Recinella, L.; Chiavaroli, A.; Orlando, G.; Ferrante, C.; Marconi, G.D.; Gesmundo, I.; Granata, R.; Cai, R.; Sha, W.; Schally, A.V.; et al. Antinflammatory, Antioxidant, and Behavioral Effects Induced by Administration of Growth Hormone-Releasing Hormone Analogs in Mice. *Sci. Rep.* **2020**, *10*, 732. [CrossRef]

27. Recinella, L.; Micheli, L.; Chiavaroli, A.; Libero, M.L.; Orlando, G.; Menghini, L.; Acquaviva, A.; Di Simone, S.; Ferrante, C.; Ghelardini, C.; et al. Anti-Inflammatory Effects Induced by a Polyphenolic Granular Complex from Olive (Olea Europaea, Mainly Cultivar Coratina): Results from In Vivo and Ex Vivo Studies in a Model of Inflammation and MIA-Induced Osteoarthritis. *Nutrients* **2022**, *14*, 1487. [CrossRef]
28. Fujisawa, H.; Suma, K.; Origuchi, K.; Seki, T.; Ariga, T. Thermostability of Allicin Determined by Chemical and Biological Assays. *Biosci. Biotechnol. Biochem.* **2008**, *72*, 2877–2883. [CrossRef]
29. Fujisawa, H.; Suma, K.; Origuchi, K.; Kumagai, H.; Seki, T.; Ariga, T. Biological and Chemical Stability of Garlic-Derived Allicin. *J. Agric. Food Chem.* **2008**, *56*, 4229–4235. [CrossRef]
30. Recinella, L.; Chiavaroli, A.; Orlando, G.; Menghini, L.; Ferrante, C.; Di Cesare Mannelli, L.; Ghelardini, C.; Brunetti, L.; Leone, S. Protective Effects Induced by Two Polyphenolic Liquid Complexes from Olive (Olea Europaea, Mainly Cultivar Coratina) Pressing Juice in Rat Isolated Tissues Challenged with LPS. *Molecules* **2019**, *24*, 3002. [CrossRef]
31. Recinella, L.; Libero, M.L.; Veschi, S.; Piro, A.; Marconi, G.D.; Diomede, F.; Chiavaroli, A.; Orlando, G.; Ferrante, C.; Florio, R.; et al. Effects of GHRH Deficiency and GHRH Antagonism on Emotional Disorders in Mice. *Cells* **2023**, *12*, 2615. [CrossRef] [PubMed]
32. Livak, K.J.; Schmittgen, T.D. Analysis of Relative Gene Expression Data Using Real-Time Quantitative PCR and the 2(-Delta Delta C(T)) Method. *Methods* **2001**, *25*, 402–408. [CrossRef]
33. Hormaechea-Agulla, D.; Gahete, M D.; Jiménez-Vacas, J.M.; Gómez-Gómez, E.; Ibáñez-Costa, A.; L-López, F.; Rivero-Cortés, E.; Sarmento-Cabral, A.; Valero-Rosa, J.; Carrasco-Valiente, J.; et al. The Oncogenic Role of the In1-Ghrelin Splicing Variant in Prostate Cancer Aggressiveness. *Mol. Cancer* **2017**, *16*, 146. [CrossRef]
34. Fuentes-Fayos, A.C.; G-García, M.E.; Pérez-Gómez, J.M.; Montero-Hidalgo, A.J.; Martín-Colom, J.; Doval-Rosa, C.; Blanco-Acevedo, C.; Torres, E.; Toledano-Delgado, Á.; Sánchez-Sánchez, R.; et al. Metformin and Simvastatin Exert Additive Antitumour Effects in Glioblastoma via Senescence-State: Clinical and Translational Evidence. *eBioMedicine* **2023**, *90*, 104484. [CrossRef] [PubMed]
35. Jiménez-Vacas, J.M.; Herrero-Aguayo, V.; Gómez-Gómez, E.; León-González, A.J.; Sáez-Martínez, P.; Alors-Pérez, E.; Fuentes-Fayos, A.C.; Martínez-López, A.; Sánchez-Sánchez, R.; González-Serrano, T.; et al. Spliceosome Component SF3B1 as Novel Prognostic Biomarker and Therapeutic Target for Prostate Cancer. *Transl. Res.* **2019**, *212*, 89–103. [CrossRef]
36. Del Rio-Moreno, M.; Alors-Perez, E ; Borges de Souza, P.; Prados-Gonzalez, M.E.; CastaÑo, J.P.; Luque, R.M.; Gahete, M.D. Peptides Derived from the Extracellular Domain of the Somatostatin Receptor Splicing Variant SST5TMD4 Increase Malignancy in Multiple Cancer Cell Types. *Transl Res.* **2019**, *211*, 147–160. [CrossRef]
37. León-González, A.J.; Sáez-Martínez, P.; Jiménez-Vacas, J.M.; Herrero-Aguayo, V.; Montero-Hidalgo, A.J.; Gómez-Gómez, E.; Madrona, A.; Castaño, J.P.; Espartero, J.L.; Gahete, M.D.; et al. Comparative Cytotoxic Activity of Hydroxytyrosol and Its Semisynthetic Lipophilic Derivatives in Prostate Cancer Cells. *Antioxidants* **2021**, *10*, 1348. [CrossRef]
38. Kang, H. Sample Size Determination and Power Analysis Using the G*Power Software. *J. Educ. Eval. Health Prof.* **2021**, *18*, 17. [CrossRef] [PubMed]
39. Sun, Y.; Liu, W.-Z.; Liu, T.; Feng, X.; Yang, N.; Zhou, H.-F. Signaling Pathway of MAPK/ERK in Cell Proliferation, Differentiation, Migration, Senescence and Apoptosis. *J. Recept. Signal Transduct. Res.* **2015**, *35*, 600–604. [CrossRef]
40. Jang, Y.-G.; Ko, E.-B.; Choi, K.-C. Gallic Acid, a Phenolic Acid, Hinders the Progression of Prostate Cancer by Inhibition of Histone Deacetylase 1 and 2 Expression. *J. Nutr. Biochem.* **2020**, *84*, 108444. [CrossRef]
41. Horoszewicz, J.S.; Leong, S.S.; Chu, T.M.; Wajsman, Z.L.; Friedman, M.; Papsidero, L.; Kim, U.; Chai, L.S.; Kakati, S.; Arya, S.K.; et al. The LNCaP Cell Line--a New Model for Studies on Human Prostatic Carcinoma. *Prog. Clin. Biol. Res.* **1980**, *37*, 115–132. [PubMed]
42. Sramkoski, R.M.; Pretlow, T.G.; Giaconia, J.M.; Pretlow, T.P.; Schwartz, S.; Sy, M.S.; Marengo, S.R.; Rhim, J.S.; Zhang, D.; Jacobberger, J.W. A New Human Prostate Carcinoma Cell Line, 22Rv1. *In Vitro Cell Dev. Biol. Anim.* **1999**, *35*, 403–409. [CrossRef]
43. Jikihara, H.; Qi, G.; Nozoe, K.; Hirokawa, M.; Sato, H.; Sugihara, Y.; Shimamoto, F. Aged Garlic Extract Inhibits 1,2-Dimethylhydrazine-Induced Colon Tumor Development by Suppressing Cell Proliferation. *Oncol. Rep.* **2015**, *33*, 1131–1140. [CrossRef] [PubMed]
44. BenSaad, L.A.; Kim, K.H.; Quah, C.C.; Kim, W.R.; Shahimi, M. Anti-Inflammatory Potential of Ellagic Acid, Gallic Acid and Punicalagin A&B Isolated from Punica Granatum. *BMC Complement. Altern. Med.* **2017**, *17*, 47. [CrossRef]
45. Tai, S.; Sun, Y.; Squires, J.M.; Zhang, H ; Oh, W.K.; Liang, C.-Z.; Huang, J. PC3 Is a Cell Line Characteristic of Prostatic Small Cell Carcinoma. *Prostate* **2011**, *71*, 1668–1679. [CrossRef]
46. Siddiqui, I.A.; Malik, A.; Adhami, V.M ; Asim, M.; Hafeez, B.B.; Sarfaraz, S.; Mukhtar, H. Green Tea Polyphenol EGCG Sensitizes Human Prostate Carcinoma LNCaP Cells to TRAIL-Mediated Apoptosis and Synergistically Inhibits Biomarkers Associated with Angiogenesis and Metastasis. *Oncogene* **2008**, *27*, 2055–2063. [CrossRef]
47. Recinella, L.; Chiavaroli, A.; Masciulli, F.; Fraschetti, C.; Filippi, A.; Cesa, S.; Cairone, F.; Gorica, E.; De Leo, M.; Braca, A.; et al. Protective Effects Induced by a Hydroalcoholic Allium Sativum Extract in Isolated Mouse Heart. *Nutrients* **2021**, *13*, 2332. [CrossRef]
48. Xin, P.; Xu, X.; Deng, C.; Liu, S.; Wang, Y.; Zhou, X.; Ma, H.; Wei, D.; Sun, S. The Role of JAK/STAT Signaling Pathway and Its Inhibitors in Diseases. *Int. Immunopharmacol.* **2020**, *80*, 106210. [CrossRef]
49. Senturk, S.; Mumcuoglu, M.; Gursoy-Yuzugullu, O.; Cingoz, B.; Akcali, K.C.; Ozturk, M. Transforming Growth Factor-Beta Induces Senescence in Hepatocellular Carcinoma Cells and Inhibits Tumor Growth. *Hepatology* **2010**, *52*, 966–974. [CrossRef]

50. Yoshida, K.; Miki, Y. The Cell Death Machinery Governed by the P53 Tumor Suppressor in Response to DNA Damage. *Cancer Sci.* **2010**, *101*, 831–835. [CrossRef]
51. Yu, G.; Lee, Y.-C.; Cheng, C.-J.; Wu, C.-F.; Song, J.H.; Gallick, G.E.; Yu-Lee, L.-Y.; Kuang, J.; Lin, S.-H. RSK Promotes Prostate Cancer Progression in Bone through ING3, CKAP2, and PTK6-Mediated Cell Survival. *Mol. Cancer Res.* **2015**, *13*, 348–357. [CrossRef] [PubMed]
52. Saxton, R.A.; Sabatini, D.M. mTOR Signaling in Growth, Metabolism, and Disease. *Cell* **2017**, *168*, 960–976. [CrossRef]
53. Morita, M.; Gravel, S.-P.; Hulea, L.; Larsson, O.; Pollak, M.; St-Pierre, J.; Topisirovic, I. mTOR Coordinates Protein Synthesis, Mitochondrial Activity and Proliferation. *Cell Cycle* **2015**, *14*, 473–480. [CrossRef] [PubMed]
54. Wang, K.; Wang, K.; Ma, Q. The Expression and Significance of p4E-BP1/4E-BP1 in Prostate Cancer. *J. Clin. Lab. Anal.* **2022**, *36*, e24332. [CrossRef]
55. Ougolkov, A.V.; Billadeau, D.D. Targeting Gsk-3: A Promising Approach For Cancer Therapy? *Future Oncol.* **2006**, *2*, 91–100. [CrossRef]
56. González-García, A.; Garrido, A.; Carrera, A.C. Targeting PTEN Regulation by Post Translational Modifications. *Cancers* **2022**, *14*, 5613. [CrossRef]
57. Nemoto, K.; Vogt, A.; Oguri, T.; Lazo, J.S. Activation of the Raf-1/MEK/Erk Kinase Pathway by a Novel Cdc25 Inhibitor in Human Prostate Cancer Cells. *Prostate* **2004**, *58*, 95–102. [CrossRef] [PubMed]
58. Li, R.; Wheeler, T.M.; Dai, H.; Sayeeduddin, M.; Scardino, P.T.; Frolov, A.; Ayala, G.E. Biological Correlates of P27 Compartmental Expression in Prostate Cancer. *J. Urol.* **2006**, *175*, 528–532. [CrossRef]
59. Keerthana, C.K.; Rayginia, T.P.; Shifana, S.C.; Anto, N.P.; Kalimuthu, K.; Isakov, N.; Anto, R.J. The Role of AMPK in Cancer Metabolism and Its Impact on the Immunomodulation of the Tumor Microenvironment. *Front. Immunol.* **2023**, *14*, 1114582. [CrossRef]
60. Nam, S.; Kim, D.; Cheng, J.Q.; Zhang, S.; Lee, J.-H.; Buettner, R.; Mirosevich, J.; Lee, F.Y.; Jove, R. Action of the Src Family Kinase Inhibitor, Dasatinib (BMS-354825), on Human Prostate Cancer Cells. *Cancer Res.* **2005**, *65*, 9185–9189. [CrossRef]
61. Chang, Y.-M.; Bai, L.; Liu, S.; Yang, J.C.; Kung, H.-J.; Evans, C.P. Src Family Kinase Oncogenic Potential and Pathways in Prostate Cancer as Revealed by AZD0530. *Oncogene* **2008**, *27*, 6365–6375. [CrossRef] [PubMed]
62. Jiang, Q.; Li, J.; Wang, J.; Zhang, W. Inhibition of CDKL3 Downregulates STAT1 Thus Suppressing Prostate Cancer Development. *Cell Death Dis.* **2023**, *14*, 189. [CrossRef] [PubMed]
63. Canar, J.; Darling, K.; Dadey, R.; Gamero, A.M. The Duality of STAT2 Mediated Type I Interferon Signaling in the Tumor Microenvironment and Chemoresistance. *Cytokine* **2023**, *161*, 156081. [CrossRef]
64. Gu, L.; Vogiatzi, P.; Puhr, M.; Dagvadorj, A.; Lutz, J.; Ryder, A.; Addya, S.; Fortina, P.; Cooper, C.; Leiby, B.; et al. Stat5 Promotes Metastatic Behavior of Human Prostate Cancer Cells in Vitro and in Vivo. *Endocr. Relat. Cancer* **2010**, *17*, 481–493. [CrossRef]
65. Mendoza-Rodríguez, M.G.; Sánchez-Barrera, C.Á.; Callejas, B.E.; García-Castillo, V.; Beristain-Terrazas, D.L.; Delgado-Buenrostro, N.L.; Chirino, Y.I.; León-Cabrera, S.A.; Rodríguez-Sosa, M.; Gutierrez-Cirlos, E.B.; et al. Use of STAT6 Phosphorylation Inhibitor and Trimethylglycine as New Adjuvant Therapies for 5-Fluorouracil in Colitis-Associated Tumorigenesis. *Int. J. Mol. Sci.* **2020**, *21*, 2130. [CrossRef]
66. Tam, L.; McGlynn, L.M.; Traynor, P.; Mukherjee, R.; Bartlett, J.M.S.; Edwards, J. Expression Levels of the JAK/STAT Pathway in the Transition from Hormone-Sensitive to Hormone-Refractory Prostate Cancer. *Br. J. Cancer* **2007**, *97*, 378–383. [CrossRef]
67. Gu, L.; Talati, P.; Vogiatzi, P.; Romero-Weaver, A.L.; Abdulghani, J.; Liao, Z.; Leiby, B.; Hoang, D.T.; Mirtti, T.; Alanen, K.; et al. Pharmacologic Suppression of JAK1/2 by JAK1/2 Inhibitor AZD1480 Potently Inhibits IL-6-Induced Experimental Prostate Cancer Metastases Formation. *Mol. Cancer Ther.* **2014**, *13*, 1246–1258. [CrossRef] [PubMed]
68. Ide, H.; Nakagawa, T.; Terado, Y.; Kamiyama, Y.; Muto, S.; Horie, S. Tyk2 Expression and Its Signaling Enhances the Invasiveness of Prostate Cancer Cells. *Biochem. Biophys. Res. Commun.* **2008**, *369*, 292–296. [CrossRef]
69. Zhang, J.; Zhang, F.; Niu, R. Functions of Shp2 in Cancer. *J. Cell Mol. Med.* **2015**, *19*, 2075–2083. [CrossRef]
70. Wu, J.; Zhang, M.; Faruq, O.; Zacksenhaus, E.; Chen, W.; Liu, A.; Chang, H. SMAD1 as a Biomarker and Potential Therapeutic Target in Drug-Resistant Multiple Myeloma. *Biomark. Res.* **2021**, *9*, 48. [CrossRef]
71. Miyaki, M.; Kuroki, T. Role of Smad4 (DPC4) Inactivation in Human Cancer. *Biochem. Biophys. Res. Commun.* **2003**, *306*, 799–804. [CrossRef] [PubMed]
72. Ma, J.; Chang, K.; Peng, J.; Shi, Q.; Gan, H.; Gao, K.; Feng, K.; Xu, F.; Zhang, H.; Dai, B.; et al. SPOP Promotes ATF2 Ubiquitination and Degradation to Suppress Prostate Cancer Progression. *J. Exp. Clin. Cancer Res.* **2018**, *37*, 145. [CrossRef] [PubMed]
73. Thomsen, M.K.; Bakiri, L.; Hasenfuss, S.C.; Wu, H.; Morente, M.; Wagner, E.F. Loss of JUNB/AP-1 Promotes Invasive Prostate Cancer. *Cell Death Differ.* **2015**, *22*, 574–582. [CrossRef] [PubMed]

nutrients

MDPI

Article

Effects of *Castanopsis echinocarpa* on Sensorineural Hearing Loss via Neuronal Gene Regulation

Isabel Rodriguez [1,†], Youn Hee Nam [2,†], Sung Woo Shin [1], Gyeong Jin Seo [1], Na Woo Kim [2], Wanlapa Nuankaew [1], Do Hoon Kim [1], Yu Hwa Park [1], Hwa Yeon Lee [1], Xi Hui Peng [3], Bin Na Hong [2,*] and Tong Ho Kang [1,*]

[1] Department of Oriental Medicine Biotechnology, Graduate School of Biotechnology, Kyung Hee University, Global Campus, Yongin 17104, Republic of Korea; isabelula3r@gmail.com (I.R.); 01073205620@khu.ac.kr (S.W.S.); seogj115@gmail.com (G.J.S.); wanlapa.nuankaew@gmail.com (W.N.); kdh2@dkpharm.co.kr (D.H.K.); pyh@dkpharm.co.kr (Y.H.P.); lllhy8024@naver.com (H.Y.L.)

[2] Invivotec Co., Ltd., Seongnam 13449, Republic of Korea; 01030084217@hanmail.net (Y.H.N.); nawookim@invivotec.com (N.W.K.)

[3] Department of Garden, Xishuangbanna Tropical Botanical Garden, Chinese Academy of Sciences, Menglun 666303, China; xihuipeng@xtbg.ac.cn

* Correspondence: habina22@hanmail.net (B.N.H.); panjae@khu.ac.kr (T.H.K.)

† These authors contributed equally to this work.

Abstract: Sensorineural hearing loss (SNHL), characterized by damage to the inner ear or auditory nerve, is a prevalent auditory disorder. This study explores the potential of *Castanopsis echinocarpa* (CAE) as a therapeutic agent for SNHL. In vivo experiments were conducted using zebrafish and mouse models. Zebrafish with neomycin-induced ototoxicity were treated with CAE, resulting in otic hair cell protection with an EC_{50} of 0.49 μg/mL and a therapeutic index of 1020. CAE treatment improved auditory function and protected cochlear sensory cells in a mouse model after noise-induced hearing loss (NIHL). RNA sequencing of NIHL mouse cochleae revealed that CAE upregulates genes involved in neurotransmitter synthesis, secretion, transport, and neuronal survival. Real-time qPCR validation showed that NIHL decreased the mRNA expression of genes related to neuronal function, such as *Gabra1*, *Gad1*, *Slc32a1*, *CaMK2b*, *CaMKIV*, and *Slc17a7*, while the CAE treatment significantly elevated these levels. In conclusion, our findings provide strong evidence that CAE protects against hearing loss by promoting sensory cell protection and enhancing the expression of genes critical for neuronal function and survival.

Keywords: sensorineural hearing loss; *Castanopsis echinocarpa*; ototoxicity; noise-induced hearing loss; neuronal function and survival

1. Introduction

Sensorineural hearing loss (SNHL) is a major global health concern, with its prevalence significantly increasing over the past decade. This rise appears to be correlated with increased exposure to hazardous noise levels in daily life, ototoxic agents, and aging [1]. Currently, more than 466 million people worldwide suffer from hearing loss, which is projected to keep rising. Notably, excessive occupational noise exposure is a critical health hazard, accounting for 16% of adult hearing loss cases, as reported by the World Health Organization [2].

Auditory functions require complex interactions among the sensory cells in the inner ear, specifically involving otic hair cells and spiral ganglion neurons. In noise-induced hearing loss (NIHL), high-frequency sounds damage the cochlear sensory cells, which lack the capacity to regenerate [3]. Therefore, hearing loss prevention strategies are crucial to attenuate cochlear sensory cell loss by blocking several cellular mechanisms that contribute to premature hearing impairment [4–6]. Recently, neuroprotective drugs, antioxidants, anti-inflammatory, and anti-apoptotic agents have been widely used to improve hearing deficits in NIHL [7]. Specifically, polyphenols have been shown to protect sensory cells and improve hearing function [8,9]. However, natural products have not been studied extensively as potential treatments. Thus, we have been studying natural products with high polyphenol content as candidates for hearing loss prevention [10,11].

Recently, growing research has focused on herbal species as multi-target approaches to treat sensorineural hearing loss in vitro and in vivo. Currently, clinical trials have been carried out using different traditional herbs, including *Ginkgo biloba*, *Panax ginseng*, and *Astragalus propinquus* [12]. The molecular mechanisms of natural products on protection and recovery from auditory insults involve targeting several pathophysiological states such as oxidative damage, inflammation, disruption of ion homeostasis, pro-apoptotic and apoptotic mediators, and decreased survival regulation. Such a multi-target approach on the inner ear makes natural products important for drug discovery on hearing impairments [12]. We previously demonstrated SNHL amelioration by using natural products. To name a few, *Curculigo orchioides* showed protective efficacy from ototoxicity through a reduction in oxidative stress and increased scavenging activity against free radicals in vitro [13] and improved auditory function on NIHL in vivo [14]; *Scutellaria baicalensis* showed improved auditory function on different models of SNHL in vivo through lipoxygenase inhibition [11]; and avocado oil (*Persea ameriacana*) demonstrated efficacy against SNHL in vitro and in vivo by reducing the altered gene expression related to oxidative stress, cytokine production, and protein synthesis [15].

After extensive screening, we identified *Castanopsis echinocarpa* (CAE)'s potential as a therapy for SNHL. Despite recent interest in Castanopsis species, they have not yet been widely studied. The leaves of these species are reported to be rich in polyphenols, such as galloyl quinic acids, triterpene hexahydroxydiphenoyl esters, ellagitannins, phenol glucosides, condensed tannins, and flavonol glycosides. Some species have already been reported to possess powerful antioxidant properties, effective against oxidative stress and inflammation and preventive against apoptosis [16–19]. Currently, no studies have investigated Castanopsis species in the context of SNHL, and specifically, CAE has not reported any pharmacological activity. Therefore, our aim is to demonstrate CAE's efficacy on different models of SNHL in vivo and to elucidate its mode of action.

In this study, we investigated the protective effect of CAE on different models of SNHL in vivo, using the neomycin (NM)-induced ototoxicity model in zebrafish and the NIHL model in mice. CAE demonstrated significant improvement in auditory function and protective effects on auditory structures. To further assess CAE's mechanism of action, we identified differentially expressed genes in the cochlea of NIHL mice treated with CAE using RNA sequencing. Then, for data validation, we performed real-time quantitative PCR. We found that the protective effect of CAE on SNHL might be explained by the up-regulation of gene expression related to neural functions, such as genes involved in neurotransmitter synthesis, transport and release, and neuronal survival.

Recent research has demonstrated that the loss of hearing function is also related to the damage in synaptic connections among cochlear hair cells and spiral ganglion neurons; such damage can occur much earlier than otic hair cell death [20]. This study thus proposes a therapeutic approach based on recent perspectives to treat hearing impairments.

2. Materials and Methods

2.1. Plant Collection and Voucher Specimen Information

The plant extract of *Castanopsis echinocarpa* Miq. (FBM070-066) used in this research was obtained from the International Biological Material Research Center at the Korea Research Institute of Bioscience and Biotechnology (Daejeon, Republic of Korea). The plant was collected in Menglun Mengla district, Xishuangbanna, Yunnan province of China, in December 2009. A voucher specimen (KRIB 0062375) is kept in the herbarium of the Korea Research Institute of Bioscience and Biotechnology.

2.2. Extraction Procedure for Castanopsis Echinocarpa (CAE)

The raw material was stored at room temperature until extraction. The extraction process comprised two phases. Initially, we placed 1 kg of the aerial parts in a commercial extractor (KS220, Kyungseo E&P Co., Ltd., Incheon, Republic of Korea) with 8 L of 70% ethanol for 2 h. Subsequently, an additional 4 L of 70% ethanol was added, and the extraction continued for another hour. The extract was filtered and concentrated, then frozen at −50 °C for 24 h and freeze-dried in a rotary evaporator (HS-2001NS, Hahanshin Scientific, Gimpo-si, Republic of Korea) for 7 days. The final yield of CAE was 15.5%, and the product was stored at −20 °C.

2.3. Animals

Adult zebrafish (*Danio rerio*), wild-type strain, were housed in an S-type 1500(W) × 400(D) × 2050(H) mm system (WoojungBio, Inc., Suwon, Republic of Korea). Spawning and egg collection followed established protocols [15]. Embryos were maintained under a 14 h light/10 h dark cycle at 28.5 °C ± 0.5 until 6 days post-fertilization, after which they were randomly selected for experiments.

Six-week-old male mice, ICR strain, were obtained from Orient Bio, Inc. (Seongnam, Republic of Korea). They were housed under a 12 h light/dark cycle with food and water ad libitum and environmental conditions as follows: 23.0 ± 2.0 °C temperature and 50.0 ± 5.0% humidity. Following a week of acclimation, mice were evaluated by auditory brainstem response (ABR) test to confirm normal hearing (≤25 dB), representing the inclusion criteria as described in previous studies [15].

2.4. Ethical Statement

All the procedures involving zebrafish and mice were conducted following protocols approved by the Animal Care and Use Committee of Kyung Hee University [KHUASP-21-230 and KHUASP-21-229, respectively].

2.5. Neomycin-Induced Ototoxicity in a Zebrafish Model

Zebrafish larvae were exposed to Neomycin sulfate (MB Cell Co., Irvine, CA, USA) to induce ototoxicity, following established methods [15]. Post-exposure, larvae were first rinsed and then treated with 0.03% sea salt solution and CAE for 6 h at 28 °C, respectively. Post-treatment, larvae were stained with 0.1% YO-PRO-1 (Thermo Fisher Scientific Inc., Waltham, Massachusetts, USA) for 30 min for otic hair cell visualization, anesthetized with 0.04% tricaine, and examined using a fluorescence microscope (Olympus 1 × 70; Olympus Co., Tokyo, Japan). Images were analyzed with Focus Lite software (Focus Co., Daejeon, Republic of Korea).

2.6. The 50% Effective Concentration (EC_{50})

Varying concentrations (0.01 to 10 μg/mL) of CAE were defined to treat zebrafish larvae. EC_{50} values were determined by non-linear regression using GraphPad Prism version 5.01 software (Graph Pad Software, San Diego, CA, USA).

2.7. The 50% Lethal Concentration (LC_{50})

Varying concentrations (50 to 1000 μg/mL) of CAE were defined to treat zebrafish larvae. LC_{50} values were determined by non-linear regression using GraphPad Prism version 5.01 software (Graph Pad Software, San Diego, CA, USA).

2.8. Therapeutic Index (TI)

The therapeutic index (TI) was calculated to define the safety margin of CAE.

$$TI = LC_{50}/EC_{50}$$

2.9. Noise-Induced Hearing Loss (NIHL) in Mice

NIHL procedures were performed as previously described [15]. Briefly, mice were exposed to 115 dB sound pressure level (SPL) broadband noise (100 Hz to 10 kHz) for 90 min. Post-exposure, mice were divided into four groups (n = 10/group) and treated orally once a day, as follows: control (0.3 mL distilled water), 100 mg/kg (CAE 100), 300 mg/kg (CAE 300), and 500 mg/kg (CAE 500) of CAE in distilled water, starting one day after noise exposure.

2.10. Auditory Brainstem Response (ABR) Test

Auditory function was measured using channel recording (Intelligent Hearing Systems, Miami, FL, USA) as previously described [15]. Hearing thresholds were evaluated with ABR using clicks, 8 kHz, and 16 kHz stimuli at 1, 10, and 20 days post-noise exposure.

2.11. Evaluation of Otoprotective Effects of Cochlear Hair Cells

After 20 days of drug administration, the cochleae were harvested, fixed, decalcified, and microdissected as described previously [15]. Cochleae were stained for hair cell visualization with 5 U/mL rhodamine phalloidin (Thermo Fisher Scientific Inc., Gainesville, FL, USA), and outer hair cells (OHCs) at the apex, middle, and base of the cochlea were identified and counted in a 1 mm strip. Hair cells were evaluated in three groups: control, NIHL, and NIHL + CAE (n = 6 per group) using fluorescence microscopy.

2.12. mRNA Sequencing and Pathway Analysis

Twenty days post-administration, the cochleae were harvested for RNA extraction using TRIzol™ reagent (Thermo Fisher Scientific Korea Ltd., Seoul, Republic of Korea) and purified with a RNeasy mini kit (QIAGEN, Hilden, Germany). For sampling, both right and left cochleae were collected from 3 animals in each group. RNA quality and quantity were assessed using an Agilent 2100 Bioanalyzer (Agilent, Santa Clara, CA, USA). Sequencing libraries were prepared with the TruSeq Stranded mRNA Sample Preparation kit (Illumina, San Diego, CA, USA) per the manufacturer's instructions. Libraries were evaluated with an Agilent 2100 bioanalyzer and quantified by qPCR using the CFX96 Real Time System (Bio-Rad, Hercules, CA, USA), then sequenced on a NextSeq500 sequencer (Agilent, Santa Clara, CA, USA) with a paired-end 75 bp plus single 8 bp index read run. The raw data from the RNA analysis were converted into sequence data and stored as FASTQ files. Differentially expressed genes (DEGs) were determined based on an absolute fold change (FC) greater than 1.4 and a $p < 0.05$. Reactome Pathway analysis was performed to identify significant DEGs using Enrichr (2016) [21]. The 3 animals per group were pooled into 1 biological replicate.

2.13. Quantitative PCR (qPCR)

Twenty days post-administration, total RNA was extracted from mice cochleae using TRIzol™ reagent (Thermo Fisher Scientific Korea Ltd., Seoul, Republic of Korea) per the manufacturer's protocol. Briefly, 1 μg of total RNA was reverse-transcribed using the RevertAid First Strand cDNA Synthesis Kit (Thermo Fisher Scientific Korea Ltd., Seoul, Republic of Korea). Relative mRNA expression was measured by qPCR, normalized to *β-actin*. qPCR reactions contained 5 μL SYBR Select Master Mix (Applied Biosystems, Thermo Fisher Scientific Korea Ltd., Seoul, Republic of Korea), 1 μL cDNA template, 1 μL each of forward and reverse primers (10 pmol each), and 2 μL RNAse-free water. The qPCR parameters were initial denaturation at 95 °C for 5 min, followed by 45 cycles of 95 °C for 15 s, 60 °C for 15 s, and 72 °C for 20 s, with a melting step at 73 °C for 5 min. Gene expression was analyzed using the $2-\Delta\Delta Ct$ method. Primer sequences are listed in Table 1.

Table 1. Primers for qPCR.

Gene Name	Forward Sequence	Reverse Sequence
β-Actin	GAAGAGCTATGAGCTGCCTGA	TGATCCACATCTGCTGGAAGG
Gabra1	AATGGGCGGATTGGTGTC	TCATCTTGGGAGGGCTGT
Gad1	GCCTGGAAGAGAAGAGTCGT	TCCCCGTTCTTAGCTGGAAG
Slc17a7	TGGCTGTGTCATCTTCGTGAGG	TTGCCAGCCGACTCCGTTCTAA
Camk4	GGAGAAGGGATACTACAGTGAGC	CTGGTTTGAGGTCACGATGGAC
Camk2b	CCTACGGCAAACCTGTGGACAT	GCCTTGATCTGCTGGTACAGCT
Slc32a1	GGCTGGAACGTGACAAATGCCA	TACAGGCACGCGATGAGGATCT

2.14. Statistical Analyses

Statistical analyses were performed using GraphPad Prism version 5.01 software (GraphPad Software, San Diego, CA, USA). All data are expressed as the mean ± standard error of the mean (SEM). The statistical significance between groups was determined using a paired *t*-test or a one-way repeated measures ANOVA followed by Tukey's post hoc test. Statistical significance was set at $p < 0.05$.

3. Results

3.1. CAE's Efficacy on Otic Hair Cell Protection after NM-Induced Ototoxicity in Zebrafish

The efficacy of CAE on otic neuromast hair cell protection was assessed following exposure to the ototoxic drug neomycin (NM) using zebrafish. Hair cells within the otic (O1) neuromast were damaged after NM exposure (Figure 1). NM exposure significantly reduced ($p < 0.001$) the number of otic hair cells. In contrast, the CAE treatment significantly promoted hair cell protection in a dose-dependent manner ($p < 0.05$, $p < 0.01$, and $p < 0.001$) compared to the control. These findings indicate that CAE is effective in facilitating otic hair cell protection following ototoxicity induced by NM.

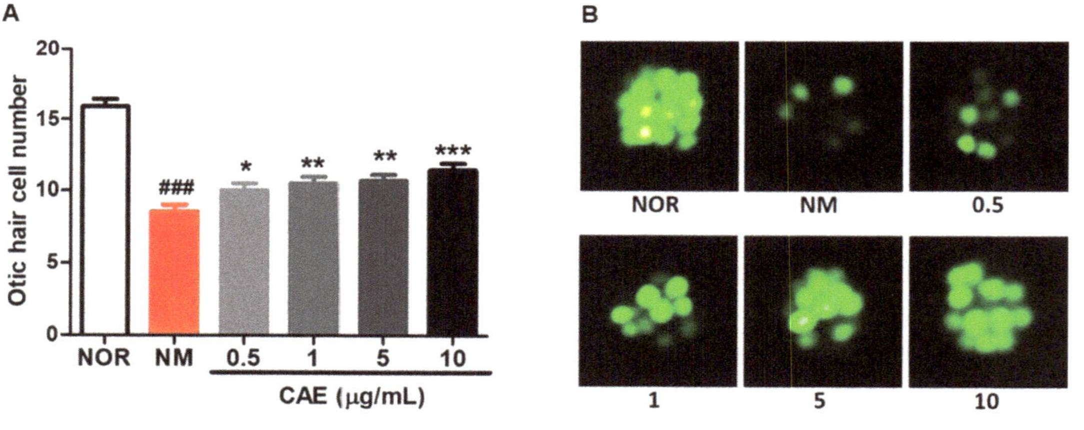

Figure 1. CAE's efficacy on otic hair cell protection after neomycin-induced ototoxicity in zebrafish model. (**A**) Number of otic hair cells in the untreated group (NM) and the treated groups (0.5, 1, 5, and 10 μg/mL of CAE). (**B**) Fluorescence images of otic hair cells in the normal (NOR), control (NM), and treated groups. Hair cells were stained with YO-PRO-1 at 0.1%. Data are presented as means ± SEM. * $p < 0.05$, ** $p < 0.01$, *** $p < 0.001$ (control vs. treated groups). ### $p < 0.001$ (normal vs. control group). $n = 10$ per group.

3.2. EC_{50}, LC_{50}, and TI Values of CAE in Zebrafish

To determine the EC_{50} value of CAE in NM-induced ototoxicity, a dose–response curve was generated for CAE-treated zebrafish at varying concentrations (0.01 to 10 μg/mL). The EC_{50} value of CAE was defined as 0.497 μg/mL (Figure 2A).

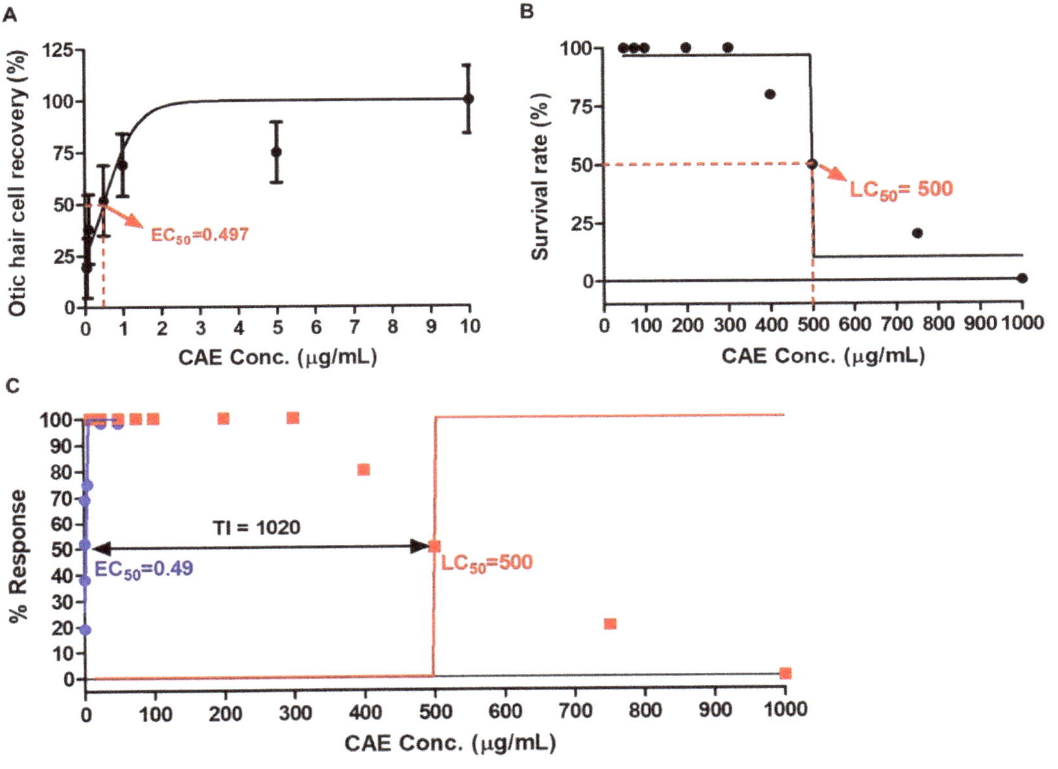

Figure 2. Dose–response curves and therapeutic index of CAE. (**A**) The EC_{50} value of CAE in neomycin (NM)-induced ototoxicity was defined as 0.497 μg/mL. (**B**) The LC_{50} value of zebrafish embryos exposed to CAE for 48 h was defined as 500 μg/mL. (**C**) The therapeutic index (TI) of CAE was calculated to be 1020, indicating a high level of drug safety. Data are presented as means ± SEM. Conc. = concentration; EC_{50} = 50% effective concentration; LC_{50} = 50% lethal concentration. $n = 10$ per group for EC_{50}; $n = 20$ per group for LC_{50}.

To assess the LC_{50} value, mortality rates were examined in zebrafish exposed to CAE at varying concentrations (50 to 1000 μg/mL). The LC_{50} value of CAE was defined as 500 μg/mL (Figure 2B).

The therapeutic index (TI) of CAE was then calculated; TI is defined as the ratio of LC_{50} to EC_{50} (LC_{50}/EC_{50}). The TI is an index of drug safety, with higher TI values indicating greater safety. The TI of CAE was calculated to be 1020, indicating a high level of therapeutic safety for the use of CAE (Figure 2C).

3.3. Toxicity Evaluation of CAE

To evaluate CAE toxicity in zebrafish embryos, we investigated the hatching rate, heartbeat, body length, and morphological changes in zebrafish embryos after 48 h of exposure (Figure 3). A significant decrease in the hatching rate was observed in zebrafish treated with CAE at concentrations of 500 μg/mL or higher. However, no significant differences were detected between the CAE-treated and non-treated groups at concentrations up to 400 μg/mL (Figure 3A). Additionally, no significant differences were found in the heartbeat and body length of zebrafish treated with CAE compared to the non-treated group at concentrations up to 400 μg/mL (Figure 3B,C). These results indicate that CAE does not exhibit toxicity at concentrations up to 400 μg/mL.

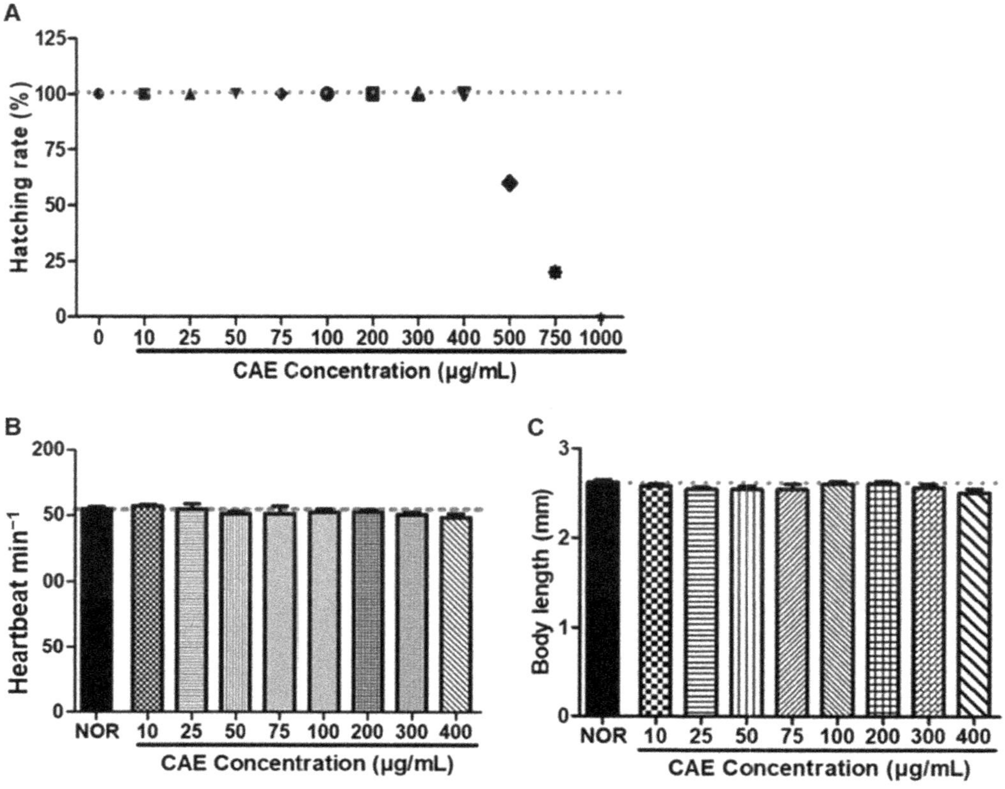

Figure 3. Toxicity evaluation of CAE based on zebrafish embryo testing. Data represent 48 h of exposure. (**A**) Hatching rate of zebrafish embryos exposed to CAE at varying concentrations: 10–1000 μg/mL. (**B**) Heartbeat rate (beats per minute) of zebrafish treated with CAE at varying concentrations: 10–400 μg/mL. (**C**) Body length of zebrafish treated with CAE at varying concentrations: 10–400 μg/mL. Data are presented as means ± SEM. $n = 20$ per group.

3.4. CAE Effects on Auditory Function in NIHL Mouse Model

We assessed the impact of CAE on auditory function using the auditory brainstem response (ABR) test (Figure 4). The ABR thresholds prior to noise exposure were within normal ranges across the evaluated frequencies for all mice included in this study. Threshold shifts were elevated on day 1 post-noise exposure. However, 20 days post-administration of CAE treatment at various concentrations, the threshold shifts significantly decreased ($p < 0.05$, $p < 0.01$, and $p < 0.001$) compared to the control group in response to click, 8 kHz, and 16 kHz stimuli. Additionally, CAE exhibited a dose-dependent efficacy for click thresholds (Figure 4A). In contrast, at 8 and 16 kHz, the 100 μg/mL CAE treatment demonstrated a greater effect than higher concentrations (Figure 4B,C).

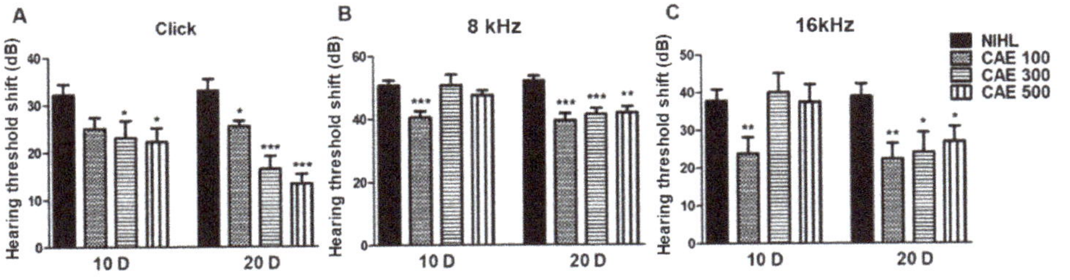

Figure 4. Effects of CAE on auditory function in NIHL mouse model. No-treatment (NIHL) and CAE-treated groups were compared. Auditory brainstem response (ABR) threshold shifts with click stimulus (**A**), 8 kHz tone burst (**B**), and 16 kHz tone burst (**C**) in mouse model at 10 days (10 D) and 20 days (20 D) after noise insult. Data are presented as means ± SEM. * $p < 0.05$, ** $p < 0.01$, *** $p < 0.001$ (NIHL group vs. CAE-treated groups). CAE 100, 100 mg/kg; CAE 300, 300 mg/kg; CAE 500, 500 mg/kg. $n = 10$ per group.

3.5. CAE Alleviation of Cochlear Hair Cell Damage in NIHL Mice

Given that CAE at 100 mg/kg demonstrated superior efficacy in improving hearing function, we evaluated its effects on cochlear hair cells at the apex, middle, and base following noise-induced damage (Figure 5). Noise exposure resulted in a significant loss of outer hair cells (OHCs) in the NIHL group ($p < 0.01$, $p < 0.001$), particularly in the base of the cochlea (Figure 5A). In contrast, CAE administration after NIHL substantially protected hair cells from noise-induced damage (Figure 5B). As shown in Figure 5A, the quantification of OHCs revealed significantly higher numbers of OHCs ($p < 0.05$, $p < 0.01$) in the CAE-treated mice compared to the untreated NIHL group. These results indicate that CAE has therapeutic potential in hair cell protection.

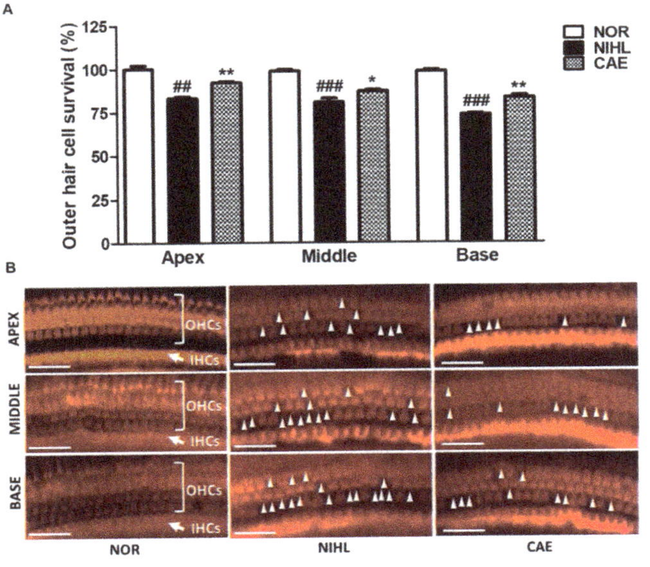

Figure 5. CAE alleviated cochlear hair cell damage in NIHL mice. (**A**) Outer hair cell (OHC) survival in 1 mm segments from the apex, middle, and base of the cochlea ($n = 6$ per group). (**B**) Fluorescence images of the outer (OHC) and inner (IHC) hair cells at the apex, middle, and base of the cochlea by Rhodamine phalloidin staining. Scale bar = 50 µm. ## $p < 0.01$, ### $p < 0.001$ (normal group vs. NIHL group). * $p < 0.05$, ** $p < 0.01$ (NIHL group vs. CAE-treated group). NOR = normal. CAE 100, 100 mg/kg. White triangles indicate the locations where the loss of outer hair cells occurred.

3.6. Differential Gene Expression by CAE Treatment in the Cochlea of NIHL Mice

To further investigate the protective mechanism of CAE in noise-induced hair cell damage, we conducted a transcriptome analysis to identify genes affected by CAE. RNA sequencing was performed to monitor differential gene expression in the cochlea of NIHL mice treated with CAE 100 mg/kg. Of the total genes expressed in the cochlea, 211 genes were differentially expressed (with false discovery rate (FDR) adjusted $Q < 0.01$, $|\text{fold change}| \geq 2.0$) by the CAE treatment. Among these, 204 genes were up-regulated and 7 genes were down-regulated (Figure 6).

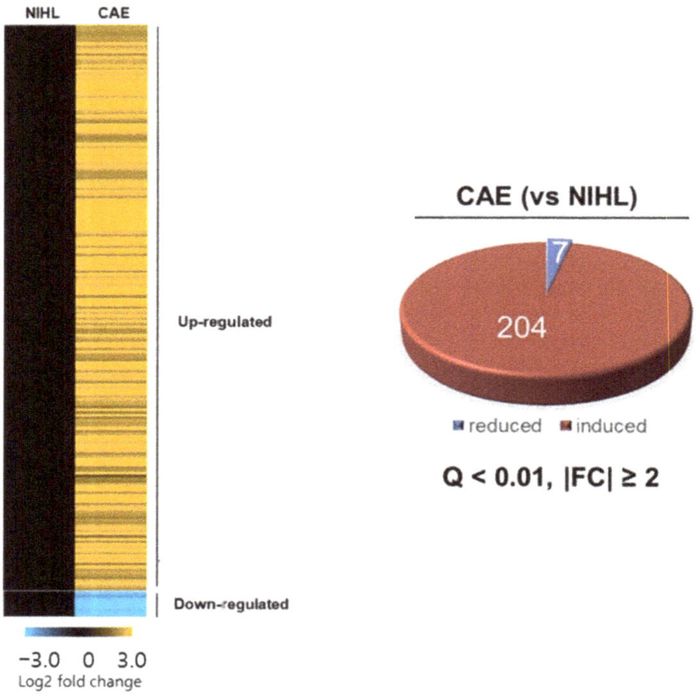

Figure 6. Differential gene expression induced by CAE treatment in the cochlea of NIHL mice ($n = 3$ per group) using Reactome Pathway analysis. Heat map based on RNA-seq analysis of gene expression in the mouse cochlea and Venn diagram showing the overlap of RNA-seq results for the regulated gene set of CAE vs. NIHL group. Genes were categorized into CAE-induced and CAE-repressed groups. Of the total genes, 211 were significantly altered by CAE treatment (false discovery rate (FDR) adjusted $Q < 0.01$, $|\text{fold change}| \geq 2.0$).

A Reactome Pathway analysis was performed to identify the functional pathways (Figure 7). We focused on the genes up-regulated by the CAE treatment that were enriched in the transmission across chemical synapses (p value 8.74×10^{-21}; Q value 1.21×10^{-18}; Enrichment score 101.5087) and the neuronal system (p value 2.92×10^{-22}; Q value 8.09×10^{-20}; Enrichment score 110.3959) pathways.

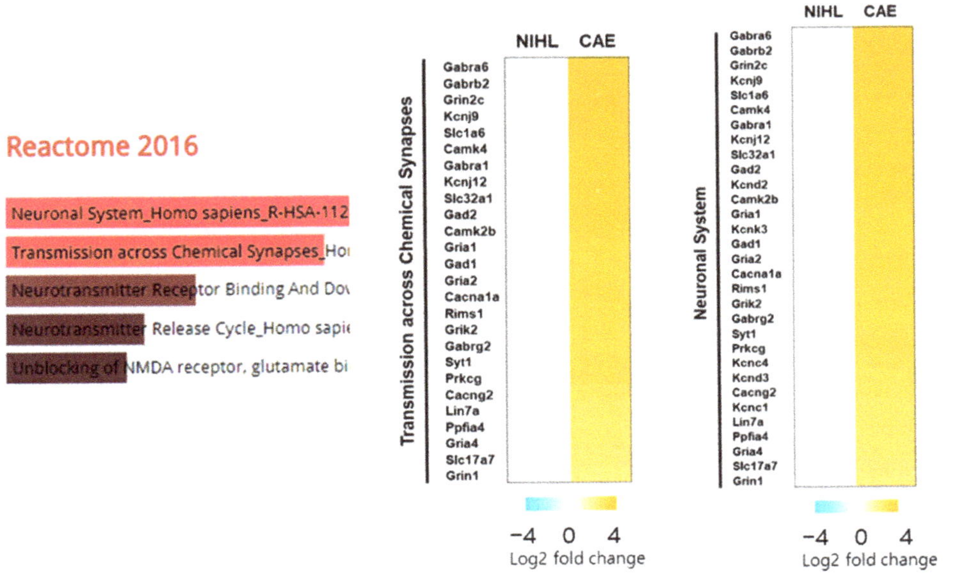

Figure 7. Functional categorization of genes up-regulated by CAE 100 mg/kg using Reactome Pathway analysis (n = 3 per group). Heat map generated from RNA-seq data showing gene sets involved in transmission across chemical synapses (p value 8.74×10^{-21}; Q value 1.21×10^{-18}; Enrichment score 101.5087) and the neuronal system (p value 2.92×10^{-22}; Q value 8.09×10^{-20}; Enrichment score 110.3959).

3.7. CAE Effects on Neurotransmitter Synthesis, Secretion, Transport, and Neuronal Survival Gene Expression in NIHL Mice

To validate the RNA-seq results, we examined the effect of NIHL on the expression of genes affected by the CAE treatment (Figure 8). NIHL mice showed decreased expression of genes related to neuronal function compared to normal mice. Specifically, the expression of genes related to inhibitory synaptic transmission (*Gabra1*, *Gad1*, and *Slc32a1*), neuronal survival (*CaMK2b* and *CaMKIV*), and synaptic function (*CaMK2b* and *Slc17a7*) were significantly decreased by NIHL, suggesting that noise exposure reduces markers of neuronal function and survival. Moreover, these genes' expression was significantly increased by CAE compared to the NIHL group. These results corroborate the RNA-seq findings and suggest that the protective mechanism of CAE may involve the enhancement of neuronal function and survival.

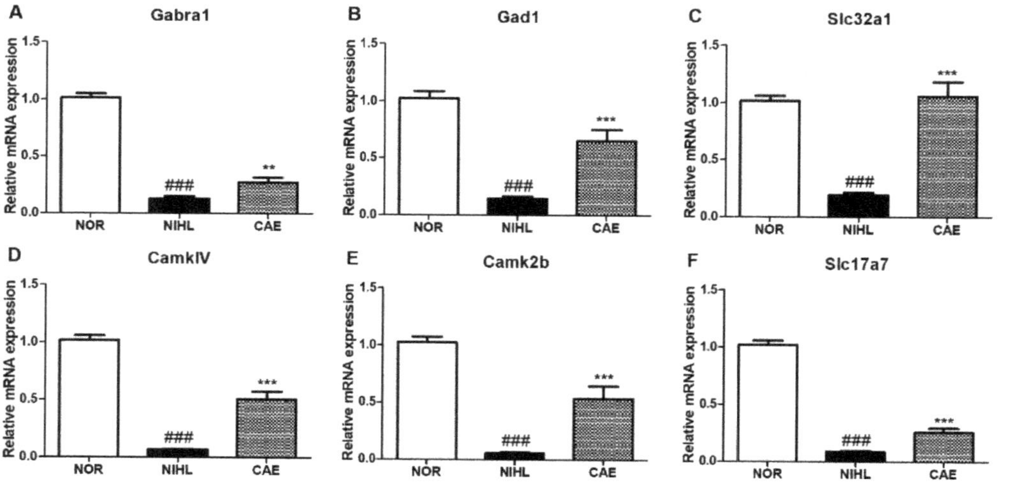

Figure 8. Changes in the expression of neuronal function-related genes in NIHL mice treated with CAE 100 mg/kg. Gene expression changes were evaluated by qPCR 20 days after noise insult. The effects of CAE treatment on genes related to inhibitory synaptic transmission (**A**–**C**), neuronal survival (**D**,**E**), and synaptic function (**E**,**F**) are shown. Data are presented as means ± SEM. ### $p < 0.001$ (NOR group vs. NIHL group); ** $p < 0.01$, *** $p < 0.001$ (NIHL group vs. CAE-treated group). NOR = normal.

4. Discussion

In the present study, we evaluated the potential efficacy of CAE, given that certain species of the genus Castanopsis are known to be rich in polyphenols such as flavonoids and have demonstrated activity against oxidative stress, inflammation, and apoptosis [16–19], which are key pharmacological targets in SNHL. However, there are no studies of Castanopsis species effects on SNHL. Specifically, CAE has not been reported to have any pharmacological activity. Therefore, we assessed the efficacy of CAE in two models of SNHL: one induced by ototoxic agents and the other by noise exposure. Additionally, we sought to elucidate its possible mode of action.

Protecting sensory hair cells has become a crucial target in the treatment of SNHL, as the condition often results from hair cell loss [6,22,23]. The zebrafish lateral line has gained prominence as a model system due to its morphological and physiological similarities to mammalian cochlear hair cells. This model is valuable for investigating the underlying mechanisms of pathology and for easily screening new candidates with potential activity as SNHL treatments [24,25]. In this study, we evaluated the effect of CAE on otic hair cell protection following ototoxicity induced by neomycin. Aminoglycoside ototoxicity, such as that caused by neomycin, is well known to damage sensory hair cells through mechanisms like those observed in NIHL [26]. Our results demonstrated that CAE significantly promotes otic hair cell protection, with an EC_{50} value of 0.497 µg/mL. Additionally, our investigation into the toxicity of CAE revealed that it is a safe drug, as indicated by its high therapeutic index (TI) value of 1020.

Because noise exposure is one of the most prevalent forms of SNHL [23], we evaluated CAE's activity on auditory function in an NIHL mouse model. It is well known that NIHL causes an increase in auditory thresholds and alterations in the waveforms of the ABR, indicating a reduced response in different regions of the auditory pathway [27]. Our results demonstrated that different doses of CAE were effective at the click, 8 kHz, and 16 kHz frequencies, as evidenced by decreased hearing thresholds in the ABR. CAE significantly improved auditory function after 20 days of treatment and also exhibited a protective effect on sensory hair cells in the apex, middle, and base of the cochlea, as shown by rhodamine phalloidin staining. Specifically, the effect of CAE was greater with the click stimulus. The click stimulus contains several frequencies along the cochlear traveling wave [28]. In contrast, tone bursts specifically represent 8 and 16 kHz. Our findings in the click stimulus may also be related to higher frequencies not considered in this study. As shown in the ABR data, the effect of CAE was greater at 16 kHz tone burst thresholds than at 8 kHz, which could support the hypothesis of its efficacy at higher frequencies. This study provides compelling evidence for the potential of CAE as a treatment for SNHL.

To elucidate the mode of action of CAE, we assessed the differential expression of genes in NIHL mice following CAE treatment using RNA-seq. Among the genes affected by CAE, we focused specifically on those involved in hearing impairments. The up-regulated genes of interest were enriched in pathways related to chemical synaptic transmission and the neuronal system.

Interestingly, we observed that the enriched genes were involved in neuronal function, neuronal survival, and GABA inhibitory mechanisms. CAE up-regulated genes involved in GABAergic inhibition, including GABA receptor genes (*Gabrd*, *Gabra6*, *Gabrb2*, *Gabra1*, *Gabrg2*); glutamate decarboxylase genes (*Gad1*, *Gad2*), which catalyze the production of GABA from L-glutamic acid; and a GABA transporter-related gene (*Slc32a1*). Impairments in GABA-mediated synaptic transmission have been implicated in the pathogenesis of auditory disorders [29]. A significant reduction in GABA receptors has been reported in both noise-induced and age-related hearing loss, and increasing the expression of GABA receptors has been suggested as a potential target for NIHL treatment to enhance auditory function [30–32]. Additionally, *Gad1* expression has been reported to decrease in the cochlear nucleus and the inferior colliculus in hearing loss models [33].

Furthermore, CAE up-regulated genes related to synaptic function, such as *Slc17a7* and *CaMK2b*. Synaptic transmission at cochlear hair cells and spiral ganglion neurons is crucial for normal hearing function. The *Slc17a7* gene, also known as *Vglut1*, encodes the vesicular glutamate transporter 1 (VGLUT1) protein, which is required for the transmission of sound-induced signals from the cochlea to the central auditory pathway. Cochlear damage induced by noise or ototoxic drugs results in decreased *Vglut1* expression [34,35]. The *CaMK2b* gene encodes the calcium/calmodulin-dependent protein kinase II beta (CaMKIIβ) protein. Genes related to calcium homeostasis, such as *CaMK2b*, are important in ototoxic insults, including cisplatin exposure, which leads to the decreased expression of genes related to neurotransmitter secretion and transport [36]. The up-regulation of these genes has been associated with increased survival of cochlear hair cells and spiral ganglion neurons after cisplatin ototoxicity, making this an interesting pharmacological approach [36].

As mentioned previously, SNHL results from damage to otic hair cells and cochlear spiral ganglion neurons. In vivo studies have demonstrated that it is possible to counteract this damage by enhancing survival mechanisms, such as growth factors [34]. Both Ca^{2+}/calmodulin-dependent protein kinases II and IV (*CaMKII* and *CaMKIV*) have shown survival-promoting effects on spiral ganglion neurons in vitro [37–39]. CAE up-regulated both *CaMKII* and *CaMKIV*, suggesting that its mechanism of action might also involve improved survival of cochlear spiral ganglion neurons.

To validate the RNA-seq results, we selected six neuronal function-related genes identified in the cochlea of CAE-treated mice for qPCR analysis. The target genes were related to GABA inhibitory action (*Gabra1*, *Gad1*, and *Slc32a1*), neuronal survival (*CaMK2b* and *CaMKIV*), and synaptic function (*CaMK2b* and *Slc17a7*). As expected, NIHL mice showed significantly decreased mRNA expression of genes related to neuronal function and survival compared to normal mice, whereas the CAE treatment significantly increased the mRNA levels of these genes.

5. Conclusions

Our data suggest that auditory function improvement and protection of sensory cells by CAE might be explained through increased genes related to synthesis, secretion, and transport of neurotransmitters and neuronal survival. In addition, this study provides more evidence about changes in genes related to neuronal function in the mice cochlea after noise-induced hearing loss. Thus, we propose a therapeutic approach based on recent perspectives to treat hearing impairments by improving neuronal function and survival. However, a limitation of this study is the lack of sufficient evidence to support proceeding to clinical trials, necessitating additional research on toxicity, pharmacokinetics, pharmacodynamics, and dosage optimization. Another limitation in this study is the lack of data demonstrating the difference in gene expression between the normal and NIHL groups, which represents an opportunity for further studies. It would be necessary to conduct a timeline study of the up-regulated and down-regulated genes in NIHL compared to normal mice to better understand the optimal intervention with natural products, mainly to translate these studies into clinical trials. Additionally, in subsequent studies, we will characterize this extract to find the main compounds responsible for the therapeutic efficacy of CAE and their potential synergistic effects.

Author Contributions: Conceptualization, B.N.H. and T.H.K.; methodology, I.R., Y.H.N. and X.H.P.; validation, I.R. and Y.H.N.; formal analysis, I.R., Y.H.N. and S.W.S.; investigation, I.R., Y.H.N., S.W.S., G.J.S., N.W.K., W.N., D.H.K., Y.H.P., H.Y.L. and X.H.P.; writing—original draft preparation, I.R. and Y.H.N.; writing—review and editing, S.W.S. and G.J.S.; supervision, B.N.H. and T.H.K. All authors have read and agreed to the published version of the manuscript.

Funding: This work was supported by the Technology Development Program (S3033322) funded by the Ministry of SMEs and Startups (MSS, Republic of Korea).

Institutional Review Board Statement: The animal study protocol was approved by the Animal Care and Use Committee of Kyung Hee University (KHUASP-21-230, 2021.05.14, and KHUASP-21-229, 4 June 2021).

Data Availability Statement: Data are contained within this article.

Acknowledgments: We would like to express our sincere gratitude to Kwang Won Jeong for his contribution to this study by performing the RNA sequencing and providing the necessary data.

Conflicts of Interest: Authors Y.H.N., N.W.K., and B.N.H. were employed by Invivotec Co., Ltd. The remaining authors declare that this research was conducted in the absence of any commercial or financial relationships that could be construed as a potential conflict of interest.

References

1. Shargorodsky, J.; Curhan, S.G. Change in prevalence of hearing loss in US adolescents. *JAMA* **2010**, *304*, 772–778. [CrossRef]
2. Hong, O.; Kerr, M.J. Understanding and preventing noise-induced hearing loss. *Disease-a-Month* **2013**, *59*, 110–118. [CrossRef]
3. Poirrier, A.L.; Pincemail, J. Oxidative Stress in the Cochlea: An Update. *Curr. Med. Chem.* **2010**, *17*, 3591–3604. [CrossRef] [PubMed]
4. Kurabi, A.; Keithley, E.M. Cellular mechanisms of noise-induced hearing loss. *Hear. Res.* **2017**, *349*, 129–137. [CrossRef] [PubMed]
5. Menardo, J.; Tang, Y. Oxidative Stress, Inflammation, and Autophagic Stress as the Key Mechanisms of Premature Age-Related Hearing Loss in SAMP8 Mouse Cochlea. *Antioxid. Redox Signal.* **2012**, *16*, 263–274. [CrossRef] [PubMed]
6. Rossini, B.A.A.; Penido, N.O. Sudden Sensorineural Hearing Loss and Autoimmune Systemic Diseases. *Int. Arch. Otorhinolaryngol.* **2017**, *21*, 213–223. [PubMed]
7. Prell, C.G.L.; Yamashita, D. Mechanisms of noise-induced hearing loss indicate multiple methods of prevention. *Hear. Res.* **2007**, *226*, 22–43. [CrossRef] [PubMed]
8. Sánchez-Rodríguez, C.; Martín-Sanz, E. Protective effect of polyphenols on presbycusis via oxidative/nitrosative stress suppression in rats. *Exp. Gerontol.* **2016**, *83*, 31–36. [CrossRef] [PubMed]
9. Tian, C.J.; Kim, Y.J. A combination of cilostazol and Ginkgo biloba extract protects against cisplatin-induced Cochleo-vestibular dysfunction by inhibiting the mitochondrial apoptotic and ERK pathways. *Cell Death Dis.* **2013**, *4*, 509. [CrossRef]
10. Kang, T.H.; Hong, B.N. Effect of baicalein from *Scutellaria baicalensis* on prevention of noise-induced hearing loss. *Neurosci. Lett.* **2009**, *469*, 298–302. [CrossRef]
11. Rodriguez, I.; Hong, B.N. Bioconversion of *Scutellaria baicalensis* extract can increase recovery of auditory function in a mouse model of noise-induced hearing loss. *Biomed. Pharmacother.* **2017**, *93*, 1303–1309. [CrossRef] [PubMed]
12. Castañeda, R.; Natarajan, S.; Jeong, S.Y.; Hong, B.N.; Kang, T.H. Traditional oriental medicine for sensorineural hearing loss: Can ethnopharmacology contribute to potential drug discovery? *J. Ethnopharmacol.* **2019**, *231*, 409–428. [CrossRef]

13. Kang, T.H.; Hong, B.N.; Jung, S.Y.; Lee, J.H.; So, H.S.; Park, R.; You, Y.O. *Curculigo orchioides* protects cisplatin-induced cell damage. *Am. J. Chin. Med.* **2013**, *41*, 425–441. [CrossRef] [PubMed]
14. Hong, B.N.; You, Y.O.; Kang, T.H. *Curculigo orchioides*, natural compounds for the treatment of noise-induced hearing loss in mice. *Arch. Pharm. Res.* **2011**, *34*, 653–659. [CrossRef]
15. Nam, Y.H.; Rodriguez, I. Avocado Oil Extract Modulates Auditory Hair Cell Function through the Regulation of Amino Acid Biosynthesis Genes. *Nutrients* **2019**, *11*, 113. [CrossRef] [PubMed]
16. Alkandahri, M.Y.; Berbudi, A. Antimalarial activity of extract and fractions of *Castanopsis costata* (Blume) A.DC. *Avicenna J. Phytomed.* **2019**, *9*, 474–481. [PubMed]
17. Gao, Y.; Zhang, X. *Castanopsis lamontii* Water Extract Shows Potential in Suppressing Pathogens, Lipopolysaccharide-Induced Inflammation and Oxidative Stress-Induced Cell Injury. *Molecules* **2019**, *24*, 273. [CrossRef] [PubMed]
18. Huang, Y.L.; Tsujita, T. Triterpene hexahydroxydiphenoyl esters and a quinic acid purpurogallin carbonyl ester from the leaves of *Castanopsis fissa*. *Phytochemistry* **2011**, *72*, 2006–2014. [CrossRef] [PubMed]
19. Huang, Y.L.; Wang, Y.F. Phenolic Compounds from the Leaves of *Castanopsis fargesii*. *Molecules* **2017**, *22*, 162. [CrossRef]
20. Liberman, M.C. Noise-induced and age-related hearing loss: New perspectives and potential therapies. *F1000Research* **2017**, *6*, 927. [CrossRef]
21. Chen, E.Y.; Tan, C.M. Enrichr: Interactive and collaborative HTML5 gene list enrichment analysis tool. *BMC Bioinform.* **2013**, *14*, 128. [CrossRef]
22. Furness, D.N. Molecular basis of hair cell loss. *Cell Tissue Res.* **2015**, *361*, 387–399. [CrossRef] [PubMed]
23. Sara, S.A.; Teh, B.M. Bilateral sudden sensorineural hearing loss: Review. *J. Laryngol. Otol.* **2014**, *128*, 8–15. [CrossRef] [PubMed]
24. Stawicki, T.M.; Esterberg, R. Using the zebrafish lateral line to uncover novel mechanisms of action and prevention in drug-induced hair cell death. *Front. Cell Neurosci.* **2015**, *9*, 46. [CrossRef] [PubMed]
25. Stengel, D.; Zindler, F. An optimized method to assess ototoxic effects in the lateral line of zebrafish (Danio rerio) embryos. *Comp. Biochem. Physiol. C Toxicol. Pharmacol.* **2017**, *193*, 18–29. [CrossRef]
26. Yu, X.; Liu, W. c-Myb knockdown increases the neomycin-induced damage to hair-cell-like HEI-OC1 cells in vitro. *Sci. Rep.* **2017**, *7*, 41094. [CrossRef]
27. Ingham, N.J.; Pearson, S.A. Mouse screen reveals multiple new genes underlying mouse and human hearing loss. *PLoS Biol.* **2019**, *17*, e3000194. [CrossRef]
28. Olson, E.S. Mechanics of the Cochlea. In *The Senses: A Comprehensive Reference*; Academic Press: Cambridge, MA, USA, 2020.
29. Balaram, P.; Hackett, T.A. Synergistic Transcriptional Changes in AMPA and GABAA Receptor Genes Support Compensatory Plasticity Following Unilateral Hearing Loss. *Neuroscience* **2019**, *407*, 108–119. [CrossRef]
30. Murashita, H.; Tabuchi, K. The effect of a GABAA agonist muscimol on acoustic injury of the mouse cochlea. *Neurosci. Lett.* **2007**, *418*, 18–21. [CrossRef]
31. Qu, J.; Liao, Y.H. Puerarin alleviates noise-induced hearing loss via affecting PKCγ and GABAB receptor expression. *J. Neurol. Sci.* **2015**, *349*, 110–116. [CrossRef]
32. Tang, X.; Zhu, X. Age-related hearing loss: GABA, nicotinic acetylcholine and NMDA receptor expression changes in spiral ganglion neurons of the mouse. *Neuroscience* **2014**, *259*, 184–193. [CrossRef] [PubMed]
33. Dong, S.; Mulders, W.H. Changes in neuronal activity and gene expression in guinea-pig auditory brainstem after unilateral partial hearing loss. *Neuroscience* **2009**, *159*, 1164–1174. [CrossRef] [PubMed]
34. Heeringa, A.N.; Stefanescu, R.A. Altered vesicular glutamate transporter distributions in the mouse cochlear nucleus following cochlear insult. *Neuroscience* **2016**, *315*, 114–124. [CrossRef] [PubMed]
35. Kurioka, T.; Lee, M.Y. Selective hair cell ablation and noise exposure lead to different patterns of changes in the cochlea and the cochlear nucleus. *Neuroscience* **2016**, *332*, 242–257. [CrossRef]
36. Wang, P.; Zhang, P. Trichostatin A protects against cisplatin-induced ototoxicity by regulating expression of genes related to apoptosis and synaptic function. *Neurotoxicology* **2013**, *37*, 51–62. [CrossRef] [PubMed]
37. Bok, J.; Wang, Q. CaMKII and CaMKIV mediate distinct prosurvival signaling pathways in response to depolarization in neurons. *Mol. Cell Neurosci.* **2007**, *36*, 13–26. [CrossRef]
38. Hansen, M.R.; Bok, J. Ca^{2+}/calmodulin-dependent protein kinases II and IV both promote survival but differ in their effects on axon growth in spiral ganglion neurons. *J. Neurosci. Res.* **2003**, *72*, 169–184. [CrossRef]
39. Zha, X.M.; Bishop, J.F. BDNF synthesis in spiral ganglion neurons is constitutive and CREB-dependent. *Hear. Res.* **2001**, *156*, 53–68. [CrossRef]

nutrients

MDPI

Article

Selaginella tamariscina Ethanol Extract Attenuates Influenza A Virus Infection by Inhibiting Hemagglutinin and Neuraminidase

Won-Kyung Cho *, Hee-Jeong Choi and Jin Yeul Ma *

Korean Medicine (KM) Application Center, Korea Institute of Oriental Medicine, 70 Chemdanro, Dong-gu, Daegu 41062, Republic of Korea; chj1901@kiom.re.kr

* Correspondence: wkcho@kiom.re.kr (W.-K.C.); jyma@kiom.re.kr (J.Y.M.); Tel.: +82-53-940-3870 (W.-K.C.); +82-53-940-3812 (J.Y.M.); Fax: +82-53-940-3899 (J.Y.M.)

Abstract: *Selaginella tamariscina* is a perennial plant that is used for diverse diseases. This study investigated whether *Selaginella tamariscina* has an antiviral effect against influenza A virus (IAV) infection. We used green fluorescent protein (GFP)-tagged influenza A virus (IAV) to examine the effect of *Selaginella tamariscina* ethanol extract (STE) on influenza viral infection. Fluorescence microscopy and flow cytometry showed that STE potently represses GFP expression by the virus, dose-dependently. STE significantly inhibited the expression of the IAV M2, NP, HA, NA, NS1, and PB2 proteins. Time-of-addition and hemagglutination inhibition assays showed that STE has an inhibitory effect on hemagglutinin and viral binding on the cells at an early infection time. In addition, STE exerted a suppressive effect on the neuraminidase activity of the H1N1 and H3N2 IAVs. Furthermore, dose-dependently, STE inhibited the cytopathic effect induced by H3N2, as well as by H1N1 IAV. Especially in the presence of 200 μg/mL STE, the cytopathic effect was completely blocked. Our findings suggest that STE has antiviral efficacy against IAV infection; thus, it could be developed as a natural IAV inhibitor.

Keywords: *Selaginella tamariscina*; influenza A virus; cytopathic effect; hemagglutinin; neuraminidase

1. Introduction

Influenza viruses are responsible for respiratory diseases that cause symptoms such as coughing, fever, sore throat, chills, muscle pain, and fatigue. Millions of people become infected with the influenza viruses, resulting in up to 650,000 deaths in the world every year [1]. Influenza viruses have segmented negative single-strand RNA and belong to the Orthomyxoviridae family [2]. Influenza A virus (IAV) is the major causing agent of human flu and is classified into subtypes based on hemagglutinin (HA) and neuraminidase (NA) [2,3]. The segmented genome of IAV frequently produces gene reassortment events such as antigenic drift and shift during viral RNA gene expression [4]. Antigenic drift and shift in the HA and NA of IAV make new types of viruses unpredictable each year [5]. NA inhibitors, such as zanamivir, oseltamivir, and peramivir, and PA inhibitors, such as baloxavir, are used to treat IAV infections. Still, the variants caused by mutations in viral RNA replication or resistance to NA inhibitors pose a challenge in the treatment of IAV-related diseases [6–8]. To date, many types of natural herbs have been reported to have the potential to prevent IAV infection by targeting IAV proteins, including NA, NS1, HA, NP, PA, and PB [9–13]. However, a perfect natural antiviral agent that can overcome the shortcomings of NA inhibitors has still not been developed.

Selaginella tamariscina (ST), an evergreen perennial plant widely grown in East Asia, has long been utilized to treat various diseases, including hemoptysis in pulmonary disease, traumatic and gastrointestinal bleeding, leukorrhea, and cancer [14]. ST is currently used as a component of traditional Chinese medicine to treat rhinitis/sinusitis, arthritis, and hemorrhoids in China [14]. In addition to medicine, ST is used as an ingredient in cosmetics, food, and tea. Several studies have reported that ST has antiviral effects against the respiratory syncytial virus [15], hepatitis B [16], and coxsackie viruses [17]. However, the inhibitory effect of ST on IAV has not been investigated so far. Here, we report for the first time that *Selaginella tamariscina* ethanol extract directly inhibits influenza A virus infection, by not only interfering with hemagglutinin but also by inhibiting neuraminidase activities.

2. Materials and Methods

2.1. Herbal Extract Preparation and HPLC Analysis

The preparation of *Selaginella tamariscina* ethanol extract (STE) and the HPLC analysis to verify STE were described in a previous report [18] by our research group. Briefly, dried ST was obtained from YeongCheon Hyundai Herbal Market (Yeongcheon, Republic of Korea) and verified by Professor Ki Hwan Bae of the College of Pharmacy, Chungnam National University (Daejeon, Republic of Korea). An amount of 50 g of ST was extracted by shaking in 70% ethanol at 40 °C for 24 h. After filtration with 150 μm testing sieves (Retsch, Haan, Germany), the solution was freeze-dried to evaporate the ethanol solution and stored at −20 °C. For antiviral experiments, STE was dissolved at 100 mg/mL in 50% DMSO. To identify the main compound in STE, an HPLC analysis was conducted as described in the previous report [18]. Amentoflavone was detected as a major compound at 43.00 min in an HPLC chromatogram. The content of amentoflavone was 4.65%.

2.2. Cell Culture and Influenza Viruses

The RPMI (Le Roswell Park Memorial Institute medium, Hyclone, Logan, UT, USA), containing fetal bovine serum (10%) and penicillin and streptomycin (100 U/mL), was used for the culture of RAW 264.7 cells (ATCC TIB-71). The influenza A/PR8/34 (H1N1) and green fluorescent protein (GFP)-expressing influenza A/PR8/34 viruses were kindly provided by Professor Jong-Soo Lee (Chungnam National University, Daejeon, Republic of Korea), and the HBPV-VR-32 (H3N2) influenza virus was obtained from the Korea Bank for Pathogenic Viruses (KBPV). The viruses were propagated using the allantoic fluid of a 10-day-old chicken embryo.

2.3. Cytotoxicity Assays

CCK-8 assay was used to check the toxicity of STE on the cells according to the manufacturer's instructions (Dojindo, Rockville, MD, USA). RAW 264.7 cells grown in a 96-well plate (1×10^5 cells/well) were treated with STE (1 to 1000 μg/mL) and incubated for 24 h at 37 °C. After the addition of 10 μL of the CCK-8 reagent to the cells for 2 h, the absorbance at 450 nm was determined by a spectrophotometer (Promega, Madison, WI, USA).

2.4. Anti-Influenza Viral Assay

The PR8-GFP, H1N1, or H3N2 IAVs were mixed with STE for 1 h at 4 °C. The mixtures were added to the cells for 2 h at 37 °C and the cells were washed with PBS to remove the remaining virus. The cells were further incubated until the formation of the cytopathic effect (CPE) or the expression of GFP. GFP expression was evaluated using FACS analysis, and CPE reduction was examined using a CCK-8 assay.

2.5. Immunofluorescence Staining

The RAW 264.7 cells, cotreated with a mixture of STE (100 μg/mL) and PR8-GFP IAV (10 MOI), were fixed with methanol for 10 min and 4% paraformaldehyde at room temperature. The cells were washed three times with PBS and blocked with PBS containing 1% BSA for 30 min. The cells were incubated with primary antibodies specific for IAV proteins, including M2, NP, NS1, HA, NA, and PB2 (GeneTex, Irvine, CA, USA), overnight at 4 °C. After washing with 0.05% Tween 20-containing PBS (PBST), the cells were incubated with an Alexa Fluor 594-conjugated secondary antibody (Thermo Fisher Scientific, Waltham, MA, USA) for 1 h in the dark. The cells were further incubated with Hoechst 33342 for

5 min in the dark. The images of the red color of the IAV proteins and the blue color of the nuclei were obtained by fluorescence microscopy.

2.6. Flow Cytometry

The cells coinfected with PR8-GFP IAV and STE were collected and washed three times with PBS. The cells fixed in 4% paraformaldehyde were analyzed by a CytoPLEX flow cell counter (Beckman Coulter Inc., Pasadena, CA, USA).

2.7. Time-of-Addition Assay

A time-of-addition assay was conducted as described in a previous study [19]. Briefly, for the virus attachment step, RAW 264.7 cells in 12 wells (5×10^5 cells/well) were coincubated with 100 μg/mL STE and 10 MOI PR8-GFP IAV for 30 min at 4 °C. After removing the mixture with PBS washing, the cells were incubated for 24 h at 37 °C. For the virus entry step, STE was added to the cells, which were preincubated with PR8-GFP IAV for 30 min at 4 °C. After further incubation for 30 min at 37 °C, the cells were washed with PBS and further incubated for 24 h at 37 °C. For the virucidal effect, STE, PR8-GFP IAV and STE were preincubated for 30 min at 4 °C, and the cells were coinfected with the mixtures for 30 min at 37 °C. After washing with PBS, the cells were further incubated for 24 h at 37 °C. The images of the cells were captured by fluorescence microscopy (200× magnification). The expression of GFP was analyzed using flow cytometry with paraformaldehyde-fixed cells.

2.8. Hemagglutination (HA) Assay

The H1N1 IAV (10 MOI) and STE were mixed for 1 h at 4 °C. The cells were cotreated with the mixtures and incubated for 2 h at 37 °C. After the removal of the remaining virus and STE with PBS washing, the cells were incubated for 24 h at 37 °C. Serially diluted supernatant and 1% chicken RBCs (Innovative Research, Inc., Southfield, MI, USA) were mixed and incubated in a round-bottomed 96-well plate for 1 h at room temperature. The images of the plates with red blood cell agglutination were obtained photographically.

2.9. Neuraminidase (NA) Inhibition Assay

The neuraminidase (NA) inhibition assay was performed using the NA-Fluor influenza Neuraminidase Assay Kit (Life Technologies, Carlsbad, CA, USA). Briefly, STE or oseltamivir carboxylate (as a positive control), which was serially diluted with buffer, was added to a 96-well black plate. The H1N1 or H3N2 IAV was added to each well, mixed, and incubated for 30 min at 37 °C. Each sample was incubated with NA-Fluor substrate for 1 h at 37 °C and terminated using the stop solution. NA activity was measured using a fluorescence spectrometer (Promega, Madison, WI, USA), with an excitation of 365 nm and an emission of 445 nm.

3. Results

3.1. STE Inhibits Influenza A Viral Infection in a Dose-Dependent Manner

Before investigating the effect of STE on influenza virus infection, we examined the toxicity on the RAW 264.7 cells. As presented in Figure 1A, STE was found to be nontoxic up to 500 μg/mL in the cells; therefore, we explored the effect of STE on IAV infection up to 200 μg/mL. The anti-viral effect of STE was examined in RAW 264.7 cells using the GFP-tagged influenza A virus (PR8-GFP IAV). Most studies use MDCK or A549 cells for influenza virus infection experiments. However, in this study, we used RAW 264.7 cells because they are also readily infected with IAV and their small cell size facilitates relative comparisons in dose-dependent experiments. As shown in Figure 1B, PR8-GFP IAV expressed high levels of GFP in the absence of STE. However, GFP expression was significantly reduced by STE, in a concentration-dependent manner. The effect of STE on PR8-GFP IAV infection was confirmed by FACS analysis. Figure 1C shows that STE significantly reduces GFP expression by viral infection, consistent with Figure 1B. STE showed a 50% effective concentration (EC_{50}) of 14.5 ± 2.0 μg/mL on GFP expression by viral infection. We also confirmed dose-dependent the anti-influenza viral effect of STE in MDCK and A549 cells after checking the cytotoxicity on them (Figures S1 and S2). These results suggest that STE has a potent anti-viral effect against PR8-GFP IAV infection.

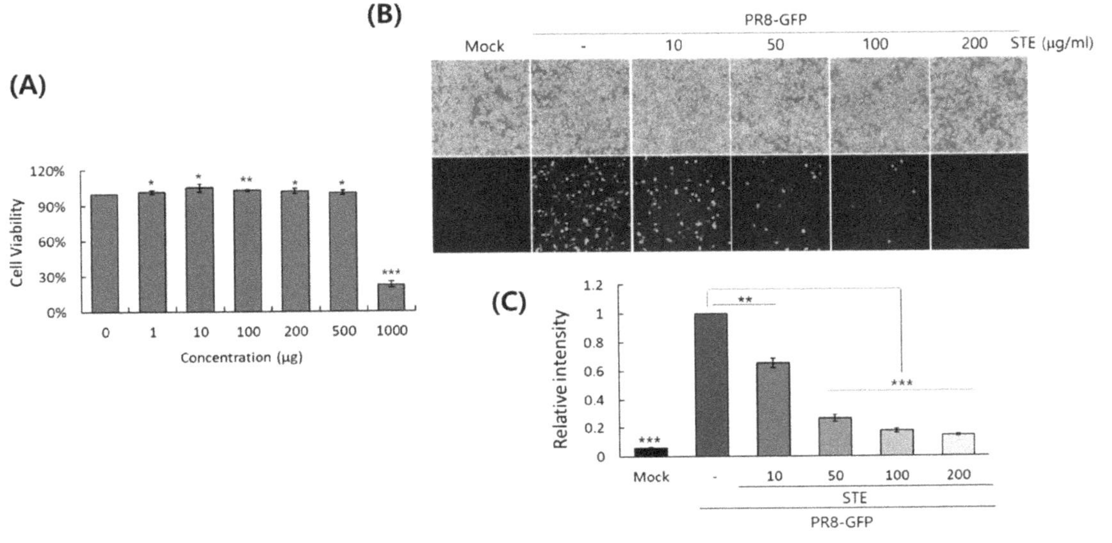

Figure 1. Cytotoxicity and antiviral effect of *Selaginella tamariscina* ethanol extract (STE) in RAW 264.7 cells. (**A**) The toxicity of STE in the cells was evaluated using a CCK-8 assay. The data represent the mean ± SD from three independent experiments. The unpaired Student *t*-test was used to assess the statistical significance. * $P < 0.5$, ** $P < 0.05$, and *** $P < 0.005$, compared with the untreated control. (**B**,**C**) The cells were cotreated with PR8-GFP IAV and STE. The effect of STE on PR8-GFP IAV infection was evaluated by comparing GFP expression using a fluorescence microscope (**B**) and FACS analysis (**C**). The data represent the mean ± SD from three independent experiments. The unpaired Student *t*-test was used to assess the statistical significance. ** $P < 0.005$, and *** $P < 0.0005$, compared with the virus-infected control.

3.2. Inhibitory Effect of STE on Influenza H1N1 and H3N2 Viruses

To investigate whether STE could inhibit other types of influenza viral infection, we checked the effect of STE on wild-type IAV infection by comparing the cytopathic effect. In the absence of STE, the H1N1 and H3N2 IAVs induced cytopathic effects in the cells (Figure 2). The viability of cells infected with H1N1 or H3N2 IAV was reduced to 30%, compared to the uninfected cells. However, in the presence of STE, the cell viability was significantly increased through the blockage of the cytopathic effect by viral replication, dose-dependently. Especially at a concentration of 200 µg/mL of STE, the cell viabilities in the cells infected with the H1N1 or H3N2 IAV were recovered up to 100%, compared to the uninfected cells. These results indicate that STE has a potent inhibitory effect against both H1N1 and H3N2 influenza virus infections.

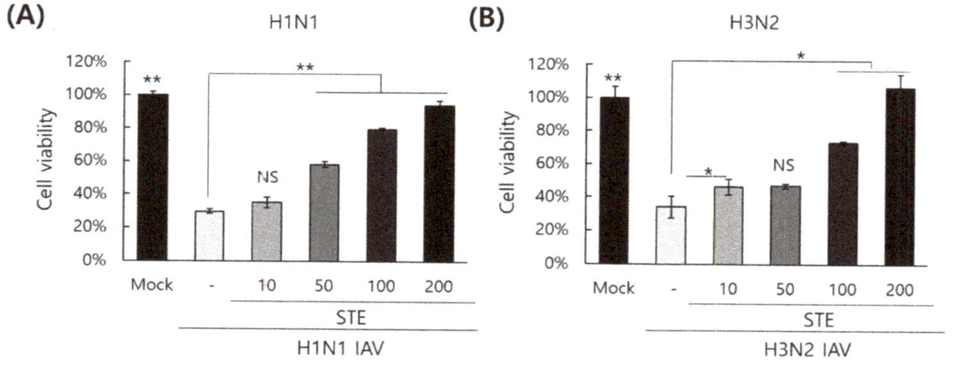

Figure 2. STE protects the cells from the cytopathic effect induced by H1N1 (**A**) and H3N2 (**B**) influenza virus infection. STE at the indicated concentrations or medium (mock) was mixed with H1N1 or H3N2 IAV before infection of the cells. The cells infected with the mixture were incubated until the cytopathic effect formed. The cell viability was determined via a CCK-8 assay. The data represent the mean ± SD from three independent experiments. The unpaired Student *t*-test was used to assess the statistical significance. * $P < 0.05$, ** $P < 0.005$; NS, no significance.

3.3. STE Represses Influenza Viral Protein Expression

Next, we explored the effect of STE on IAV protein expression using the cells infected with PR8-GFP IAV, with or without STE. Immunofluorescence analysis with antibodies specific for IAV proteins showed that STE significantly decreased IAV proteins, including M2, NP, NS1, HA, NA, and PB2 (Figure 3). This result suggests that STE strongly represses influenza A viral protein expression.

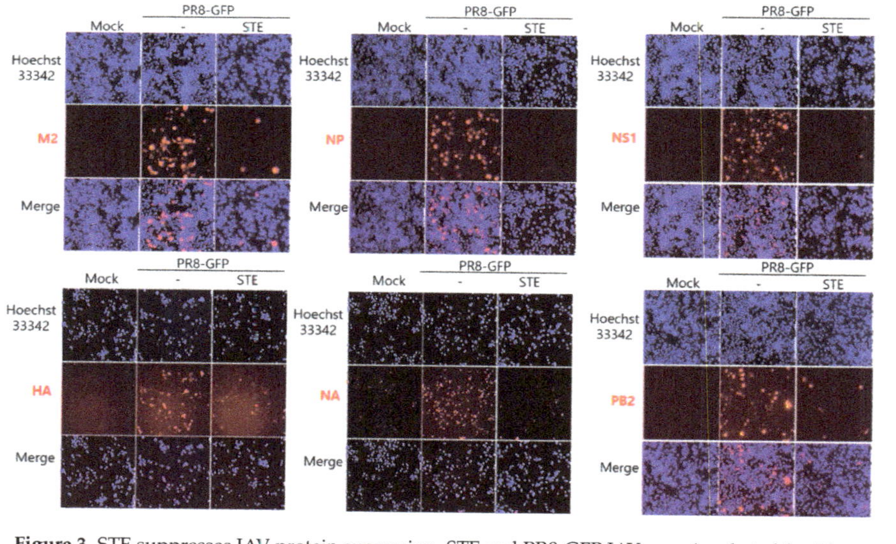

Figure 3. STE suppresses IAV protein expression. STE and PR8-GFP IAV were incubated for 1 h at 4 °C. The cells were coinfected with the mixture for 24 h at 37 °C. The cells were fixed and detected with antibodies against IAV proteins, including M2, NP, NS1, NA, HA, and PB2 (red color). To detect the nuclei, the cells were stained with Hoechst 33342 (blue color). The co-localization images of red viral proteins and blue nuclei were captured using a fluorescence microscope.

3.4. Effect of STE on Viral Attachment, Entry, or Virucidal Stages

Because STE exhibited a potent inhibitory effect against IAV infection in the cotreatment condition, we conducted a time-of-addition experiment to elucidate whether STE could affect viral binding and entry on the cells at an early infection time. In addition, we checked whether STE has a virucidal activity on IAV. FACS analysis and fluorescence microscopy results showed that, in the presence of STE, the IAV attachment was significantly suppressed and that the viral entry was slightly reduced (Figure 4). In addition, STE exerted moderate virucidal activity. These results imply that STE has a substantial inhibitory effect against IAV infection by hindering viral binding to the cells and inducing virucidal action.

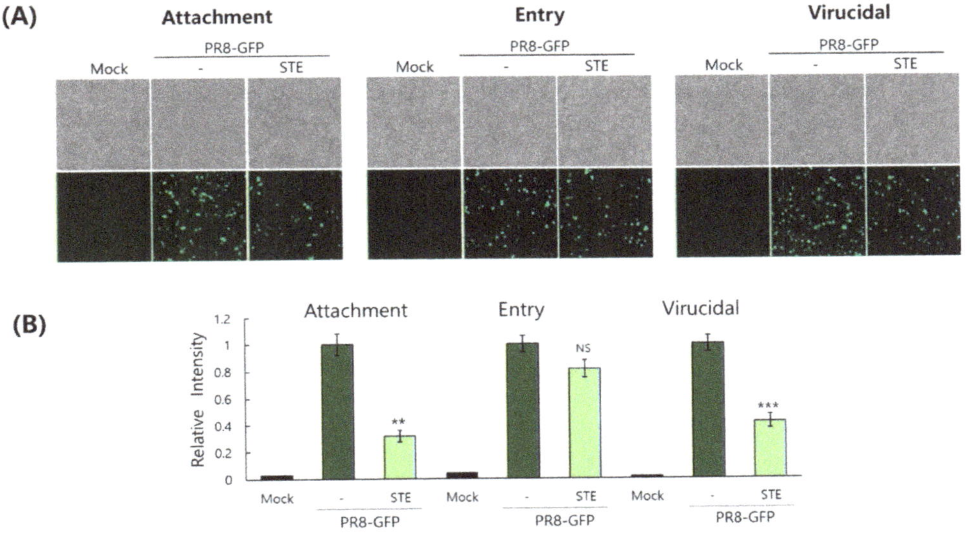

Figure 4. STE affects the virus attachment and entry and directly kills the virus at an early phase. The cells were cotreated with STE (100 μg/mL) and PR8-GFP IAV (10 MOI) to examine the effect of STE on viral attachment, entry, or virucidal stage. The detailed time-of-addition methods were described in the Materials and Methods Section. The images of GFP-expressing cells were obtained using brightfield and fluorescence microscopy (**A**). The cells fixed with paraformaldehyde were analyzed by flow cytometry (**B**). The data represent the mean ± SD from three independent experiments. The unpaired Student *t*-test was used to assess the statistical significance. ** $P < 0.005$, *** $P < 0.0005$; NS, no significance.

3.5. STE Inhibits Hemagglutination

Hemagglutination induced by IAV hemagglutinin, which is closely related to viral binding to the cells, is a main target for anti-influenza viral drugs. As we found that STE has an inhibitory effect on IAV binding to the cells, we next explored whether STE could repress IAV hemagglutination on red blood cells (RBCs). As presented in Figure 5, STE dose-dependently decreased the HA units of the H1N1 IAV. The HA units of the control H1N1 IAV were 8 units. However, in the presence of 100 μg/mL or 200 μg/mL of STE, the HA units of the virus were 4 or 2 units, respectively. STE decreased the HA units by 2- or 4-fold compared to the virus-infected control. These results imply that STE exerts an inhibitory effect on hemagglutination at concentrations of 100 or 200 μg/mL.

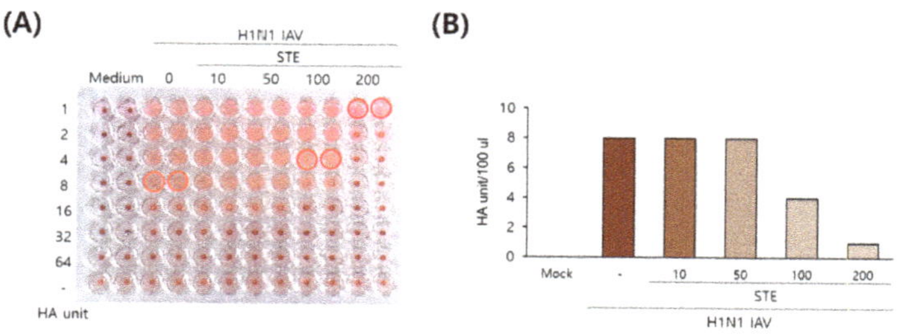

Figure 5. STE reduces the HA unit of influenza viruses (**A**,**B**). The cells were cotreated with STE at the indicated concentrations and H1N1 IAV for 24 h at 37 °C. The 2-fold serially diluted supernatants and chicken RBC cells were mixed in round 96-well plates for 1 h at room temperature. The red circle indicates hemagglutination (HA) units.

3.6. STE Represses Neuraminidase Activity of H1N1 and H3N2 IAVs

Since the neuraminidase activity is indispensable for viral progeny release from the cells after replication, we next examined whether STE could inhibit the NA activities of H1N1 and H3N2 influenza viruses. Figure 6A presents that STE dose-dependently reduces the NA activities of H1N1 and H3N2 IAVs. In particular, STE at 500 μg/mL potently inhibited the NA activities of more than 50% of the virus-infected control. Oseltamivir carboxylate, a positive control, exerted a potent inhibitory effect on the NA activities of H1N1 and H3N2, dose-dependently (Figure 6B).

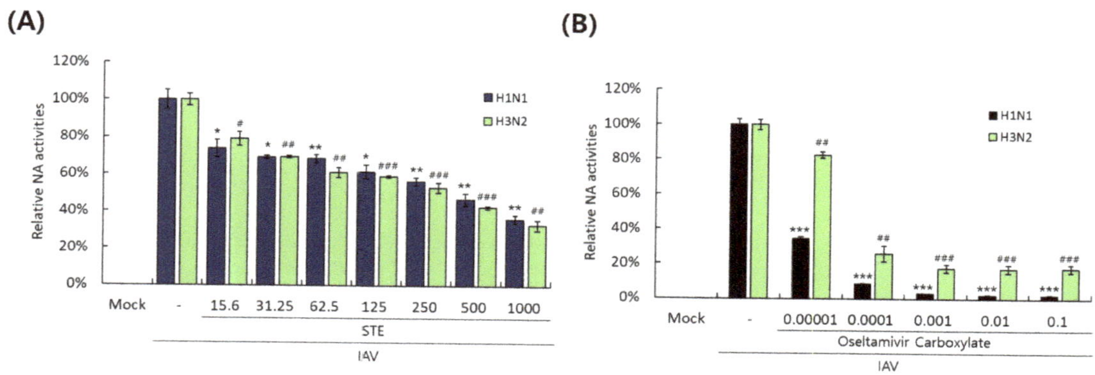

Figure 6. STE dose-dependently represses the neuraminidase activities of H1N1 and H3N2 IAVs. Serially diluted STE (**A**) or oseltamivir carboxylate (**B**) was mixed with H1N1 or H3N2 IAV in 96-well black plates. The detailed neuraminidase activity assay was described in materials and methods. The data represent the mean ± SD from three independent experiments. The unpaired Student *t*-test was used to assess the statistical significance. * $P < 0.05$, ** $P < 0.005$, and *** $P < 0.0005$, compared with the H1N1 virus-infected group. # $P < 0.05$, ## $P < 0.005$, and ### $P < 0.0005$, compared with the H3N2 virus-infected group.

4. Discussion

ST is known as a medicinal herb effective on various ailments. Our research group has demonstrated that ST has a neuroprotective effect and an inhibitory effect on osteoclastogenesis in previous reports. Several research groups have demonstrated that ST has antiviral efficacy against herpes and coxsackie viruses. However, the inhibitory effect of STE against the influenza virus was not revealed until now. In this study, we discovered that STE has an inhibitory impact against influenza virus infection. The CPE inhibition assay showed that STE significantly protected the cells from the H1N1 and H3N2 IAVs, as well as from

PR8-GFP IAV infection. The time-of-addition assay showed that the anti-viral effect of STE arises from blocking viral binding to the cells and inducing the direct killing of the virus at an early phase upon infection. When we conducted the hemagglutination inhibition assay to address whether ST could affect HA, which is critical for IAV binding to the cells, we found that STE significantly blocked the HA of IAV. These results imply that STE inhibits the virus binding to the cells by interfering with the HA of IAV. Several reports have shown that the inhibitory effect of herbal extracts, such as *Eupatorium perfoliatum* L., *Paeonia lactiflora*, *Isatidis Radix*, *Alpinia katsumadai*, *Alchemilla mollis*, *Jatropha curcas Linn.* leaf, against NA of IAV, is closely related to viral binding to the cell membrane [20–27]. We also demonstrated that medicinal herbal extracts, including *Thuja orientalis folium* [19] and *Hoveniae Semen Seu Fructus* [28], attenuate IAV infection by modulating HA. STE dose-dependently repressed the neuraminidase activities of H1N1 and H3N2 IAVs. Neuraminidase is the key enzyme for the release of viral progeny in the later stages of IAV infection. Most antiviral drugs for IAV, including oseltamivir or zanamivir, target the NA of IAV. Natural products such as *Geranii* herba [10], *Rhus verniciflua* [29], *Salvia plebeia R. Br.* [30], and chemicals, including chlorogenic acid, catechin, fucoidan, isoimperatorin, and oroxylin A [31–35], were reported to repress the neuraminidase of IAV. STE also exhibited the direct killing effect at the early stage of IAV infection. The virucidal effect has been reported to be related to certain components in the extract that directly bind to viruses and block viral particles from attaching to cells [25,36,37]. In the previous report, amentoflavone was identified as the main compound of ST in HPLC analysis [18]. Additionally, we found that amentoflavone was one of the anti-influenza viral components of *Thuja orientalis folium* [19]. These results suggest that amentoflavone may play a role in anti-influenza viral activity in ST. Bailly C. reported that ST, which contains many phenolic compounds, is used in traditional medicine and in cosmetics to protect the skin and has applications in vegetable dishes and beverages [14]. Although further studies are needed to determine which ingredients in ST are involved in inhibiting influenza virus infection, ST has the potential to be utilized as a material to inhibit the influenza virus. In summary, ST exerts its antiviral activity by inhibiting HA and NA, thereby impairing the attachment and release of influenza viruses.

5. Conclusions

STE exerted a potent anti-influenza A viral activity. STE significantly blocked influenza virus infection via the inhibition of hemagglutinin, which is involved in virus attachment. Further, STE inhibited the activity of the IAV neuraminidase. Our results suggest that STE could be used as an anti-influenza viral ingredient in vegetable dishes, beverages, or teas, as well as a natural agent against influenza virus infection.

Supplementary Materials: The following supporting information can be downloaded at: https://www.mdpi.com/article/10.3390/nu16142377/s1. Figure S1: Cytotoxicity of STE on MDCK and A549 cells; Figure S2: The inhibitory effect of STE against PR8-GFP IAV infection in MDCK and A549 cells.

Author Contributions: W.-K.C. designed and performed the experiments, analyzed the data, and wrote the manuscript. H.-J.C. carried out the experiment. J.Y.M. designed and supervised the study. All authors have read and agreed to the published version of the manuscript.

Funding: This work was supported by grant numbers KSN1823233 and KSN2411013 from KIOM (Korea Institute of Oriental Medicine), funded by the Ministry of Science and ICT, and by the National Research Foundation of Korea (NRF) (grant no. 2018R1D1A1B07042559), funded by the Korea government (MSIT), Republic of Korea.

Data Availability Statement: Data are contained within the article and Supplementary Materials.

Acknowledgments: We thank Jong-Soo Lee (Chungnam National University, Republic of Korea) for providing the GFP-tagged influenza A/PR/8/34 and H1N1 influenza viruses.

Conflicts of Interest: The authors declare no conflicts of interest.

References

1. Atkins, N.; Harikar, M.; Duggan, K.; Zawiejska, A.; Vardhan, V.; Vokey, L.; Dozier, M.; de Los Godos, E.F.; McSwiggan, E.; McQuillan, R.; et al. What are the characteristics of participatory surveillance systems for influenza-like-illness? *J. Glob. Health* **2023**, *13*, 04130. [CrossRef] [PubMed]
2. Paules, C.; Subbarao, K. Influenza. *Lancet* **2017**, *390*, 697–708. [CrossRef]
3. Gerber, M.; Isel, C.; Moules, V.; Marquet, R. Selective packaging of the influenza A genome and consequences for genetic reassortment. *Trends Microbiol.* **2014**. *22*, 446–455. [CrossRef] [PubMed]
4. Bouvier, N.M.; Palese, P. The biology of influenza viruses. *Vaccine* **2008**, *26* (Suppl. S4), D49–D53. [CrossRef] [PubMed]
5. Sautto, G.A.; Kirchenbaum, G.A.; Ross, T.M. Towards a universal influenza vaccine: Different approaches for one goal. *Virol. J.* **2018**, *15*, 17. [CrossRef] [PubMed]
6. Wu, W.L.; Lau, S.Y.; Chen, Y.; Wang, G.; Mok, B.W.; Wen, X.; Wang, P.; Song, W.; Lin, T.; Chan, K.H.; et al. The 2008–2009 H1N1 influenza virus exhibits reduced susceptibility to antibody inhibition: Implications for the prevalence of oseltamivir resistant variant viruses. *Antivir. Res.* **2012**, *93*, 144–153. [CrossRef] [PubMed]
7. Ren, X.W.; Ju, L.W.; Yang, J.X.; Lv, X.H.; Jiang, L.F.; Zhao, N.Q.; Jiang, Q.W. Antigenic and genetic variation in the hemagglutinins of H1N1 and H3N2 human influenza a viruses in the Shanghai area from 2005 to 2008. *J. Med. Virol.* **2011**, *83*, 1113–1120. [CrossRef]
8. Bouvier, N.M.; Rahmat, S.; Pica, N. Enhanced mammalian transmissibility of seasonal influenza A/H1N1 viruses encoding an oseltamivir-resistant neuraminidase. *J. Virol.* **2012**, *86*, 7268–7279. [CrossRef] [PubMed]
9. Moradi, M.T.; Karimi, A.; Shahrani, M.; Hashemi, L.; Ghaffari-Goosheh, M.S. Anti-Influenza Virus Activity and Phenolic Content of Pomegranate (*Punica granatum* L.) Peel Extract and Fractions. *Avicenna J. Med. Biotechnol.* **2019**, *11*, 285–291.
10. Choi, J.G.; Kim, Y.S.; Kim, J.H.; Chung, H.S. Antiviral activity of ethanol extract of Geranii Herba and its components against influenza viruses via neuraminidase inhibition. *Sci. Rep.* **2019**, *9*, 12132. [CrossRef]
11. Luganini, A.; Terlizzi, M.E.; Catucci, G.; Gilardi, G.; Maffei, M.E.; Gribaudo, G. The Cranberry Extract Oximacro((R)) Exerts in vitro Virucidal Activity Against Influenza Virus by Interfering with Hemagglutinin. *Front. Microbiol.* **2018**, *9*, 1826. [CrossRef]
12. Shirayama, R.; Shoji, M.; Sriwilaijaroen, N.; Hiramatsu, H.; Suzuki, Y.; Kuzuhara, T. Inhibition of PA endonuclease activity of influenza virus RNA polymerase by Kampo medicines. *Drug Discov. Ther.* **2016**, *10*, 109–113. [CrossRef] [PubMed]
13. Lo, C.W.; Pi, C.C.; Chen, Y.T.; Chen, H.W. *Vigna radiata* (L.) R. Wilczek Extract Inhibits Influenza A Virus by Targeting Viral Attachment, Penetration, Assembly, and Release. *Front. Pharmacol.* **2020**, *11*, 584973. [CrossRef]
14. Bailly, C. The traditional and modern uses of *Selaginella tamariscina* (P.Beauv.) Spring, in medicine and cosmetic: Applications and bioactive ingredients. *J. Ethnopharmacol.* **2021**, *280*, 114444. [CrossRef] [PubMed]
15. Ma, S.C.; But, P.P.; Ooi, V.E.; He, Y.H.; Lee, S.H.; Lee, S.F.; Lin, R.C. Antiviral amentoflavone from *Selaginella sinensis*. *Biol. Pharm. Bull.* **2001**, *24*, 311–312. [CrossRef]
16. Cao, Y.; Tan, N.H.; Chen, J.J.; Zeng, G.Z.; Ma, Y.B.; Wu, Y.P.; Yan, H.; Yang, J.; Lu, L.F.; Wang, Q. Bioactive flavones and biflavones from *Selaginella moellendorffii* Hieron. *Fitoterapia* **2010**, *81*, 253–258. [CrossRef] [PubMed]
17. Yin, D.; Li, J.; Lei, X.; Liu, Y.; Yang, Z.; Chen, K. Antiviral Activity of Total Flavonoid Extracts from *Selaginella moellendorffii* Hieron against Coxsackie Virus B3 In Vitro and In Vivo. *Evid. Based Complement. Alternat Med.* **2014**, *2014*, 950817. [CrossRef]
18. Jeong, Y.H.; Kim, T.I.; Oh, Y.C.; Ma, J.Y. Selaginella tamariscina Inhibits Glutamate-Induced Autophagic Cell Death by Activating the PI3K/AKT/mTOR Signaling Pathways. *Int. J. Mol. Sci.* **2022**, *23*, 1445. [CrossRef]
19. Lee, M.M.; Cho, W.K.; Cha, M.H.; Yim, N.H.; Yang, H.J.; Ma, J.Y. The antiviral activity of *Thuja orientalis folium* against Influenza A virus. *Virus Res.* **2023**, *335*, 199199. [CrossRef]
20. Derksen, A.; Kuhn, J.; Hafezi, W.; Sendker, J.; Ehrhardt, C.; Ludwig, S.; Hensel, A. Antiviral activity of hydroalcoholic extract from *Eupatorium perfoliatum* L. against the attachment of influenza A virus. *J. Ethnopharmacol.* **2016**, *188*, 144–152. [CrossRef]
21. Hamauzu, Y.; Yasui, H.; Inno, T.; Kume, C.; Omanyuda, M. Phenolic profile, antioxidant property, and anti-influenza viral activity of Chinese quince (*Pseudocydonia sinensis* Schneid.), quince (*Cydonia oblonga* Mill.), and apple (*Malus domestica* Mill.) fruits. *J. Agric. Food Chem.* **2005**, *53*, 928–934. [CrossRef] [PubMed]
22. Ho, J.Y.; Chang, H.W.; Lin, C.F.; Liu, C.J.; Hsieh, C.F.; Horng, J.T. Characterization of the anti-influenza activity of the Chinese herbal plant *Paeonia lactiflora*. *Viruses* **2014**, *6*, 1861–1875. [CrossRef] [PubMed]
23. Ke, L.; Wen, T.; Bradshaw, J.P.; Zhou, J.; Rao, P. Antiviral Decoction of *Isatidis Radix* (ban lan gen) Inhibited Influenza Virus Adsorption on MDCK Cells by Cytoprotective Activity. *J. Tradit. Complement. Med.* **2012**, *2*, 47–51. [CrossRef]
24. Kwon, H.J.; Kim, H.H.; Yoon, S.Y.; Ryu, Y.B.; Chang, J.S.; Cho, K.O.; Rho, M.C.; Park, S.J.; Lee, W.S. In vitro inhibitory activity of *Alpinia katsumadai* extracts against influenza virus infection and hemagglutination. *Virol. J.* **2010**, *7*, 307. [CrossRef]
25. Makau, J.N.; Watanabe, K.; Kobayashi, N. Anti-influenza activity of *Alchemilla mollis* extract: Possible virucidal activity against influenza virus particles. *Drug Discov. Ther.* **2013**, *7*, 189–195. [CrossRef] [PubMed]
26. Patil, D.; Roy, S.; Dahake, R.; Rajopadhye, S.; Kothari, S.; Deshmukh, R.; Chowdhary, A. Evaluation of *Jatropha curcas* Linn. leaf extracts for its cytotoxicity and potential to inhibit hemagglutinin protein of influenza virus. *Indian. J. Virol.* **2013**, *24*, 220–226. [CrossRef]
27. Song, J.M.; Lee, K.H.; Seong, B.L. Antiviral effect of catechins in green tea on influenza virus. *Antiviral Res.* **2005**, *68*, 66–74. [CrossRef]

28. Cho, W.K.; Cha, M.H.; Yim, N.H.; Choi, H.J.; Ma, J.Y. *Hoveniae Semen Seu Fructus* water extract inhibits influenza A virus infection. *J. Funct. Foods* **2024**, *112*, 105940. [CrossRef]
29. Kim, Y.S.; Li, W.; Kim, J.H.; Chung, H.S.; Choi, J.G. Anti-Influenza Activity of an Ethyl Acetate Fraction of a *Rhus verniciflua* Ethanol Extract by Neuraminidase Inhibition. *Oxid. Med. Cell Longev.* **2020**, *2020*, 8824934. [CrossRef]
30. Bang, S.; Li, W.; Ha, T.K.Q.; Lee, C.; Oh, W.K.; Shim, S.H. Anti-influenza effect of the major flavonoids from *Salvia plebeia* R.Br. via inhibition of influenza H1N1 virus neuraminidase. *Nat. Prod. Res.* **2018**, *32*, 1224–1228. [CrossRef]
31. Ding, Y.; Cao, Z.; Cao, L.; Ding, G.; Wang, Z.; Xiao, W. Antiviral activity of chlorogenic acid against influenza A (H1N1/H3N2) virus and its inhibition of neuraminidase. *Sci. Rep.* **2017**, *7*, 45723. [CrossRef] [PubMed]
32. Jin, J.; Chen, S.; Wang, D.; Chen, Y.; Wang, Y.; Guo, M.; Zhou, C.; Dou, J. Oroxylin A suppresses influenza A virus replication correlating with neuraminidase inhibition and induction of IFNs. *Biomed. Pharmacother.* **2018**, *97*, 385–394. [CrossRef] [PubMed]
33. Lai, Y.; Han, T.; Zhan, S.; Jiang, Y.; Liu, X.; Li, G. Antiviral Activity of Isoimperatorin against Influenza A Virus in vitro and its Inhibition of Neuraminidase. *Front. Pharmacol.* **2021**, *12*, 657826. [CrossRef] [PubMed]
34. Muller, P.; Downard, K.M. Catechin inhibition of influenza neuraminidase and its molecular basis with mass spectrometry. *J. Pharm. Biomed. Anal.* **2015**, *111*, 222–230. [CrossRef] [PubMed]
35. Wang, W.; Wu, J.; Zhang, X.; Hao, C.; Zhao, X.; Jiao, G.; Shan, X.; Tai, W.; Yu, G. Inhibition of Influenza A Virus Infection by Fucoidan Targeting Viral Neuraminidase and Cellular EGFR Pathway. *Sci. Rep.* **2017**, *7*, 40760. [CrossRef]
36. Li, Y.H.; Lai, C.Y.; Su, M.C.; Cheng, J.C.; Chang, Y.S. Antiviral activity of *Portulaca oleracea* L. against influenza A viruses. *J. Ethnopharmacol.* **2019**, *241*, 112013. [CrossRef]
37. Watanabe, K.; Rahmasari, R.; Matsunaga, A.; Haruyama, T.; Kobayashi, N. Anti-influenza viral effects of honey in vitro: Potent high activity of manuka honey. *Arch. Med. Res.* **2014**, *45*, 359–365. [CrossRef]

nutrients

MDPI

Article

Antithrombotic Effect of Oil from the Pulp of Bocaiúva—*Acrocomia aculeata* (Jacq.) Lodd. ex Mart. (Arecaceae)

Isabelly Teixeira Espinoça [1], Denise Caroline Luiz Soares Basilio [1], Anna Júlia Papa de Araujo [1], Rafael Seiji Nakano Ota [1], Kamylla Fernanda Souza de Souza [2], Nadla Soares Cassemiro [1,3], Davi Campos Lagatta [1], Edgar Julian Paredes-Gamero [1,2], Maria Lígia Rodrigues Macedo [1], Denise Brentan Silva [1,3], Janaina de Cássia Orlandi Sardi [4], Danilo Wilhelm-Filho [5], Ana Cristina Jacobowski [1] and Eduardo Benedetti Parisotto [1,*]

1 Faculty of Pharmaceutical Sciences, Food and Nutrition (FACFAN), Federal University of Mato Grosso do Sul (UFMS), Campo Grande 79070-900, MS, Brazil; isabellyteixeira237@gmail.com (I.T.E.); denise.carolineluiz@hotmail.com (D.C.L.S.B.); anna.julia.papa@ufms.br (A.J.P.d.A.); rafa.seiji21@gmail.com (R.S.N.O.); nadla.cassemiro@ufms.br (N.S.C.); davi_campos@ufms.br (D.C.L.); edgar.gamero@ufms.br (E.J.P.-G.); ligia.macedo@ufms.br (M.L.R.M.); denise.brentan@ufms.br (D.B.S.); anacristinaj@gmail.com (A.C.J.)

2 Department of Biochemistry, Federal University of São Paulo, São Paulo 4044-020, SP, Brazil; kamylla.bio@outlook.com

3 Laboratory of Natural Products and Mass Spectrometry (LAPNEM), Faculty of Pharmaceutical Sciences, Food and Nutrition (FACFAN), Federal University of Mato Grosso do Sul (UFMS), Campo Grande 79080-190, MS, Brazil

4 Dental Research Division, Guarulhos University, Guarulhos 07023-070, SP, Brazil; janasardi@gmail.com

5 Department of Ecology and Zoology, Center for Biological Sciences (CCB), Federal University of Santa Catarina, Florianópolis 88040-900, SC, Brazil; danilowilhelmfilho@gmail.com

* Correspondence: eduardo.parisotto@ufms.br or parisotto.edu@gmail.com; Tel.: +55-(067)-3345-7641

Abstract: The study aimed to evaluate the antithrombotic action of *Acrocomia aculeata* pulp oil (AAPO) in natura, in an in vitro experimental model. AAPO was obtained by solvent extraction, and its chemical characterization was performed by gas chromatography coupled to a mass spectrometer (GC-MS). In vitro toxicity was evaluated with the Trypan Blue exclusion test and in vivo by the *Galleria mellonella* model. ADP/epinephrine-induced platelet aggregation after treatment with AAPO (50, 100, 200, 400, and 800 μg/mL) was evaluated by turbidimetry, and coagulation was determined by prothrombin activity time (PT) and activated partial thromboplastin time (aPTT). Platelet activation was measured by expression of P-selectin on the platelet surface by flow cytometry and intraplatelet content of reactive oxygen species (ROS) by fluorimetry. The results showed that AAPO has as major components such as oleic acid, palmitic acid, lauric acid, caprylic acid, and squalene. AAPO showed no toxicity in vitro or in vivo. Platelet aggregation decreased against agonists using treatment with different concentrations of AAPO. Oil did not interfere in PT and aPTT. Moreover, it expressively decreased ROS-induced platelet activation and P-selectin expression. Therefore, AAPO showed antiplatelet action since it decreased platelet activation verified by the decrease in P-selectin expression as well as in ROS production.

Keywords: *Acrocomia aculeata*; toxicity; cardiovascular disease; reactive oxygen species; antiaggregant; antioxidant

1. Introduction

Cardiovascular diseases are one of the main causes of death in the world, and platelets play an important role in thrombosis and atherosclerosis [1]. Platelets are small cellular fragments derived from medullary polyploid megakaryocytes responsible for controlling processes related to health and disease [2], and reactive oxygen species (ROS) play an important role in regulating their function [3]. An imbalanced ROS production and deficits of antioxidants lead to hemostatic instabilities, which are responsible for increasing the risk of developing thrombotic and cardiovascular diseases [3,4].

Platelet activity differs among various human populations, which could explain the variability in cardiovascular diseases [5]. Moreover, antiplatelet therapy presents numerous difficulties and limitations, such as drug and nutritional interactions and a narrow therapeutic window, resulting in the need to investigate antiplatelet agents with greater efficacy and safety [6,7].

Brazil has one of the greatest biodiversities in the world and may be a source of natural bioactive compounds [8]. Among the promising plants for the development of natural products is *Acrocomia aculeata* (Jacq.) Lodd. ex Mart., popularly known as bocaiúva or macaúba [9]. It is a palm tree belonging to the Arecaceae family, native to tropical regions, and prevalently occurs in South America, mainly in the Brazilian Cerrado and Pantanal [9,10].

The bocaiúva pulp has great economic, industrial, and nutritional importance [11]. Traditionally, bocaiúva pulp is consumed in natura or in the form of sweets, ice cream, and flour [11]. In addition, it is widely recognized in folk medicine for its analgesic, healing, and laxative effects [12]. The pulp oil of *A. aculeata* (AAPO) is rich in compounds with antioxidant action [8,11], such as β-carotene, tocopherols, and fatty acids, such as oleic and palmitic acid [8,12].

Several studies have already demonstrated the beneficial effects of bioactive compounds derived from *A. aculeata*, such as hypoglycemic [13], neuroprotective [14], and antioxidant effects [15,16]. However, the antiaggregant and anticoagulant action of AAPO lacks additional studies. Thus, due to its antioxidant activity, we hypothesize that AAPO may have effects on human hemostasis, and these properties were investigated by using an in vitro experimental model.

2. Materials and Methods

2.1. Obtaining the Oil from the Pulp of A. aculeata (AAPO)

Ripe fruits of *A. aculeata*, intact and without signs of contamination and/or physical damage, were collected in January 2019, the period of greatest fruiting, in Campo Grande, Mato Grosso do Sul (20°27′54°39″ S54°38′43.732″ O), under authorization from the National System for the Management of Genetic Heritage and Associated Traditional Knowledge (SISGEN; n° A0F9FD6).

The fruit pulp was dehydrated (50 °C) in a tray dryer at an airflow of 0.5 m/s for 18 h, and AAPO was obtained by solvent extraction using the exhaust method for 48 h with petroleum ether and hexane (2:1). The extracted oil was evaporated in a rotary evaporator, placed under a nitrogen flow (30 min), kept in a desiccator for 2 h, and stored in an amber bottle, protected from light in a cool place (10 °C) until analysis [14,17]. For the tests, dimethyl sulfoxide (DMSO 0.5%) was used as a vehicle.

2.2. Gas Chromatography–Mass Spectrometry (GC-MS) Analysis

AAPO was analyzed by gas chromatography (Shimadzu QP2010, Shimadzu®, Tokyo, Japan) coupled to a mass spectrometer (GC-MS) equipped with a COA-20i autoinjector (Shimadzu, Kyoto, Japan). The carrier gas was helium and the pressure was 79.7 kPa. The injection temperature was 250 °C, and the temperature program was the following: 60–240 °C increasing 3 $°C.min^{-1}$, 240–310 °C increasing 15 $°C.min^{-1}$, and 310 °C for 10 min (isothermic). An RTx-5MS capillary column (30 mm × 0.25 mm × 0.25 μm) was used, and the mass spectra were obtained by electron ionization (EI), applying the energy 70 eV. The retention indices (RIs) were calculated using C8–C40 alkane standards (Sigma-Aldrich®, Cotia, São Paulo, Brazil). Identification of constituents was performed by comparing the mass spectra registered with NIST, WILEY, and FFNSC libraries, and retention indices described according to the literature [18].

2.3. Blood Collection and Obtaining Plasma

Human blood samples (5 mL) were collected in the same proportion by venipuncture from 20 healthy men and women, aged between 18 and 40 years, with no history of bleeding or thrombosis, after prior consent. Blood collection was performed using trisodium citrate (nine parts of blood and one part of 3.8% trisodium citrate) as an anticoagulant. PRP (platelet-rich plasma) was obtained after centrifugation for 10 min at 123× g at room temperature, and a PPP (platelet-poor plasma) containing approximately 10,000 platelets was obtained by diluting PRP in saline. The study protocol was approved by the Ethics Committee of the Federal University of Mato Grosso do Sul (CAAE protocol No. 57842022.2.0000.0021, approval opinion No. 5.445.802), in accordance with national and international standards for research involving human subjects.

2.4. Toxicity Assays

2.4.1. Evaluation of In Vitro Toxicity by the Trypan Blue Exclusion Test

For the experiment, 400 µL of PRP pool was incubated (37 °C for 5 min) with 5 µL of different AAPO concentrations (50, 100, 200, 400, and 800 µg/mL) and controls; positive control: Triton X100 (1%, v/v) and negative control: DMSO (0.6%). Then, 50 µL of Trypan blue (0.4%) was added to an equal volume of PRP incubated with compounds and controls. Subsequently, they were transferred to a Neubauer chamber, and the viable and non-viable platelets were quantified. The results were expressed as the mean percentage of platelet viability. All experiments were performed in triplicate, not exceeding 3 h after collection [19].

2.4.2. Evaluation of In Vivo Systemic Toxicity in Galleria Mellonella Model

For the experiment, 10 µL of AAPO of the two smallest and the two largest concentrations, yielding a final amount of 0.5, 1.0, 4.0, and 8.0 µg per larvae, or controls was injected into the hemocoel of each larva through the last left proleg using a Hamilton® syringe (Hamilton Inc.®, Reno, NV, USA). Ten larvae weighing between 0.2 and 0.3 g without signs of melanization were used per group. Saline and DMSO (100%) were used as negative and positive controls, respectively. The larvae were incubated in the dark at 37 °C, and their survival was recorded at selected intervals for 72 h, where larvae that showed no movement to touch and high levels of melanization were counted as dead [20].

2.5. Determination of Platelet Aggregation

Platelet aggregation was assessed by turbidimetry using a semi-automatic aggregometer (EasyAgreg 4.0, Qualiterm®, São Paulo, Brazil) [21]. Platelets were counted in automatic counting equipment (Sysmex XP-300, Sysmex, Kobe, Japan) and adjusted with saline solution, obtaining a value between 200,000 and 250,000 platelets/mm^3. Aliquots of 400 and 600 µL of the PRP pool were used for aggregation with adenosine diphosphate (ADP, 30 µM; Calbiochem®, Burlington, ON, Canada) or epinephrine (5 µg/mL; Hipolabor®, Belo Horizonte, Minas Gerais, Brazil), respectively. ADP is diluted in purified distilled water. The PRP pool was pre-incubated with 5 µL of AAPO (50, 100, 200, 400, and 800 µg/mL) at 37 °C for 5 min. Aggregation was measured in percentage (%) and recorded continuously for 5 or 10 min after the addition of agonists. DMSO (0.6%) was used as a negative control, and its average aggregation percentage was assumed to be 100%. PPP was used to adjust the baseline turbidity of the sample and Ticlopidine (10 µM) as a positive control. All tests were performed in triplicate on three independent days, not exceeding 3 h after collection.

2.6. Evaluation of Blood Coagulation

For coagulation evaluation, prothrombin time (PT) and activated partial thromboplastin time (aPTT) were measured following the manufacturer's guidelines (Wiener Lab®, Rosario, Argentina) in triplicate and using a semi-automated coagulation system (CLOTimer®, Quick Timer, São Paulo, Brazil). Briefly, a PPP pool was obtained after centrifugation for 15 min at 1107× g and 8 °C of human blood samples collected with sodium citrate (3.8%) (9:1; *m*/*v*). About 100 μL of PPP was pre-incubated with 1.3 μL of AAPO at different concentrations (50–1000 μg/mL) or controls for 5 min at 37 °C. For normal (standard) and positive controls, plasma without added vehicle and/or treatment and heparin (17 IU/mL blood) were used, respectively. DMSO (0.6%) was used as a negative control [21].

2.7. Platelet Activation

2.7.1. Expression of Platelet Surface P-Selectin

Platelet surface P-selectin expression was determined after incubation of PRP (400 μL) pool with 5 μL of AAPO (50, 100, 200, 400, and 800 μg/mL) or DMSO (0.6%) for 5 min at room temperature. Subsequently, the samples were stimulated with ADP (30 μM) and incubated for 5 min. Activated platelets were then labeled with fluorescein isothiocyanate (FITC) mouse anti-human CD42b (5 μL) and P-selectin with phycoerythrin (PE) mouse anti-human CD62P (5 μL) and remained in the shelter of light for 15 min. Unlabeled controls, samples labeled only with CD42b-FITC, and only CD62P-PE were used for data calibration. The assay was performed on a CytoFLEX flow cytometer (CytoFLEX, Beckman Coulter®, Brea, CA, USA), and 10,000 events were collected; the data were analyzed in FlowJo® v10.8 software (BD Life Sciences, Franklin Lakes, NJ, USA) [22].

2.7.2. Assessment of Platelet Activation by Intraplatelet Content of ROS

To evaluate platelet activation by intraplatelet content of ROS, concentrations of 50, 100, 200, 400, and 800 μg/mL of AAPO were used. DMSO (vehicle, 0.6%) was used as a negative control, and hydrogen peroxide (H_2O_2) as a positive control. A pool of PRP (200 μL) was incubated with 2.5 μL of AAPO concentrations or controls for 5 min. ROS content was determined by fluorescence intensity at 485 nm (excitation) and 520 nm (emission) using a multimode microplate reader (Synergy™ H1, BioTek Instruments®, Winooski, VT, USA) after 30 min of incubation with 10 μL 2′,7′dichlorodihydrofluorescein-diacetate (DCFH-DA, 10 μM) [23].

2.8. Statistical Analysis

Statistical analysis was performed using multiple comparisons of analysis of variance (ANOVA), complemented by the Tukey–Kramer test, when necessary, assuming a minimum significance level of $p < 0.05$ between different concentrations of AAPO and controls. For the *G. mellonella* model, differences in survival were compared using the log-rank test. The software used was GraphPad® Prism version 8.0.2.

3. Results and Discussion

3.1. Chemical Analyses of AAPO

Oilseed plants can be affected by different environmental, climatic, cultivation, harvesting, processing, and storage factors, consequently changing the chemical composition of the extracted oils [24,25]. Despite this, the main compounds observed in AAPO by GC-MS were similar to those found in the literature [26,27] and are summarized in Table 1. Oleic acid (51.25%) was predominant, followed by palmitic acid (21.51%), and other fatty acids were also observed to a minor extent, such as ethyl oleate (8.45%), lauric acid (3.58%), caprylic acid (3.09%), and squalene (2.37%).

Recently, SANT'ANA and collaborators (2023) [15] observed an oleic acid content of approximately 49.32% in AAPO, which reflected a greater total antioxidant capacity in C57Bl/6 mice [15]. In addition, the study by PERDOMO and collaborators (2015) [28] suggested that oleic acid reduces PAI-1 levels (plasminogen activator-1 inhibitor) induced by TNF-α in vascular smooth muscle cells, thereby protecting the endothelium and modulating inflammation.

In addition, pre-treatment with physiological concentrations of oleic and palmitic acid maintains glutathione (GSH) levels and protects human endothelial cells from oxidative stress [29]. Palmitic acid is a fatty acid responsible for the palmitoylation of proteins (a reversible process involving the addition of palmitic acid to specific cysteines through a thioester bond, which provides dynamic regulation of protein functions, including processes such as phosphorylation and ubiquitination) and the biosynthesis of palmitoylethanolamine, which has neuroprotective and anti-inflammatory capacity [30]. Our findings corroborate those found by COSTA and collaborators (2020), where a concentration of approximately 15.80% palmitic acid was observed in AAPO [12].

Although less prevalent, medium-chain fatty acids lauric and caprylic, as well as squalene, a triterpene present in several vegetable oils, such as soybean oil, have already been reported to have the ability to attenuate oxidative stress [31–33]. Furthermore, a previous study demonstrated a concentration of approximately 31.2 mg/100 g of ascorbic acid, 46.9 mg/100 g of β-carotene, and 12.6 mg/100 g of α-tocopherol in the pulp oil of *A. aculeata* [14].

Table 1. Constituents identified from AAPO by GC-MS.

Peak	[1]RT (min)	Compound	Area (%)	[2]RI
1	6.66	Caproic acid	2.00	991
2	6.87	β-Myrcene	0.27	1002
3	8.05	β-phellandrene	1.73	1034
4	13.58	Caprylic acid	3.09	1186
5	14.21	Ethyl octanoate	0.16	1200
6	21.36	Capric acid	0.38	1375
7	29.24	Lauric acid	3.58	1573
8	36.35	Myristic acid	1.01	1768
9	39.82	Isobutyl phthalate	0.30	1870
10	41.47	β-Springene	0.55	1920
11	42.32	Palmitoleic acid	1.45	1947
12	43.16	Palmitic acid	21.51	1973
13	43.91	Ethyl palmitate	0.28	1996
14	49.19	Linoleic acid	0.24	2137
15	48.66	Oleic acid	51.25	2154
16	49.13	Ethyl oleate	8.45	2169
17	61.15	Hexacosane	0.77	2619
18	62.76	Heptacosane	0.14	2700
19	65.20	Squalene	2.37	2831
20	66.37	Nonacosane	0.46	2901

[1]RT: retention time; [2]RI: retention indices on RTx-5MS capillary column.

3.2. In Vitro and In Vivo Toxicity

The panoply of bioactive compounds present in different plant products may impact positively or negatively human and animal health [34]. The hematopoietic system is one of the most sensitive targets for toxic substances [34]; for this reason, the in vitro and in vivo toxicological assays have been performed to establish the safety criteria, quality, and efficacy, as well as to select the suitable concentrations for their therapeutic use [35].

The in vitro toxicity results showed no toxicity to human platelets at the tested AAPO concentrations (50, 100, 200, 400, and 800 µg/mL) (Figure 1A). There was no significant difference between concentrations and the negative control (NC), and the percentage range of platelet viability obtained fell between 97.4% and 99.1%. The in vivo toxicity test using *G. mellonella* larvae confirmed the absence of systemic toxicity at the concentrations tested (50, 100, 400, and 800 µg/mL), being equivalent to the NC (Figure 1B), without high levels of melanization or larvae death.

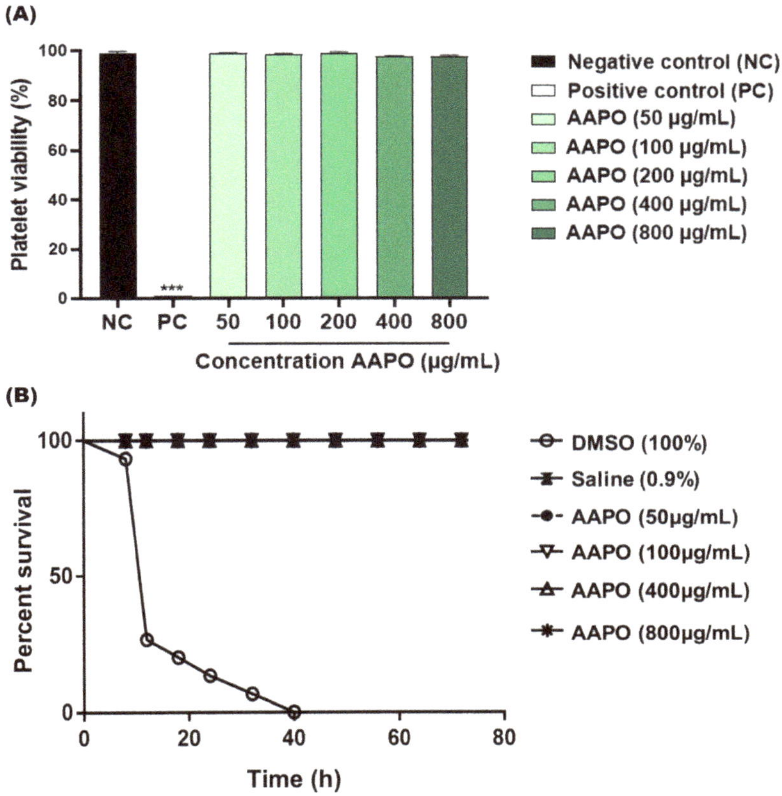

Figure 1. Toxicity in human platelets and systemic in *G. mellonella*. (**A**) Percentage (%) of human platelet viability obtained in PRP treated with *Acrocomia aculeata* (AAPO) pulp oil at different concentrations (50, 100, 200, 400, and 800 μg/mL); negative control (NC): vehicle (DMSO, 0.6%) and positive control (PC): Triton X100 (1%). (***) indicates statistical difference with $p < 0.001$ compared to NC. (**B**) In vivo systemic toxicity in *G. mellonella* model treated with different concentrations (50, 100, 400, and 800 μg/mL) of AAPO. The percentage of survival was evaluated for 72 h; negative control (NC): saline and positive control: DMSO (100%). Difference estimates in survival were compared using a $p < 0.05$ log-rank test.

These results corroborate the data found by Traesel and colleagues (2014) [17], who demonstrated through an in vivo model using Wistar rats, low acute and subacute (28 days) toxicity of AAPO on blood cells, suggesting toxicity only at high concentrations of AAPO (50% oral lethal dose higher than 2000 mg/kg).

3.3. *Effect of AAPO on Human Platelet Aggregation*

ADP is concentrated in the dense granules of platelets, when released it binds to two purinergic receptors, P2Y12 and P2Y1 [36]. The first mediates the inhibition of adenylyl cyclase activity, activates phosphatidylinositol 3-kinase (PI3-K), and promotes the activation and amplification of platelet aggregation, forming stable thrombi [36]. On the other hand, P2Y1 leads to increased intracellular calcium, altered platelet shape, and reversible aggregation [37]. The results obtained in this study demonstrated significant inhibition of this aggregation pathway in AAPO-treated PRP, with the highest inhibitory percentage (34%) at a concentration of 800 μg/mL (Figure 2A,B).

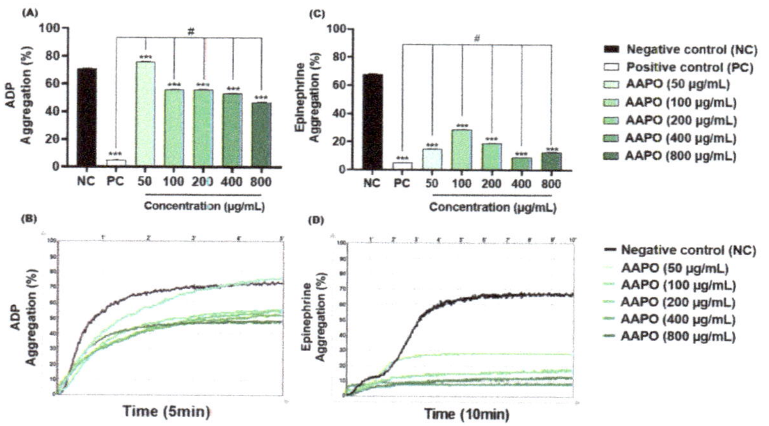

Figure 2. Effect of AAPO on platelet aggregation induced by ADP and epinephrine. Percentage (%) of platelet aggregation at different concentrations of AAPO (50, 100, 200, 400, and 800 µg/mL), induced by ADP (30 µM) (**A**,**B**) and epinephrine (5 µg/mL) (**C**,**D**) for 5 and 10 min, respectively; negative control—NC (DMSO 0.6%) and positive control—PC (Ticlopidine 10 µM). (***) The statistical difference with $p < 0.001$ compared to negative control (NC). (#) The statistical difference with $p < 0.001$ compared to positive control (PC).

Like ADP, AAPO showed antithrombotic action when epinephrine was used as an agonist. In addition to acting synergistically with other platelet agonists, epinephrine may assist in decreasing the concentration of cyclic adenosine monophosphate (cAMP) and activation of PI3-K, facilitating the thrombus formation process by binding to the adrenergic receptor (α2A) exposed on the platelet membrane [38]. Aggregation induced by this pathway was inhibited by more than 50% at all concentrations tested, with the highest percentage of inhibition (≈87%) in platelets treated with 400 µg/mL of bocaiúva pulp oil (Figure 2C,D).

No previous investigations on the antiplatelet effects of AAPO were found, making it difficult to compare the data with other studies. Nevertheless, antiaggregant effects have been previously reported in platelets treated with oil extract of the buriti fruit peel (*Mauritia flexuosa* L. F.), a palm species of the Arecaceae family, with 50% inhibitory concentrations (IC50) of 0.65 mg/mL for ADP and 0.93 mg/mL with collagen [39]. In our study, CI50 of AAPO against ADP-induced aggregation was 590 µg/mL (or 0.59 mg/mL), showing to be more potent than the oil extracts tested in those previous works. On the other hand, AAPO IC50 against epinephrine-induced aggregation was not possible to calculate, since all concentrations are capable of inhibiting more than 50% of platelet aggregation, showing an even more potent antiplatelet effect when compared to ADP.

However, the ability of oleic acid to modulate the action of receptors coupled to G proteins, mainly adrenoreceptors, and consequently its influence on adenylyl cyclase activity, has been previously reported [40]. In our study, we can observe that oleic acid is the most significant compound of AAPO (Table 1), thus, corroborating the antiplatelet activity of bocaiúva oil, especially when epinephrine is used as an agonist.

3.4. Effect of AAPO on Blood Coagulation

The anticoagulant activity of AAPO was analyzed by aTTP, which evaluates the integrity of the intrinsic and common coagulation pathways, and by PT, which evaluates changes in the coagulation factors of the extrinsic pathway [41].

Although prolongation in PT and aTTP was reported in the plasma of mice treated with flour from the mesocarp of a palm tree of the Arecaceae, *Orbignya phalerata* Mart. [42],

AAPO in natura did not significantly increase PT time and aTTP at any of the concentrations tested (Table 2).

Table 2. PT and aPTT coagulation parameters measured in human plasma treated with heparin and AAPO.

Sample [1]	Blood Coagulation Test [2]			
	PT		aPTT	
	Time (s)	IRN [3]	Time (s)	Ratio [4]
Normal control (Standard)	14 ± 0.32	-	28 ± 2.20	-
Negative control	15 ± 0.22	1.1	26 ± 1.53	0.9
AAPO (50 μg/mL)	16 ± 2.63	1.2	30 ± 0.62	1.1
AAPO (100 μg/mL)	17 ± 1.57	1.2	28 ± 1.24	1.0
AAPO (200 μg/mL)	17 ± 1.22	1.2	26 ± 3.93	0.9
AAPO (400 μg/mL)	17± 1.17	1.3	27 ± 1.12	1.0
AAPO (800 μg/mL)	16 ± 0.76	1.2	24 ± 2.08	0.8
Heparin (17 IU/mL of blood)	>100	-	>100	-

[1] Oil from *A. aculeata* pulp (AAPO) at different concentrations (50, 100, 200, 400, and 800 μg/mL); negative control (vehicle, 0.6% DMSO) and heparin (positive control). [2] Prothrombin time (PT) and activated partial thromboplastin time (aPTT) values in seconds (s) measured in AAPO-treated human plasma and expressed as mean ± SD. [3] International normalized ratio (INR) calculated based on PT results, used to monitor the effectiveness of anticoagulants. [4] Relationship between the time values of concentrations and the time (s) of the controls.

3.5. *Platelet Activation*

3.5.1. Effects of AAPO on Platelet Surface P-Selectin Expression

P-selectin is a transmembrane protein stored in platelet alpha granules and Weibel-Palade bodies in endothelial cells [43]. Different platelet agonists and high shear stress contribute to the exteriorization of P-selectin in the cell membrane [44]. When bound to PSGL-1 (P-selectin-1 glycoprotein ligand) and platelet glycoprotein (Gp)Ib, it plays an important role in leukocyte and platelet adhesion and rolling, microparticle release, expression of monocyte tissue factor [43], and in the size and stabilization of thrombi mediated by the Gp IIb/IIa–fibrinogen interaction [22].

We evaluated the expression of P-selectin in the membrane of activated platelets after exposure to AAPO (Figure 3) using the flow cytometry technique. As a result, we observed a significant reduction at concentrations of 400 and 800 μg/mL of AAPO. When compared to the results of platelet aggregation tests (Figure 2), it is observed that concentrations of 400 and 800 μg/mL present better results.

Furthermore, Fuentes and colleagues (2013) observed thrombin-induced inhibition of P-selectin expression in platelets treated with buriti oil extracts, where concentrations of 0.1 and 1 mg/mL inhibited approximately 18% and 29% of the expression of P-selectin, respectively [39].

3.5.2. Content of ROS Produced by Platelets after Exposure to AAPO

The results obtained showed that concentrations of 50, 100, 300, and 400 μg/mL of AAPO significantly decreased ($p < 0.001$) the production of ROS when compared to the negative control (Figure 4). However, the same result was not observed in plasma treated with a concentration of 800 μg/mL. Physiologically, ROS are necessary for the maintenance of cellular function, while an imbalance between pro-oxidants and antioxidants generates a state of oxidative stress [45]. Increased platelet activation is directly associated with ROS generation and platelet adhesion receptor expression [2], so the use of ROS scavengers preserves platelet adhesion to collagen [46].

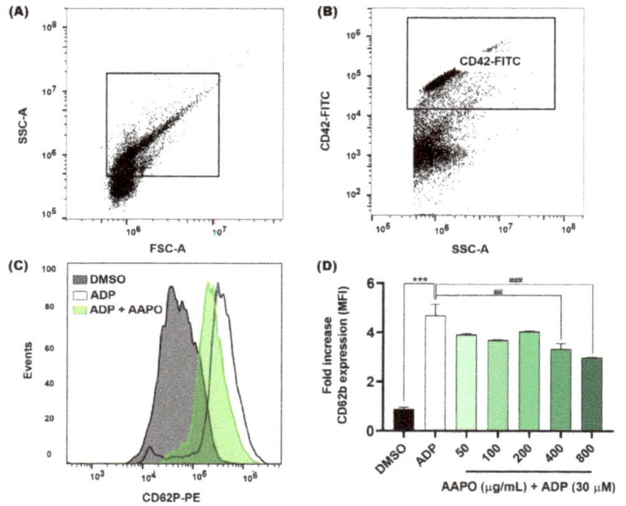

Figure 3. Expression of platelet surface P-selectin after exposure of platelets to AAPO. (**A**) Representative dot plots generated by FlowJo software. The gate shows the platelet population. (**B**) Representative dot plot showing a platelet-positive population (CD42b-FITC). (**C**) Representative histograms showing the activation of platelets incubated with AAPO and stimulated by ADP (30 μM) for 5 min. Activated platelets were labeled with CD42b-FITC (5 μL) and CD62P (CD62P-PE, 5 μL) and kept in the dark for 15 min. (**D**) Mean fluorescence intensity (MFI) of CD62P-PE expressed on the membrane of activated platelets treated with different concentrations of AAPO (50, 100, 200, 400, and 800 μg/mL). DMSO (0.6%): negative control; ADP (30 μM): positive control. Three independent experiments were performed. (***) The statistical difference with $p < 0.001$ compared to negative control. (##) The statistical difference with $p < 0.01$ and (###) statistical difference with $p < 0.001$ compared to ADP group.

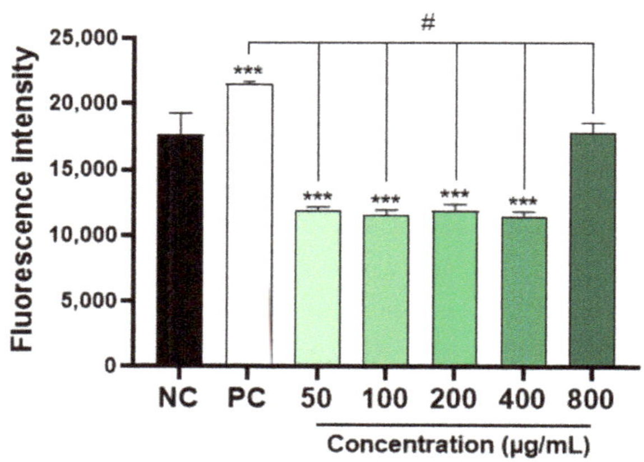

Figure 4. Intraplatelet content of ROS in AAPO-treated platelets. Intraplatelet ROS content after 30 min of incubation with DCFH-DA (10 μM), in platelets treated with 50, 100, 200, 400, and 800 μg/mL of *A. aculeata* pulp oil (AAPO) or controls; negative control—NC (DMSO 0.6%) and positive control—PC (hydrogen peroxide, H_2O_2). (***) The statistical difference with $p < 0.001$ compared to negative control (NC). (#) The statistical difference with $p < 0.001$ compared to positive control (PC).

Recently, a higher total antioxidant capacity of bocaiúva pulp oil was reported in mice fed a high-fat diet [15]. In addition, the aqueous extract of dried leaves of *Acrocomia aculeata* (EA-Aa) revealed protective and hypoglycemic effects in type 2 diabetes promoted by polyphenols present in macaúba extracts (at concentrations of 125, 250, and 500 μg.mL^{-1}) [16]. EA-Aa was able to protect against H_2O_2 at a concentration of 125 μg.mL^{-1} in human dermal microvascular endothelial cells and also in histological slices of liver, kidney, and aorta from Wistar and Goto-Kakizaki, whereas the antioxidant effect of EA-Aa on the vascular wall was also revealed in a tissue-specific manner in microvascular endothelial cell line represented by an improvement (≈22%) in cell viability [16]. Furthermore, our research group previously demonstrated that AAPO has a neuroprotective effect, being able to protect brain structures from oxidative damage induced by chronic restriction stress in Wistar rats, and effect attributable to the relatively high levels of α-tocopherol, β-carotene, and ascorbic acid found in AAPO [14].

Therefore, the data obtained here corroborate those found in the literature and highlight the present results regarding the antiaggregant potential of AAPO, which can be related to its promising ability to inhibit the production and release of ROS by platelets. This beneficial effect, as well as those demonstrated in related studies, is mainly attributable to the high concentration of compounds that possess a significant antioxidant capacity present in the macaúba fruit.

4. Conclusions

AAPO showed no toxicity in vitro or in vivo. It significantly inhibited platelet aggregation triggered by ADP and epinephrine in most of the concentrations tested, but it was unable to change coagulation parameters. In addition, AAPO decreased the expression of P-selectin on the platelet membrane and in the intraplatelet production of ROS, thus preventing platelet activation resulting in an antithrombotic effect.

Author Contributions: Conceptualization: E.B.P.; writing—original draft: E.B.P., I.T.E., N.S.C. and D.B.S.; writing—review and editing: E.B.P., I.T.E., D.C.L.S.B., D.C.L., E.J.P.-G., N.S.C. and D.B.S.; data curation: I.T.E., D.C.L.S.B., A.J.P.d.A., R.S.N.O., D.B.S., J.d.C.O.S., K.F.S.d.S., N.S.C., M.L.R.M. and A.C.J.; review and editing: D.W.-F. and E.B.P.; supervision: E.B.P. and A.C.J. All authors have read and agreed to the published version of the manuscript.

Funding: This research was funded by the Fundação de Apoio ao Desenvolvimento do Ensino, Ciência e Tecnologia do Estado de Mato Grosso do Sul (FUNDECT/ Universal/ No 31/2021), the Conselho Nacional de Desenvolvimento Científico e Tecnológico (CNPq, EDITAL UFMS/PROPP/CNPq No107/2022), the Coordenação de Aperfeiçoamento de Pessoal de Nível Superior—Brasil (CAPES, Finance Code 001), and UFMS. R.S.N.O. and A.J.P.d.A. were awarded a PIBIC scholarship by CNPq and UFMS, respectively.

Institutional Review Board Statement: The study was conducted in accordance with national and international standards for research involving human subjects and approved by the Ethics Committee of the Federal University of Mato Grosso do Sul (CAAE protocol No. 57842022.2.0000.0021, approval opinion No. 5.445.802, approval date: 6 February 2022).

Informed Consent Statement: Informed consent was obtained from all subjects involved in the study.

Data Availability Statement: The data presented in this study are available on request from the corresponding author. The data are not publicly available due to privacy.

Acknowledgments: We thank all individuals who voluntarily agreed to participate in this study. We would also like to thank the Postgraduate Programs in Pharmaceutical Sciences and Biotechnology at the Federal University of Mato Grosso do Sul for supporting the revision of the English language.

Conflicts of Interest: The authors declare no conflicts of interest.

References

1. Khodadi, E. Platelet function in cardiovascular disease: Activation of molecules and activation by molecules. *Cardiovasc. Toxicol.* **2019**, *20*, 1–10. [CrossRef] [PubMed]
2. van der Meijden, P.E.; Heemskerk, J.W. Platelet biology and functions: New concepts and clinical perspectives. *Nat. Rev. Cardiol.* **2018**, *16*, 166–179. [CrossRef] [PubMed]
3. Qiao, J.; Arthur, J.F.; Gardiner, E.F.; Andrews, R.K.; Zeng, L.; Xu, K. Regulation of platelet activation and thrombus formation by reactive oxygen species. *Redox Biol.* **2018**, *14*, 126–130. [CrossRef] [PubMed]
4. Roth, G.A.; Mensah, G.A.; Johnson, C.O.; Addolorato, G.; Ammirati, E.; Baddour, L.M.; Barengo, N.C.; Beaton, A.Z.; Benjamin, E.J.; Benziger, C.P.; et al. Global burden of cardiovascular diseases and risk factors, 1990–2019. *J. Am. Coll. Cardiol.* **2020**, *76*, 2982–3021. [CrossRef] [PubMed]
5. Montenont, E.; Echagarruga, C.; Allen, N.; Araldi, E.; Suarez, Y.; Berger, J.S. Platelet WDR1 suppresses platelet activity and is associated with cardiovascular disease. *Blood* **2016**, *128*, 2033–2042. [CrossRef] [PubMed]
6. Chan, N.; Sobieraj-Teague, M.; Eikelboom, J.W. Direct oral anticoagulants: Evidence and unresolved issues. *Lancet* **2020**, *396*, 1767–1776. [CrossRef] [PubMed]
7. Melnikova, I. The anticoagulants market. *Nat. Rev. Drug Discov.* **2009**, *8*, 353. [CrossRef]
8. Calixto, J.B. The role of natural products in modern drug discovery. *An. Acad. Bra. Ciênc.* **2019**, *91*, e20190105. [CrossRef]
9. Borges, C.E.; Santos, J.C.B.D.; Evaristo, A.B.; da Cunha, T.G.; Von dos Santos Veloso, R.; Barroso, G.M.; da Silva, R.S. Distribution and future projection of potential cultivation areas for *Acrocomia aculeata* (Arecaceae) worldwide: The emerging energy culture of the tropics. *Theor. Appl. Climatol.* **2021**, *146*, 1069–1078. [CrossRef]
10. Ciconini, G.; Favaro, S.P.; Roscoe, R.; Miranda, C.H.B.; Tapeti, C.F.; Miyahira, M.A.M.; Bearari, L.; Galvani, F.; Borsato, A.V.; Colnago, L.A.; et al. Biometry and oil contents of *Acrocomia aculeata* fruits from the Cerrados and Pantanal biomes in Mato Grosso do Sul, Brazil. *Ind. Crop. Prod.* **2013**, *45*, 208–214. [CrossRef]
11. Souza, F.G.; Araújo, F.F.; Farias, D.P.; Zanotto, A.W.; Neri-Numa, I.A.; Pastore, G.M. Brazilian fruits of Arecaceae family: An overview of some representatives with promising food, therapeutic and industrial applications. *Food Res. Int.* **2020**, *138*, 109690. [CrossRef]
12. Costa, G.L.A.; Buccini, D.F.; Arruda, A.L.A.; Favaro, S.P.; Moreno, S.E. Phytochemical profile, anti-inflammatory, antimutagenic and antioxidant properties of *Acrocomia aculeata* (Jacq.) Lodd. pulp oil. *Food Sci. Technol.* **2020**, *40*, 963–971. [CrossRef]
13. Nunes, Â.A.; Buccini, D.F.; Jaques, J.A.S.; Portugal, L.C.; Guimarães, R.C.A.; Favaro, S.P.; Caldas, R.A.; Carvalho, C.M.E. Effect of *Acrocomia aculeata* kernel oil on adiposity in type 2 diabetic rats. *Plant Foods Hum. Nutr.* **2017**, *73*, 61–67. [CrossRef]
14. Jacobowski, A.C.; Parisotto, E.B.; Aydos, L.R.; Serafim de Souza, R.; Viveros, S.; Colín-Gonzalez, A.L.; Silva, I.S.; Sanjinez-Argandoña, E.J.; Wilhelm Filho, D.; Angel, A.S.; et al. Neuroprotective Effects of *Acrocomia aculeata* Pulp Oil Microcapsules on Rats Subjected to Chronic Stress. *J. Med. Food* **2021**, *24*, 1068–1075. [CrossRef]
15. Sant' Ana, C.T.; Agrizzi Verediano, T.; Grancieri, M.; Toledo, R.C.L.; Tako, E.; Costa, N.M.B.; Martino, H.S.D.; de Barros, F.A.R. Macauba (*Acrocomia aculeata*) pulp oil prevents adipogenesis, inflammation and oxidative stress in mice fed a high-fat diet. *Nutrients* **2023**, *15*, 1252. [CrossRef]
16. Monteiro-Alfredo, T.; Oliveira, S.; Amaro, A.; Rosendo-Silva, D.; Antunes, K.; Pires, A.S.; Teixo, R.; Abrantes, A.M.; Botelho, M.F.; Castelo-Branco, M.; et al. Hypoglycaemic and antioxidant properties of *Acrocomia aculeata* (Jacq.) Lodd ex Mart. extract are associated with better vascular function of Type 2 diabetic rats. *Nutrients* **2021**, *13*, 2856. [CrossRef] [PubMed]
17. Traesel, G.K.; de Souza, J.C.; de Barros, A.L.; Souza, M.A.; Schmitz, W.O.; Muzzi, R.M.; Oesterreich, S.A.; Arena, A.C. Acute and subacute (28 days) oral toxicity assessment of the oil extracted from *Acrocomia aculeata* pulp in rats. *Food Chem. Toxicol.* **2014**, *74*, 320–325. [CrossRef]
18. Adams, R.P. *Identification of Essential Oil Components by Gas Chromatography/Mass Spectrometry*, 4th ed.; Allured Publishing Corporation: Carol Stream, IL, USA, 2007.
19. Lopez, E.; Ortega-Liébana, M.D.C.; Salido, S.; Salido, G.M.; Altarejos, J.; Rosado, J.A.; Redondo, P.C. Evaluation of the antiaggregant activity of ascorbyl phenolic esters with antioxidant properties. *J. Physiol. Biochem.* **2015**, *71*, 415–434. [CrossRef]
20. Megaw, J.; Thompson, T.P.; Lafferty, R.A; Gilmore, B.F. *Galleria mellonella* as a novel in vivo model for assessment of the toxicity of 1-alkyl-3-methylimidazolium chloride ionic liquids. *Chemosphere* **2015**, *139*, 197–201. [CrossRef] [PubMed]
21. Weber, S.S.; de Souza, A.C.S.; Soares, D.C.L.; Lima, C.C.; de Moraes, A.C.R.; Gkionis, S.V.; Arenhart, T.; Rodrigues, L.G.G.; Ferreira, S.R.S.; Pedrosa, R.C.; et al. Chemical profile, antimicrobial potential, and antiaggregant activity of supercritical fluid extract from *Agaricus bisporus*. *Chem. Pap.* **2022**, *76*, 6205–6214. [CrossRef]
22. Merten, M.; Thiagarajan, P. P-Selectin expression on platelets determines size and stability of platelet aggregates. *Circulation* **2000**, *102*, 1931–1936. [CrossRef] [PubMed]
23. Reiniers, M.J.; van Golen, R.F.; Bonnet, S.; Broekgaarden, M.; van Gulik, T.M.; Egmond, M.R.; Heger, M. Preparation and practical applications of 2′,7′-dichlorodihydrofluorescein in redox assays. *Anal. Chem.* **2017**, *89*, 3853–3857. [CrossRef]
24. Lescano, C.H.; Oliveira, I.P.; Silva, L.R.; Baldivia, D.S.; Sanjinez-Argandoña, E.J.; Arruda, E.J.; Moraes, I.C.F.; Lima, F.F. Nutrients content, characterization and oil extraction from *Acrocomia aculeata* (Jacq.) Lodd. fruits. *Afr. J. Food Sci.* **2015**, *9*, 113–119. [CrossRef]
25. Zhou, Y.; Zhao, W.; Lai, Y.; Zhang, B.; Zhang, D. Edible plant oil: Global status, health issues, and perspectives. *Front. Plant Sci.* **2020**, *11*, 1315. [CrossRef]

26. del Río, J.C.; Evaristo, A.B.; Marques, G.; Martín-Ramos, P.; Martín-Gil, J.; Gutiérrez, A. Chemical composition and thermal behavior of the pulp and kernel oils from macauba palm (*Acrocomia aculeata*) fruit. *Ind. Crop. Prod.* **2016**, *84*, 294–304. [CrossRef]
27. Hiane, P.A.; Ramos, F.M.M.; Ramos, M.I.L.; Macedo, M.L.R. Bocaiúva, *Acrocomia aculeata* (Jacq.) Lodd., pulp and kernel oils: Characterization and fatty acid composition. *Braz. J. Food Technol.* **2005**, *8*, 256–259.
28. Perdomo, L.; Beneit, N.; Otero, Y.F.; Escribano, Ó.; Díaz-Castroverde, S.; Gómez-Hernández, A.; Benito, M. Protective role of oleic acid against cardiovascular insulin resistance and in the early and late cellular atherosclerotic process. *Cardiovasc. Diabetol.* **2015**, *14*, 1–12. [CrossRef] [PubMed]
29. Palomino, O.; Giordani, V.; Chowen, J.; Fernández-Alfonso, M.; Goya, L. Physiological doses of oleic and palmitic acids protect human endothelial cells from oxidative stress. *Molecules* **2022**, *27*, 5217. [CrossRef] [PubMed]
30. Vesga-Jiménez, D.J.; Martin, C.; Barreto, G.E.; Aristizábal-Pachón, A.F.; Pinzón, A.; González, J. Fatty Acids: An insight into the pathogenesis of neurodegenerative diseases and therapeutic potential. *Int. J. Mol. Sci.* **2022**, *23*, 2577. [CrossRef]
31. Micera, M.; Botto, A.; Geddo, F.; Antoniotti, S.; Bertea, C.M.; Levi, R.; Gallo, M.P.; Querio, G. Squalene: More than a step toward sterols. *Antioxidants* **2020**, *9*, 688. [CrossRef]
32. Alves, N.F.B.; Queiroz, T.M.; Travassos, R.A.; Magnani, M.; Braga, V.A. Acute treatment with lauric acid reduces blood pressure and oxidative stress in spontaneously hypertensive rats. *Basic Clin. Pharmacol. Toxicol.* **2017**, *120*, 348–353. [CrossRef] [PubMed]
33. Cansız, D.; Ünal, İ.; Üstündağ, Ü.V.; Alturfan, A.A.; Altinoz, M.A.; Elmacı, İ.; Emekli-Alturfan, E. Caprylic acid ameliorates rotenone induced inflammation and oxidative stress in the gut-brain axis in Zebrafish. *Mol. Biol. Rep.* **2021**, *48*, 5259–5273. [CrossRef] [PubMed]
34. Li, X.; Luo, Y.; Wang, L.; Li, Y.; Shi, Y.; Cui, Y.; Xue, M. Acute and subacute toxicity of ethanol extracts from Salvia przewalskii Maxim in rodents. *J. Ethnopharmacol.* **2010**, *131*, 110–115. [CrossRef] [PubMed]
35. Yang, M.; Wu, Z.; Wang, Y.; Kai, G.; Singor Njateng, G.S.; Cai, S.; Cao, J.; Cheng, G. Acute and subacute toxicity evaluation of ethanol extract from aerial parts of Epigynum auritum in mice. *Food Chem. Toxicol.* **2019**, *131*, 110534. [CrossRef] [PubMed]
36. Bandyopadhyay, S.K.; Azharuddin, M.; Dasgupta, A.K.; Ganguli, B.; SenRoy, S.; Patra, H.K.; Deb, S. Probing ADP induced aggregation kinetics during platelet-nanoparticle interactions: Functional dynamics analysis to rationalize safety and benefits. *Front. Bioeng. Biotechnol.* **2019**, *7*, 163. [CrossRef] [PubMed]
37. Cattaneo, M. The platelet P2 receptors. In *Platelets*; Academic Press: Cambridge, MA, USA, 2019; pp. 259–277. [CrossRef]
38. Martin, A.C.; Zlotnik, D.; Bonete, G.P.; Baron, E.; Decouture, B.; Belleville-Rolland, T.; Le Bonniec, B.; Poirault-Chassac, S.; Alessi, M.C.; Gaussem, P.; et al. Epinephrine restores platelet functions inhibited by ticagrelor: A mechanistic approach. *Eur. J. Pharmacol.* **2020**, *866*, 172798. [CrossRef] [PubMed]
39. Fuentes, E.; Rodríguez-Pérez, W.; Guzmán, L.; Alarcón, M.; Navarrete, S.; Forero-Doria, O.; Palomo, I. Mauritia flexuosa presents in vitro and in vivo antiplatelet and antithrombotic Activities. *Evi. Based Complement. Alternat. Med.* **2013**, *2013*, 653257. [CrossRef]
40. Yang, Q.; Alemany, R.; Casas, J.; Kitajka, K.; Lanier, S.M.; Escribá, P.V. Influence of the membrane lipid structure on signal processing via g protein-coupled receptors. *Mol. Pharmacol.* **2005**, *68*, 210–217. [CrossRef] [PubMed]
41. Wu, Y.; Hu, S.; Ma, Y.; Zhao, B.; Yang, W.; Lu, Y.; Li, P.; Du, S. Novel Pheretima guillelmi-derived antithrombotic protein DPf3: Identification, characterization, in vitro evaluation and antithrombotic mechanisms investigation. *Int. J. Biol. Macromol.* **2020**, *154*, 545–556. [CrossRef]
42. Azevedo, A.P.; Farias, J.C.; Costa, G.C.; Ferreira, S.C.; Aragão-Filho, W.C.; Sousa, P.R.; Pinheiro, M.T.; Maciel, M.C.; Silva, L.A.; Lopes, A.S.; et al. Anti-thrombotic effect of chronic oral treatment with Orbignya phalerata Mart. *J. Ethnopharmacol.* **2007**, *111*, 155–159. [CrossRef]
43. Purdy, M.; Obi, A.; Myers, D.; Wakefield, T. P- and E-selectin in venous thrombosis and non-venous pathologies. *J. Thromb. Haemost.* **2022**, *20*, 1056–1066. [CrossRef] [PubMed]
44. Fang, J.; Sun, X.; Liu, S.; Yang, P.; Lin, J.; Feng, J.; Cruz, M.A.; Dong, J.F.; Fang, Y.; Wu, J. Shear stress accumulation enhances von willebrand factor-induced platelet P-Selectin translocation in a PI3K/Akt pathway-dependent manner. *Front. Cell Dev. Biol.* **2021**, *9*, 642108. [CrossRef] [PubMed]
45. Wang, G.; Yang, F.; Zhou, W.; Xiao, N.; Luo, M.; Tang, Z. The initiation of oxidative stress and therapeutic strategies in wound healing. *Biomed. Pharmacother.* **2023**, *157*, 114004. [CrossRef]
46. Hosseini, E.; Solouki, A.; Roudsari, Z.O.; Kargar, F.; Ghasemzadeh, M. Reducing state attenuates ectodomain shedding of GPVI while restoring adhesion capacities of stored platelets: Evidence addressing the controversy around the effects of redox condition on thrombosis. *J. Thromb. Thrombolysis* **2020**, *50*, 123–134. [CrossRef] [PubMed]

nutrients MDPI

Article

Antidiabetic Effect of *Passiflora ligularis* Leaves in High Fat-Diet/Streptozotocin-Induced Diabetic Mice

Diana P. Rey [1], Sandra M. Echeverry [1], Ivonne H. Valderrama [1], Ingrid A. Rodriguez [1], Luis F. Ospina [1], Fatima Regina Mena Barreto Silva [2] and Marcela Aragón [1,*]

[1] Departamento de Farmacia, Universidad Nacional de Colombia, Av. Carrera 30 # 45-03 Edif. 450, Bogotá 111321, Colombia; dpreyp@unal.edu.co (D.P.R.); smecheverryg@unal.edu.co (S.M.E.); ihvalderramap@unal.edu.co (I.H.V.); inarodriguezma@unal.edu.co (I.A.R.); lfospinag@unal.edu.co (L.F.O.)

[2] Departamento de Bioquímica, Centro de Ciências Biológicas, Universidade Federal de Santa Catarina, Campus Universitário, Rua João Pio Duarte Silva, 241, Sala G301, Florianópolis 88037-000, SC, Brazil; mena.barreto@ufsc.br

* Correspondence: dmaragonn@unal.edu.co; Tel.: +57-6013165000 (ext. 14630) or +57-3177488247

Abstract: Type 2 diabetes mellitus (T2DM) is a major global public health concern, prompting the ongoing search for new treatment options. Medicinal plants have emerged as one such alternative. Our objective was to evaluate the antidiabetic effect of an extract from the leaves of *Passiflora ligularis* (*P. ligularis*). For this purpose, T2DM was first induced in mice using a high-fat diet and low doses of streptozotocin. Subsequently, an aqueous extract or an ethanolic extract of *P. ligularis* leaves was administered for 21 days. The following relevant results were found: fasting blood glucose levels were reduced by up to 41%, and by 29% after an oral glucose overload. The homeostasis model assessment of insulin resistance (HOMA-IR) was reduced by 59%. Histopathologically, better preservation of pancreatic tissue was observed. Regarding oxidative stress parameters, there was an increase of up to 48% in superoxide dismutase (SOD), an increase in catalase (CAT) activity by 35% to 80%, and a decrease in lipid peroxidation (MDA) by 35% to 80% in the liver, kidney, or pancreas. Lastly, regarding the lipid profile, triglycerides (TG) were reduced by up to 30%, total cholesterol (TC) by 35%, and low-density lipoproteins (LDL) by up to 32%, while treatments increased high-density lipoproteins (HDL) by up to 35%. With all the above, we can conclude that *P. ligularis* leaves showed antihyperglycemic, hypolipidemic, and antioxidant effects, making this species promising for the treatment of T2DM.

Keywords: *Passiflora ligularis*; antidiabetic; flavonoids-O-glucoside; antihyperglycemic; antioxidant; antihyperlipidemic

1. Introduction

T2DM is considered a public health problem since it affects 6.28% of the world's population, its prevalence rate is 2.5% per year, and it is increasing at a much faster rate in developed countries; therefore, it is necessary to take prevention and treatment measures urgently [1,2]. T2DM is characterized by defective insulin secretion by pancreatic β cells and tissue resistance to insulin responses, causing hyperglycemia, hyperinsulinemia, increased reactive oxygen species (ROS), oxidative stress, and adipose tissue hypertrophy, among other metabolic changes [3,4].

Due to the previous metabolic changes, the treatment of T2DM requires not only the reduction of blood glucose but also the improvement of the lipid profile and insulin resistance index, among others, so the treatment involves lifestyle changes, oral medications, and in some cases, injectable drugs [5,6]. Despite these therapeutic alternatives, the WHO estimates that 80% of the world's population uses traditional medicine to treat diseases such as T2DM, and in recent years, studies have increased on plants with potential antidiabetic activity, their main bioactive compounds, and their possible mechanisms of action involved [7,8]. The main bioactive compounds that have shown antidiabetic activity are flavonoids, polyphenols, terpenoids, and alkaloids [9,10].

Although various authors have reported a diversity of medicinal plant species with antidiabetic activity, one of the most extensively studied genus has been Passiflora [11–13]. Specifically, our research group has focused its attention on the study of *P. ligularis* and its potential use in the treatment of T2DM [14,15]. Although the antihyperglycemic effect of the aqueous extract and ethanol fraction of *P. ligularis* leaves were demonstrated in normoglycemic animals subjected to an oral glucose tolerance test [16,17], it is important to highlight that the normoglycemic conditions are characterized by a better physiological functionality. Therefore, to demonstrate the antidiabetic effect, it is necessary to conduct tests in an animal model in which diabetes has been induced and mimic the pathogenesis of the disease [18].

Given the importance of not only studying the antidiabetic effect of a medicinal plant but also identifying its bioactive compounds, it should be noted that previously, astragalin and isoquercetin, metabolites of the extract and fraction of *P. ligularis* leaves, were shown to improve glucose homeostasis through insulin secretion in isolated rat pancreatic islets and glucose uptake in the soleus muscle, respectively [19,20]. Therefore, it is interesting to evaluate the antidiabetic effect of the extract and fraction where both compounds are found in greater proportion.

Finally, as mentioned above, given the importance of simulating the pathophysiology and symptomatology of T2DM, there are several animal biomodels that involve genetically modified rodents, but one of the most used biomodels is the induction of obesity and chemical pancreatic damage [21,22]. These models used in the present study combine a high-fat diet with low-dose streptozotocin (HFD/STZ) which mimics the generation of insulin resistance, β-cell dysfunction, the metabolic characteristics, cytokine levels, and oxidative stress similar to those observed in patients with T2DM [23,24].

This research aimed to evaluate the antidiabetic activity of the aqueous extract of *P. ligularis* leaves and its respective ethanol fraction obtained using the XAD2 resin. A chronic model of diabetes induced by HFD/STZ was selected to evaluate this pharmacological activity monitoring the blood glucose levels. Likewise, parameters related to oxidative stress and lipid profile were assessed. A histopathological evaluation of the pancreas was performed too.

2. Materials and Methods

2.1. Chemicals

Ethanol 99.5% (PanReac AppliChem, Darmstadt, Germany) was employed in the process of obtaining the ethanol fraction of *P. ligularis* extract. Formic acid reagent grade 85% (Carlo Erba, Milan, Italy), Acetonitrile HPLC Grade (Merck Rahway, NJ, USA), and ultrapure water (Milli-Q system Millipore® (Merck, Rahway, NJ, USA) were used for liquid chromatographic analysis. Regarding the analytical standards, isoquercetin (Quercetin-3-glucoside, ≥90%, HPLC), astragalin (Kaempferol 3-glucoside, ≥97.0% HPLC), and chrysin (≥98%, HPLC) were acquired from Sigma-Aldrich® (Sigma Chemical Company, St. Louis, MO, USA).

Streptozotocin (572201), glucose (G7021), carboxymethyl cellulose (CMC) (419273), Lipid Peroxidation (MDA) Assay Kit (MAK085), Catalase Assay Kit (CAT100), and SOD Assay Kit (19160) were purchased from Sigma (St. Louis, MO, USA). An ELISA kit, Monobind (2425-300A), was used to determine the serum insulin levels. Cholesterol MR kit (1118005), HDL-Cholesterol kit (1133010), Triglycerides MR kit, and LDL-Cholesterol kit (1133105) were used to measure lipid markers and were acquired from Linear Chemicals S.L.U. Pentobarbital (Montgat, Spain). (Euthanex®) used for animal sacrifice was manufactured by INVET S. A. and purchased from a veterinary establishment.

2.2. Preparation of the Extract and Fraction of Passiflora ligularis

The leaves of *P. ligularis* were collected in Anolaima, Cundinamarca-Colombia (Longitude: 74°29.97′ W; Latitude: 4°50.0172′ N; Altitude: 1850 m.a.s.l.) through the sample collection permit granted by the Autoridad Nacional de Licencias Ambientales (ANLA) and the Ministerio de Ambiente y Desarrollo, code 38024, resolution 0699 of 26 April 2018. A voucher copy was deposited in the National Herbarium of Colombia (COL 602878).

Obtaining the extract was carried out as described by Rey et al., 2020 [20]., where the leaves of *P. ligularis* were collected in the municipality of Anolaima in the Department of Cundinamarca, Colombia. After collection, the leaves were dried at room temperature and subsequently pulverized using a knife mill. The aqueous extract was prepared by steeping the plant material in water at 90 °C. To obtain the ethanol fraction, the crude extract was agitated with XAD-2 resin and then washed with ethanol.

2.3. Chemical Characterization and Quantification of Flavonoids in the Extract and Ethanolic Fraction of P. ligularis Leaves

The total flavonoid content, isoquercetin, and astragalin were quantified using high-performance liquid chromatography (HPLC) following the methodology previously described [17]. The HPLC was performed on an Agilent 1260 Infinity LC system coupled with a diode array detector (DAD). A Phenomenex-Luna® C18 column (150 × 4.6 mm × 5 µm) was used as the stationary phase at a temperature of 45 °C. Quantification was carried out at wavelengths of 260 nm, 265 nm, and 350 nm for isoquercitrin, astragalin, and total flavonoids, respectively. Chrysin was identified and detected at 267 nm using chrysin ≥ 98%, HPLC grade, as an external standard.

2.4. Induction of T2DM and Experimental Design

A total of 30 female Swiss mice between 14 and 16 weeks old, were used in the experiment. Of these, 6 animals (n = 6) were randomly selected to constitute the normoglycemic control group throughout the study period, receiving a standard diet. This group was not induced with diabetes nor administered any treatment. The remaining 24 animals were fed a high-fat diet for 8 weeks and then received two low doses of streptozotocin (STZ 40 mg/kg) intraperitoneally, dissolved in citrate buffer (pH 4.5), with a 5-day interval between doses. The animals were provided with a 5% glucose solution overnight to prevent drug-induced hypoglycemia [25]. Three days after administering the second dose of STZ, blood glucose levels (BGL) were measured using Accu-Chek Performa® equipment, collecting blood samples from the lateral tail vein through a small incision. Animals with BGLs above 150 mg/dL were considered for further experimentation. These 24 diabetic mice were then randomly divided into 4 groups (n = 6) and received the following by oral gavage for the next 21 days:

Vehicle group: Diabetic control mice receiving the vehicle (0.5% CMC *w*/*v* and 0.5% Tween 80 *w*/*v*).
Metformin group: Diabetic mice receiving metformin (250 mg/kg) as a positive control.
Aqueous extract group: Diabetic mice receiving the aqueous extract of leaves of *P. ligularis* (500 mg/kg).
Ethanolic fraction group: Diabetic mice receiving the ethanolic fraction of *P. ligularis* (250 mg/kg).

It is worth mentioning that during the 21-day treatment period, diabetic mice continued to receive a high-fat diet. Additionally, the normoglycemic group was injected with saline instead of STZ and orally administered the vehicle for 21 days to ensure they experienced the same stress conditions as the diabetic mice.

At the end of the experiment, all the animals were anesthetized with pentobarbital (60 mg/kg) and then sacrificed by cervical decapitation [26]. Once the blood samples were obtained, these were centrifuged (3500 rpm, 10 min) and the serum supernatant was collected. The blood and organ samples were conserved to −80 °C until the lipid profile analysis or serum insulin measurement.

2.5. Oral Glucose Tolerance Test

This assay was carried out on the 21st day of administering the treatments, following the methodology previously developed in our research group [27]. Animals were fasted four hours before the test. Oral glucose overload (2000 mg glucose/kg) was administered 30 min after each treatment, and BGLs were measured before and after (30, 60, and 90 min) the overload, using the Accu-Check Performa® (Roche Diagnostics, Basel, Switzerland) equipment.

2.6. Insulin Resistance Index (HOMA-IR)

For determining the serum insulin levels, an ELISA kit was used. Insulin resistance (IR) was determined according to the homeostasis model assessment index calculated using Equation (1) [28]:

$$HOMA - \mathrm{IR} = \frac{(plasma\ insulin\ level\ [\mu\mathrm{U/mL}] \times fasting\ plasma\ glucose\ [\mathrm{mg/dL}])}{405} \quad (1)$$

2.7. Histopathological Examination

After being sacrificed, the pancreas was quickly removed, weighed, and placed in a 10% phosphate-buffered formaldehyde solution in a 1:20 ratio to histopathological studies. According to the standard procedure, the samples were embedded in paraffin, cut into 5 μm thick sections, and stained with hematoxylin and eosin stain according to widely known protocols [29].

2.8. Biochemical Parameters

2.8.1. Analysis of Oxidative Stress Parameters

At the end of the bioassay, the organs collected (liver, pancreas, and kidney) were used for the estimation of biochemical parameters of superoxide dismutase (SOD) and catalase (CAT) using commercial kits. A commercial kit was employed to estimate the lipid peroxidation as the MDA (Malondialdehyde) levels in the tissue homogenate.

2.8.2. Serum Lipid Profile

The triglycerides (TG), total cholesterol (TC), high-density lipoprotein (HDL), and low-density lipoprotein (LDL) levels were estimated using diagnostic kits.

2.9. Statistical Analysis

GraphPad Prism® software (version 6, San Diego, CA, USA) was employed for data analysis. All results are expressed as mean ± SEM (blood glucose levels, oxidative stress parameters) or mean ± SD (serum lipid profile, fasting glucose, fasting insulin, and HOMA index). We use two-way analysis of variance (ANOVA) followed by Bonferroni post hoc test to analyze the data of Figures 1–3, and use a one-way ANOVA followed by post-test Dunnet for the data of Figures 4 and 5, Tables 1 and 2. Differences were considered significant at $p \leq 0.05$. The assumptions of ANOVA's test were evaluated by the software GraphPad prism 6® by the Brown–Forsythe test and Bartlett test for ANOVA.

Table 1. Effect of the aqueous extract and ethanol fraction of *P. ligularis* on fasting glucose, fasting insulin, and HOMA index.

TREATMENT	Fasting Glucose mg/dL	Insulin Levels (μUI/mL)	HOMA-IR
Normoglycemic	105.600 ± 7.579 ****	2.267 ± 0.332 ****	0.591 ± 0.086 ****
vehicle	434.000 ± 26.069	23.178 ± 2.527	24.830 ± 2.421
Metformin 250 mg/kg	347.286 ± 19.499 ****	15.877 ± 1.752 ****	13.610 ± 1.343 ****
Aqueous extract 500 mg/kg	333.800 ± 15.766 ****	12.493 ± 1.407 ****	10.294 ± 1.037 ****
Ethanol fraction 250 mg/kg	292.600 ± 27.207 ****	12.986 ± 1.217 ****	9.379 ± 0.786 ****

Data are expressed as mean ± SD. $n = 6$ animals per group. One-way ANOVA post-test Dunnet; **** $p < 0.0001$ with respect to the vehicle group.

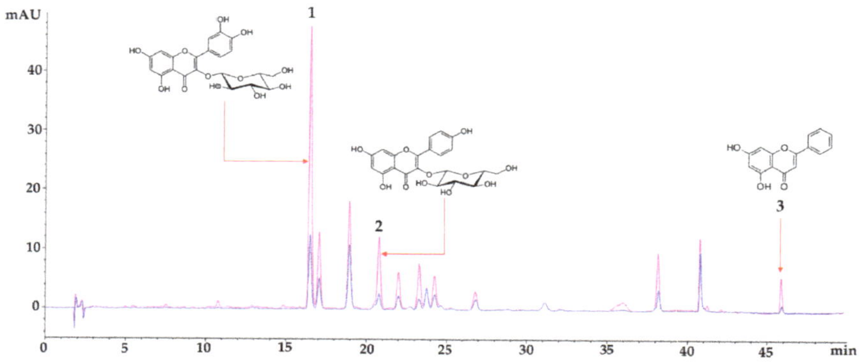

Figure 1. Chromatographic profile of aqueous extract of *Passiflora ligularis* leaves (blue) and an ethanol fraction of *Passiflora ligularis* leaves (pink) at 350 nm. Chromatographic signal 1 corresponds to isoquercetin, signal 2 corresponds to astragalin, and signal 3 corresponds to chrysin. The analytical method used was previously described in the methodology section.

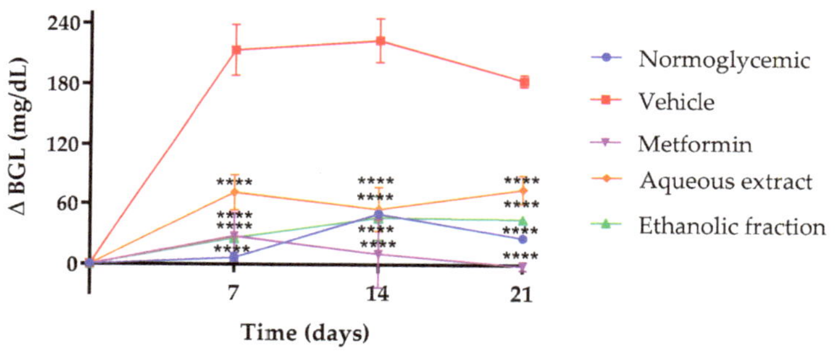

Figure 2. Difference between day 0 and 7, 14, and 21 days in blood glucose levels (BGLs) of the experimental mice. Normoglycemic (blue), vehicle (red), metformin 250 mg/kg (purple), aqueous extract 500 mg/kg (yellow), ethanol fraction 250 mg/kg (green). Data are expressed as mean ± SEM, $n = 6$ animals per group. Two-way ANOVA post-test Bonferroni; **** $p < 0.0001$ with respect to the vehicle group.

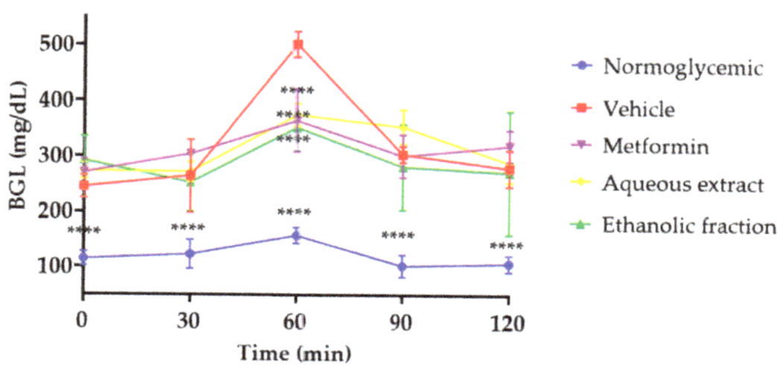

Figure 3. Oral glucose overload test. Normoglycemic (blue), vehicle (red), metformin 250 mg/kg (purple), aqueous extract of *P. ligularis* 500 mg/kg (yellow), ethanol fraction of *P. ligularis* 250 mg/kg (green). Data are expressed as mean ± SEM, $n = 6$ animals per group. Two-way ANOVA post-test Bonferroni; **** $p < 0.0001$ with respect to the vehicle group.

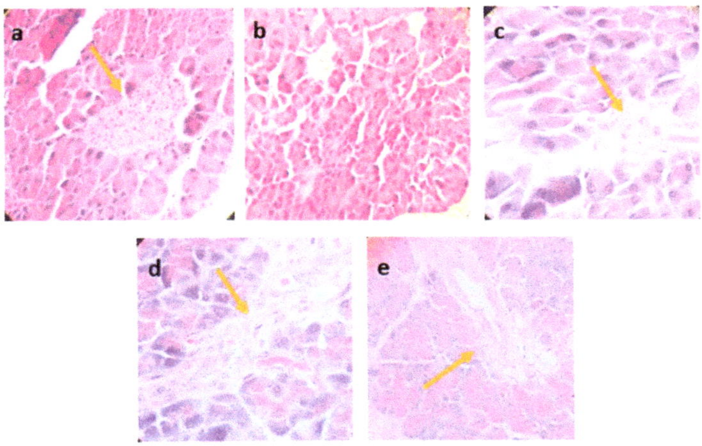

Figure 4. Photomicrographs of pancreatic tissues from different experimental groups were stained by hematoxylin and eosin (H&E) and examined with magnifying power (40×). (**a**) Normoglycemic group, (**b**) Vehicle, (**c**) Metformin, (**d**) Aqueous extract of *P. ligularis*, (**e**) Ethanol fraction of *P. ligularis*. Arrows show the presence of Langerhans islets.

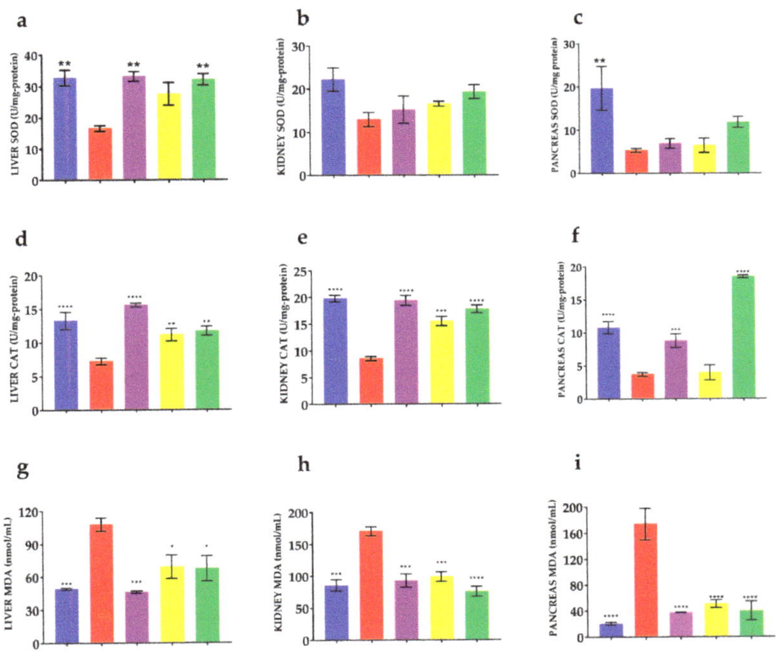

Figure 5. Effect of *P. ligularis* on oxidative stress parameters. Normoglycemic (blue), vehicle (red), metformin 250 mg/kg (purple), aqueous extract of *P. ligularis* 500 mg/kg (yellow), ethanol fraction of *P. ligularis* 250 mg/kg (green). SOD activity: (**a**) liver, (**b**) kidney, (**c**) pancreas; CAT activity: (**d**) liver, (**e**) kidney, (**f**) pancreas; MDA levels: (**g**) liver, (**h**) kidney, (**i**) pancreas. Data are expressed as mean ± SEM, $n = 6$ animals per group. One-way ANOVA post-test Dunnet; * $p < 0.05$, ** $p < 0.01$, *** $p < 0.001$ and **** $p < 0.0001$ with respect to the vehicle group.

Table 2. Effect of aqueous extract *P. ligularis* 500 mg/kg and ethanol fraction *P. ligularis* on serum lipid profile in diabetic mice.

TREATMENT	Triglyceride (TG) mg/dL	Total Cholesterol mg/dL	LDL-C mg/dL	HDL-C mg/dL
Normoglycemic	96.870 ± 2.230	140.280 ± 15.345	88.820 ± 25.778	37.843 ± 1.926
vehicle	225.506 ± 13.345	252.076 ± 5.479	174.658 ± 17.526	28.923 ± 0.081
Metformin 250 mg/kg	169.606 ± 3.615 ****	159.775 ± 4.805 ****	98.438 ± 13.633 ***	36.727 ± 4.824 **
Aqueous extract 500 mg/kg	159.450 ± 7.070 ****	207.410 ± 17.580 *	131.464 ± 25.953 *	34.263 ± 2.206 *
Extract fraction 250 mg/kg	157.160 ± 0.430 ****	162.700 ± 13.790 ****	117.336 ± 2.449 **	36.237 ± 1.980 **

LDL-C—low-density lipoprotein cholesterol, HDL-C—high-density lipoprotein cholesterol. Data are expressed as mean ± SD. $n = 6$ animals per group. One-way ANOVA post-test Dunnet; * $p < 0.05$, ** $p < 0.01$, *** $p < 0.001$ and **** $p < 0.0001$ with respect to the vehicle group.

3. Results

3.1. Chemical Characterization

Chromatographic analysis was performed for the aqueous extract and ethanol fraction. A concentration of total flavonoids of 60.983 ± 0.755 µg-equivalent of isoquercetin/mg extract was quantified for the aqueous extract, while for the ethanol fraction, the value was 134.998 ± 0.489 µg-equivalent of isoquercetin/mg fraction. As shown in Figure 1, isoquercetin, astragalin, and chrysin in the ethanol fraction showed a significant increase concerning the aqueous extract. The quantified values for isoquercetin and astragalin in the aqueous extract were 12.890 ± 0.376 µg of isoquercetin/mg extract and 4.190 ± 0.042 µg of astragalin/mg extract, respectively. In the ethanol fraction, the content of isoquercetin increased by 241.8% and astragalin by 227.3%, concerning the concentrations found in the aqueous extract of *P. ligularis*.

3.2. Effect of *P. ligularis* on Blood Glucose Levels

Figure 2 presents the fasting blood glucose levels (BGLs) at 7, 14, and 21 days of treatment. As expected, metformin reduced BGLs throughout treatment, the aqueous extract reduced the BGLs by 34%, 27%, and 31% at 7, 14, and 21 days of treatment compared to the vehicle, and the ethanolic fraction reduced BGLs by 36%, 33%, and 41% in the same days in comparison to the vehicle.

3.3. Oral Glucose Tolerance Test (OGTT)

In Figure 3, it is possible to see that the normoglycemic mice presented significant differences at all times compared to the vehicle group after oral glucose overload carried out on day 21 after diabetes induction. In contrast, all diabetic mice that received treatment presented with a decrease in BGLs at 60 min. While the vehicle group raised 500.7 ± 23 mg/dL of BGLs, treatments reduced BGLs by 27% for metformin, 25% for the aqueous extract, and 29% for the ethanol fraction of *P. ligularis* with respect to the vehicle group.

3.4. Insulin Resistance Index (HOMA-IR)

To measure insulin resistance in HFD/STZ-induced diabetes models, the homeostasis model assessment of insulin resistance (HOMA-IR) is commonly used [30].

According to the results described in Table 1, after 21 days of treatment, fasting glucose decreased by 23% with the aqueous extract and by 32% with the ethanol fraction; meanwhile, fasting insulin decreased by 46% and by 43% for the aqueous extract and ethanol fraction, respectively. The HOMA index decreased by 58% for the extract and 59% for the ethanol fraction; metformin also caused a significant decrease in the three parameters compared to the vehicle group.

3.5. Histopathological Examination

According to the photomicrograph shown in Figure 4, it can be observed that diabetic mice, after 21 days of treatment with metformin, aqueous extract, and the ethanol fraction of *P. ligularis*, showed significant preservation of pancreatic islets and exocrine tissue in comparison with the diabetic mice that did not receive treatment. Image A shows normal islets in which the insulin secretion has not been over-stimulated, keeping its structure and size. Micrograph B corresponding to the vehicle group showed cytoplasmic vacuolar degeneration, not the endocrine component. Image C shows a not proliferated islet compared with the other treatments. Image D shows endocrine tissue which is not hypertrophic compared to Figure 4e, which shows a diffused and hypertrophic structure with remarkable preservation of the pancreatic islets compared to the untreated animals. Histological analysis showed that aqueous extract and the ethanol fraction of *P. ligularis* caused a remarkable preservation of pancreatic islets compared to the untreated animals, without an endocrine component.

3.6. Analysis of Oxidative Stress Parameters

SOD activity is shown in Figure 5b,c. Significant differences were found between the normoglycemic and vehicle groups in kidney and pancreas tissues. In liver tissue (Figure 5a), the activity of this enzyme increased by 39% for the aqueous extract, 48% for the fraction, and 50% for metformin compared to the vehicle.

Respecting the CAT activity, as shown in Figure 5d, in the liver, the aqueous extract increased the catalase activity by 35%, while the ethanol fraction increased it by 38% compared to the vehicle. According to Figure 4e, in the kidney, the catalase activity increased by 44% in the aqueous extract and 51% for the ethanol fraction compared to the vehicle. Finally, according to Figure 5f, although the aqueous extract did not increase the catalase activity in the pancreas, the ethanol fraction did increase it by 80% with respect to the vehicle. Metformin improved catalase activity in all organs.

Concerning MDA levels, as shown in Figure 5g, the aqueous extract decreased the levels of MDA by 35% and the fraction by 37% compared to the vehicle group. According to Figure 5h, in the kidney, the aqueous extract decreased the levels of MDA by 42% and the fraction by 55% concerning diabetic mice without treatment. Finally, in the pancreas (Figure 5i), the aqueous extract decreased the levels of MDA by 70% and the ethanol fraction by 80% compared to the vehicle. As expected, normoglycemic mice showed higher catalase and SOD activity and lower MDA levels in all organs.

3.7. Effect of *P. ligularis* on Serum Lipid Profile

Due to the relationship between diabetes and hyperlipidemia, the quantification of total triglycerides, high-density lipoprotein cholesterol, low-density lipoprotein cholesterol, and total cholesterol were considered in this study (Table 2).

According to Table 2, TG decreased by 29% for the aqueous extract and by 30% for the ethanol fraction. The total cholesterol parameter decreased by 17% and 35% for the aqueous extract and ethanol fraction, respectively. The LDL-C levels decreased by 24% for the aqueous extract and 32% for the ethanol fraction. Finally, HDL-C increased by 18% for the aqueous extract and 25% for the ethanol fraction compared to the vehicle. For its part, metformin also showed an improvement in the lipid profile.

This effect could be related to the protective effect of the aqueous extract and the ethanol fraction of *P. ligularis* leaves on the pancreas. Figure 4d,e showed that both treatments found endocrine components associated with pancreatic islets. When insulin production or release is deficient, the lipolysis process is not inhibited, causing hyperlipidemia. However, our results showed that the animals treated with the aqueous extract and the ethanol fraction of *P. ligularis* attenuated insulin resistance, which could be related to the decrease in TG, total cholesterol, and LDL-C with the increase in HDL-C compared to diabetic animals administered with the vehicle.

4. Discussion

The effect of *P. ligularis* leaves in HFD/STZ-induced diabetic mice was evaluated. The extract and ethanol fraction were assessed for phytochemical identification purposes. According to the chromatographic analysis, isoquercetin, astragalin, and chrysin in the ethanol fraction were found in major amounts compared to the aqueous extract. These findings are in contrast with previous analyses obtained by our research group. It is evident that these flavonoids are found in greater proportion in the fraction, in which, given the nature of the XAD resin, they were expected to be enriched with these polar compounds [31,32].

Other tests were carried out in order to identify changes in diabetic mice after treatment administration. BGL differences were found from day 7. Previously, an extract of *P. glandulosa* fruit showed an antihyperglycemic effect in streptozotocin-induced diabetic mice at 15, 21, and 28 days of treatment, an effect attributed mainly to the presence of flavonoids [33]. The effect of *P. ligularis* on the control of this parameter can also be attributed to flavonoids in the aqueous extract and the ethanol fraction, especially *O*-glycosyl flavonoids such as isoquercetin, astragalin, and chrysin which have been reported previously [15].

With respect to the results obtained in the OGTT test, this test in rodents is a usual test employed to determine if a mouse is glucose intolerant and diabetic. However, this is also useful to determine the hypoglycemic or antihyperglycemic effect of drugs and extracts, among others [34]. Other species of Passiflora have been reported to have a similar antihyperglycemic effect in diabetic models, for example, ethanol extracts of *P. edulis*, methanolic extract of leaves of *P. incarnata*, and *P. foetida* maintain blood glucose levels, improving the oral glucose tolerance in streptozotocin-induced diabetic mice or alloxan diabetic rats [35,36].

In previous studies, the aqueous extract and ethanol fraction of *P. ligularis* leaves demonstrated an antihyperglycemic effect in normoglycemic rats after an oral glucose overload and an increase in glycogenesis [20]. It is noteworthy that this study confirms this effect in diabetic mice after receiving 21 days of treatment considering that the ethanol fraction had a more significant effect. It has been shown that the fraction is rich in flavonoids such as isoquercetin, astragalin, and chrysin [20,37]. This effect may be due to flavonoids since isoquercetin has been shown to decrease BGLs after an oral overload of glucose in diabetic mice associated with an inhibition of the enzyme dipeptidyl peptidase IV (DPP IV) and an increase in serum levels of glucagon-like peptide (GLP-1) and insulin [38].

Another flavonoid that may be involved in the process is astragalin, which has demonstrated a hypoglycemic effect after an oral glucose overload in normoglycemic rats linked to an insulin secretagogue [19]. On the other hand, chrysin also showed an effect of reduction of glucose levels at 60 min after an oral glucose overload in diabetic rats after 30 days of treatment, an effect associated with an increase in the sensitivity of insulin receptors, GLUT-4 glucose transporters, and an increase in muscle glycogen [39].

Given the above, we can suggest that the effects of the aqueous extract and ethanol fraction of *P. ligularis* improve glucose intolerance induced by T2DM and are associated with the presence of the flavonoids mentioned previously.

The homeostasis model assessment of insulin resistance (HOMA-IR) is the most widely used model to determine insulin resistance in rodent models of diabetes since it is a simple, accurate method and causes minimal stress to the animals. This mathematical model relates insulin and fasting plasma glucose with the hyperinsulinemic euglycemic glucose clamp (HEGC) [40]. According to the HOMA-IR results obtained, the extract and the fraction decreased insulin resistance, and this effect had already been evidenced in other passifloras species. For example, the consumption of *P. setacea* juice decreased HOMA-IR in humans, fasting as well as 3 h after consumption [41]. Likewise, the extract of *P. incarnata* leaves prevents insulin resistance, and its effect was strongly associated with the presence of flavonoids [42]. Our results are according to previous reports in the literature since the ethanol fraction decreased HOMA-IR values slightly. In addition, in previous studies, isoquercetin has been shown to decrease HOMA-IR in a dose-dependent manner in type-2-diabetes-induced hepatic injury in rats [43]. Finally, an extract with rich contents of astragalin has also been shown to decrease insulin resistance in a model of diabetes induced with a high-fat diet in rats [44].

According to the previous results, we can suggest that the aqueous extract and especially the ethanolic fraction of *P. ligularis* leaves improved the HOMA index, an effect that can be attributed to the presence of astragalin since it has been shown to increase insulin secretion in the pancreatic tissue by stimulating calcium influx through K^+_{ATP}, L-VDCC channels, and activating protein kinases PKC and PKA [19]. This effect can also be associated with glucose uptake by peripheral tissues such as skeletal muscle, given that isoquercetin, another of the major components, has an insulinomimetic effect by activating the PI3K, MAPK, and MEK/ERK pathways, and de novo protein synthesis of the GLUT-4 transporter [20].

Regarding the histopathological analysis, the disturbance of islet proliferation was observed as result of the diabetes model, which is coherent with previous studies that showed high glucose levels in mice fed with an HFD on islet proliferation but inhibited by metformin administration [45]. Previously, isoquercetin showed protective activity in pancreatic islets showing a similar morphology to normal ones [43]. The results are expected according to the concentration of this molecule within the fraction with respect to the aqueous extract of *P. ligularis.*

Regarding the analysis of the results obtained related to oxidative stress, these parameters were measured since SOD and CAT are antioxidant enzymes that decrease the production of reactive oxygen species (ROS), protect against oxidative stress, nephropathy, and other T2DM complications. CAT also protects pancreatic beta cells from damage caused by hydrogen peroxide (H_2O_2). The increase in MDA levels in diabetics suggests that peroxidative lesions are related to the development of diabetic complications and a decrease in antioxidant mechanisms [46].

In this study, only the ethanol fraction was shown to improve the activity of hepatic SOD; however, CAT showed an improvement in all the organs studied, indicating that the antioxidant effect is more related to the metabolism of H_2O_2. This effect is evidenced with a higher proportion at the pancreatic level comparable to the normoglycemic group, which confirms the results obtained at the histopathological level. Likewise, since the ethanol fraction had a more significant antioxidant effect, it can be associated with flavonoids such as chrysin, which may be responsible for this effect since it has previously shown a decrease in MDA levels and an increase in SOD and CAT activity in the liver, brain, and pancreas of diabetic rats after 4 weeks of treatment [47]. In the same way, the aqueous extract of *M. oleifera* leaves rich in flavonoids such as isoquercetin and astragalin has shown an increase in the levels of CAT and SOD, and decreased to reduce MDA levels at the liver and kidney level in diabetic rats [48]. Also, an extract of *P. incarnata* extract with flavonoids such as quercetin and kaempferol showed after 30 days of treatment a decrease in the levels of MDA at the liver level in mice that received a high-fat diet [42].

The above information leads us to conclude that *P. ligularis* treatments ameliorate oxidative stress in tissues such as the pancreas, liver, and kidney, which in turn can prevent the onset of complications such as nephropathy, which, as mentioned above, is related to ROS. This effect can be attributed to the presence of isoquercetin or astragalin, although their molecular mechanisms must be studied in depth in future research.

In relation to the results obtained in the lipid profile, is well known that defects in insulin action or hyperglycemia could be associated with changes in plasma lipid/lipoprotein metabolism in patients with diabetes [49]. Hypertriglyceridemia and reduced plasma high-density lipoprotein cholesterol are the most common lipid abnormalities in T2DM [50].

Previous reports have shown that different species of *Passiflora* generate changes in the serum lipid profile of rodents. *Passiflora incarnata* L. decreased the impact of a high-fat diet in insulin-resistant mice, reducing total cholesterol and triglycerides levels and increasing the concentration of high-density lipoproteins (HDL) [42]. Similar behavior was also reported for different extracts of *P. edulis* in diabetic rats, attributed to glycosyl flavonoids [51,52]. Improvements in the lipid profile have been demonstrated by *P. ligularis* in obese rats and is correlated with the decrease in hepatic steatosis [53]. The results of the present study are according to previous studies which demonstrated the antilipidemic activity of isoquercetin in a dependent dosage which attenuated triglycerides and cholesterol levels in diabetic mice [38]. Additionally, an extract with rich contents of astragalin has been shown to decrease cholesterol, triglycerides, LDL, and increase HDL in high-fat-induced and fructose-diet-induced diabetes in Wistar rats [43].

5. Conclusions

The results of this study suggest that the aqueous extract and the ethanolic fraction of *P. ligularis* leaves are promising as a complementary or adjuvant treatment for T2DM, since they are not only limited to controlling glucose levels in streptozotocin-induced diabetic mice, but also improve oxidative stress parameters in organs such as the kidney, pancreas, or liver, as well as improve the lipid profile by reducing levels of TG, TC, LDL-C, and increasing levels of HDL-C. Likewise, the oxidative stress parameters were improved, increasing the enzyme activity of SOD and CAT and decreasing the MDA values. It is important to highlight that this would be the first time that an extract from *P. ligularis* leaves has been determined to have a positive effect on several relevant outcomes in the control of T2DM. It is also important to keep in mind that the leaves of this species are generally discarded after the fruit has been grown, so they would also become a usable resource. For subsequent studies, it is recommended to design a formulation through which to administer the extract and carry out studies in humans.

Author Contributions: Conceptualization, M.A., L.F.O., D.P.R., I.H.V. and S.M.E.; methodology, D.P.R., I.H.V. and S.M.E.; formal analysis and data analysis, D.P.R., I.H.V., S.M.E. and I.A.R.; writing—original project, M.A. and F.R.M.B.S.; funding resources, M.A.; writing—original draft, D.P.R., S.M.E., I.H.V. and I.A.R.; writing—review and editing, M.A., L.F.O. and F.R.M.B.S. All authors have read and agreed to the published version of the manuscript.

Funding: This project was funded by the Facultad De Ciencias Sede Bogotá de la Universidad Nacional De Colombia, through the Resolución 1504 del 14 de agosto de 2020.

Institutional Review Board Statement: The bioassays were carried out following the Guide for the Care and Use of Laboratory Animals (1996, published by National Academy Press, 2101 Constitution Ave. NW, Washington, DC 20055, USA) and approved by the Ethics Committee of Universidad Nacional de Colombia (Act 04/2017 Faculty of Science, Faculty of Science, approval on 8 May 2017).

Informed Consent Statement: Not applicable.

Data Availability Statement: The original contributions presented in the study are included in the article, further inquiries can be directed to the corresponding author.

Acknowledgments: The authors D.P.R., I.H.V. and S.M.E. would like to thank COL CIENCIAS-Convocatoria 647/2014, and Programa de Becas de Excelencia doctoral del bicentenario cohorte I-2019, respectively. The ANLA and Ministerio de Ambiente y Desarrollo Sostenible granted permission to collect samples and perform this research ("BIOPROSPECCION DE ESPECIES DE SOLANUM, PASSIFLORA, PHYSALIS, HYPERICUM, CECROPIA E ILEX", código 38024, resolución 0699 de Abril 26 de 2018, Ministerio de Ambiente y Desarrollo Sostenible Otro Si No. 7 al contrato 121 del 22 de enero del 2016). FRMBS is a recipient of the CNPq fellowship #305799/2019-3.

Conflicts of Interest: The authors declare no conflicts of interest.

References

1. Khan, M.A.B.; Hashim, M.J.; King, J.K.; Govender, R.D.; Mustafa, H.; Al Kaabi, J. Epidemiology of Type 2 Diabetes—Global Burden of Disease and Forecasted Trends. *J. Epidemiol. Glob. Health* **2019**, *10*, 107. [CrossRef] [PubMed]
2. Kotwas, A.; Karakiewicz, B.; Zabielska, P.; Wieder-Huszla, S.; Jurczak, A. Epidemiological Factors for Type 2 Diabetes Mellitus: Evidence from the Global Burden of Disease. *Arch. Public Health* **2021**, *79*, 110. [CrossRef] [PubMed]

3. Galicia-Garcia, U.; Benito-Vicente, A.; Jebari, S.; Larrea-Sebal, A.; Siddiqi, H.; Uribe, K.B.; Ostolaza, H.; Martín, C. Pathophysiology of Type 2 Diabetes Mellitus. *Int. J. Mol. Sci.* **2020**, *21*, 6275. [CrossRef] [PubMed]
4. Sanches, J.M.; Zhao, L.N.; Salehi, A.; Wollheim, C.B.; Kaldis, P. Pathophysiology of Type 2 Diabetes and the Impact of Altered Metabolic Interorgan Crosstalk. *FEBS J.* **2023**, *290*, 620–648. [CrossRef] [PubMed]
5. Chaudhury, A.; Duvoor, C.; Reddy Dendi, V.S.; Kraleti, S.; Chada, A.; Ravilla, R.; Marco, A.; Shekhawat, N.S.; Montales, M.T.; Kuriakose, K.; et al. Clinical Review of Antidiabetic Drugs: Implications for Type 2 Diabetes Mellitus Management. *Front. Endocrinol.* **2017**, *8*, 6. [CrossRef] [PubMed]
6. Marín-Peñalver, J.J.; Martín-Timón, I.; Sevillano-Collantes, C.; del Cañizo-Gómez, F.J. Update on the Treatment of Type 2 Diabetes Mellitus. *World J. Diabetes* **2016**, *7*, 354. [CrossRef] [PubMed]
7. Surya, S.; Salam, A.D.; Tomy, D.V.; Carla, B.; Kumar, R.A.; Sunil, C. Diabetes Mellitus and Medicinal Plants-a Review. *Asian Pac. J. Trop. Dis.* **2014**, *4*, 337–347. [CrossRef]
8. Unuofin, J.O.; Lebelo, S.L. Antioxidant Effects and Mechanisms of Medicinal Plants and Their Bioactive Compounds for the Prevention and Treatment of Type 2 Diabetes: An Updated Review. *Oxid. Med. Cell Longev.* **2020**, *2020*, 1356893. [CrossRef] [PubMed]
9. Salehi, B.; Ata, A.; Kumar, N.V.A.; Sharopov, F.; Ramírez-Alarcón, K.; Ruiz-Ortega, A.; Ayatollahi, S.A.; Fokou, P.V.T.; Kobarfard, F.; Zakaria, Z.A.; et al. Antidiabetic Potential. of Medicinal Plants and Their Active Components. *Biomolecules* **2019**, *9*, 551. [CrossRef]
10. Salaj, N.; Kladar, N.; Srđenović Čonić, B.; Jeremić, K.; Hitl, M.; Gavarić, N.; Božin, B. Traditional Multi-Herbal Formula in Diabetes Therapy—Antihyperglycemic and Antioxidant Potential. *Arab. J. Chem.* **2021**, *14*, 103347. [CrossRef]
11. He, X.; Luan, F.; Yang, Y.; Wang, Z.; Zhao, Z.; Fang, J.; Wang, M.; Zuo, M.; Li, Y. Passiflora Edulis: An Insight Into Current Researches on Phytochemistry and Pharmacology. *Front. Pharmacol.* **2020**, *11*, 617. [CrossRef] [PubMed]
12. de Almeida, V.L.; Silva, C.G.; Campana, P.R.V. Flavonoids of Passiflora: Isolation, Structure Elucidation, and Biotechnological Application. *Stud. Nat. Prod. Chem.* **2021**, *71*, 263–310.
13. Miroddi, M.; Calapai, G.; Navarra, M.; Minciullo, P.L.; Gangemi, S. *Passiflora incarnata L.*: Ethnopharmacology, Clinical Application, Safety and Evaluation of Clinical Trials. *J. Ethnopharmacol.* **2013**, *150*, 791–804. [CrossRef]
14. Saravanan, S.; Parimelazhagan, T. In Vitro Antioxidant, Antimicrobial and Anti-Diabetic Properties of Polyphenols of Passiflora Ligularis Juss. Fruit Pulp. *Food Sci. Hum. Wellness* **2014**, *3*, 56–64. [CrossRef]
15. Aragón Novoa, D.M.; Ospina Giraldo, L.F.; Ramos Rodríguez, F.A.; Castellanos Hernández, L.; Costa Modesti, G.; Barreto Silva, F.R.M. *Passiflora Ligularis Juss. (Granadilla): Farmacológicos de Una Estudios Químicos y Planta Con Potencial Terapéutico*, 1st ed.; Aragón Novoa, D.M., Ed.; Universidad Nacional de Colombia—Sede Bogotá: Bogotá, Colombia, 2021; ISBN 9789587946420.
16. Sepúlveda, P.M.; Echeverrry, S.; Costa, G.; Aragón, M. Passiflora Ligularis Leaf Ultrasound-Assisted Extraction in the Optimization of Flavonoid Content and Enhancement of Hypoglycemic Activity. *J. Appl. Pharm. Sci.* **2020**, *10*, 086–094. [CrossRef]
17. Echeverry, S.M.; Rey, D.; Valderrama, I.H.; de Araujo, B.V.; Aragón, D.M. Development of a Self-Emulsifying Drug Delivery System (SEDDS) to Improve the Hypoglycemic Activity of Passiflora Ligularis Leaves Extract. *J. Drug Deliv. Sci. Technol.* **2021**, *64*, 102604. [CrossRef]
18. Kottaisamy, C.P.D.; Raj, D.S.; Prasanth Kumar, V.; Sankaran, U. Experimental Animal Models for Diabetes and Its Related Complications—A Review. *Lab. Anim. Res.* **2021**, *37*, 23. [CrossRef] [PubMed]
19. Rey, D.; Miranda Sulis, P.; Alves Fernandes, T.; Gonçalves, R.; Silva Frederico, M.J.; Costa, G.M.; Aragon, M.; Ospina, L.F.; Mena Barreto Silva, F.R. Astragalin Augments Basal Calcium Influx and Insulin Secretion in Rat Pancreatic Islets. *Cell Calcium* **2019**, *80*, 56–62. [CrossRef] [PubMed]
20. Rey, D.; Fernandes, T.A.; Sulis, P.M.; Gonçalves, R.; Sepúlveda, R.M.; Silva Frederico, M.J.; Aragon, M.; Ospina, L.F.; Costa, G.M.; Silva, F.R.M.B. Cellular Target of Isoquercetin from Passiflora Ligularis Juss for Glucose Uptake in Rat Soleus Muscle. *Chem. Biol. Interact.* **2020**, *330*, 109198. [CrossRef]
21. Al-Awar, A.; Kupai, K.; Veszelka, M.; Szucs, G.; Attieh, Z.; Murlasits, Z.; Török, S.; Pósa, A.; Varga, C. Experimental Diabetes Mellitus in Different Animal Models. *J. Diabetes Res.* **2016**, *2016*, 9051426. [CrossRef]
22. Dash, S.; Pattnaik, G.; Kar, B.; Sahoo, N.; Bhattacharya, S. An Approach towards Method Development to Investigate the Anti-Diabetic Activity on Experimental Animals. *Curr. Trends Biotechnol. Pharm.* **2021**, *15*, 330–348.
23. Saliu, T.P.; Kumrungsee, T.; Miyata, K.; Tominaga, H.; Yazawa, N.; Hashimoto, K.; Kamesawa, M.; Yanaka, N. Comparative Study on Molecular Mechanism of Diabetic Myopathy in Two Different Types of Streptozotocin-Induced Diabetic Models. *Life Sci.* **2022**, *288*, 120183. [CrossRef] [PubMed]
24. Guo, X.X.; Wang, Y.; Wang, K.; Ji, B.P.; Zhou, F. Stability of a Type 2 Diabetes Rat Model Induced by High-Fat Diet Feeding with Low-Dose Streptozotocin Injection. *J. Zhejiang Univ. Sci. B* **2018**, *19*, 559–569. [CrossRef] [PubMed]
25. Furman, B.L. Streptozotocin-Induced Diabetic Models in Mice and Rats. *Curr. Protoc. Pharmacol.* **2015**, *70*, 5–47. [CrossRef] [PubMed]
26. Janssen, B.J.A.; De Celle, T.; Debets, J.J.M.; Brouns, A.E.; Callahan, M.F.; Smith, T.L. Effects of Anesthetics on Systemic Hemodynamics in Mice. *Am. J. Physiol. Heart Circ. Physiol.* **2004**, *287*, 1618–1624. [CrossRef] [PubMed]
27. Echeverry, S.M.; Valderrama, I.H.; Costa, G.M.; Ospina-Giraldo, L.F.; Aragón, D.M. Development and Optimization of Microparticles Containing a Hypoglycemic Fraction of Calyces from Physalis Peruviana. *J. Appl. Pharm. Sci.* **2018**, *8*, 10–18. [CrossRef]

28. Abdelhameed, R.F.A.; Ibrahim, A.K.; Elfaky, M.A.; Habib, E.S.; Mahamed, M.I.; Mehanna, E.T.; Darwish, K.M.; Khodeer, D.M.; Ahmed, S.A.; Elhady, S.S. Antioxidant and Anti-Inflammatory Activity of *Cynanchum acutum* L. Isolated Flavonoids Using Experimentally Induced Type 2 Diabetes Mellitus: Biological and In Silico Investigation for NF-KB Pathway/MiR-146a Expression Modulation. *Antioxidants* **2021**, *10*, 1713. [CrossRef] [PubMed]
29. Kong, Y.; Ebrahimpour, P.; Liu, Y.; Yang, C.; Alonso, L.C. Pancreatic Islet Embedding for Paraffin Sections. *J. Vis. Exp.* **2018**, *2018*, 57931. [CrossRef] [PubMed]
30. Wickramasinghe, A.S.D.; Attanayake, A.P.; Kalansuriya, P. Biochemical Characterization of High Fat Diet Fed and Low Dose Streptozotocin Induced Diabetic Wistar Rat Model. *J. Pharmacol. Toxicol. Methods* **2022**, *113*, 107144. [CrossRef]
31. Hori, M. An Automatic Chromatographic Method for the Separation of Flavonoid Compounds. *Bull. Chem. Soc. Jpn.* **1969**, *42*, 2333–2336. [CrossRef]
32. Rosler, K.-H.; Goodwin, R.S. A General Use of Amberlite XAD-2 Resin for the Purification of Flavonoids from Aqueous Fractions. *J. Nat. Prod.* **1984**, *47*, 188. [CrossRef]
33. Queiroz, E.A.M.; Paim, R.T.T.; Lira, S.M.; da Silva, J.Y.G.; Lima, C.L.S.; Holanda, M.O.; Benjamin, S.R.; Vieira, Í.G.P.; Guedes, M.I.F. Antihyperglycemic Effect of Passiflora Glandulosa Cav. Fruit Rinds Flour in Streptozotocin-Induced Diabetic Mice. *Asian Pac. J. Trop. Med.* **2018**, *11*, 510–517. [CrossRef]
34. Andrikopoulos, S.; Blair, A.R.; DeLuca, N.; Fam, B.C.; Proietto, J. Evaluating the Glucose Tolerance Test in Mice. *Am. J. Physiol.-Endocrinol. Metab.* **2008**, *295*, E1323–E1332. [CrossRef] [PubMed]
35. Shanmugam, S.; Rajan, M.; de Souza Araújo, A.A.; Narain, N. Potential of Passion (Passiflora Spp.) Fruit in Control of Type II Diabetes. *Curr. Res. Diabetes Obes. J.* **2018**, *7*, CRDOJ.MS.ID.555712. [CrossRef]
36. Asir, P.J.; Hemmalakshmi, S.; Priyanga, S.; Devaki, K. Antidiabetic Activity of Aqueous and Ethanolic Extracts of *Passiflora foetida* L. in Alloxan Induced Diabetes Rats. *J. Pharm. Res.* **2014**, *3*, 1627–1641.
37. Meneses, C.; Monzón Daza, G.; Modesti Costa, G.; Aragón Novoa, M.; Ramos, R.F.; Castellanos Hernández, L. Evaluación de La Actividad Antiinflamatoria Del Extracto Acuoso, La Fracción Butanólica y Compuestos Identificados En Las Hojas de Passiflora Ligularis Juss. In *Passiflora Ligularis Juss. (Granadilla): Estudios Químicos y Farmacológicos de una Planta con Potencial Terapéutico*; Aragon, M., Ed.; Universidad Nacional de Colombia—Sede Bogotá: Bogotá, Colombia, 2021; pp. 41–54. ISBN 9789587946420.
38. Zhang, L.; Zhang, S.-T.; Yin, Y.-C.; Xing, S.; Li, W.-N.; Fu, X.-Q. Hypoglycemic Effect and Mechanism of Isoquercitrin as an Inhibitor of Dipeptidyl Peptidase-4 in Type 2 Diabetic Mice. *RSC Adv.* **2018**, *8*, 14967–14974. [CrossRef] [PubMed]
39. Satyanarayana, K.; Sravanthi, K.; Shaker, I.; Ponnulakshmi, R.; Selvaraj, J. Role of Chrysin on Expression of Insulin Signaling Molecules. *J. Ayurveda Integr. Med.* **2015**, *6*, 248. [CrossRef] [PubMed]
40. Antunes, L.C.; Elkfury, J.L.; Jornada, M.N.; Foletto, K.C.; Bertoluci, M.C. Validation of HOMA-IR in a Model of Insulin-Resistance Induced by a High-Fat Diet in Wistar Rats. *Arch. Endocrinol. Metab.* **2016**, *60*, 138–142. [CrossRef] [PubMed]
41. Duarte, I.d.A.E.; Milenkovic, D.; Borges, T.K.d.S.; Rosa, A.J.d.M.; Morand, C.; Oliveira, L.d.L.d.; Costa, A.M. Acute Effects of the Consumption of Passiflora Setacea Juice on Metabolic Risk Factors and Gene Expression Profile in Humans. *Nutrients* **2020**, *12*, 1104. [CrossRef]
42. Sarto, D.A.Q.S.; de Siqueira, A.H.D.; de Almeida Magalhaes, F.M.; de Paula Caproni, K.; Martins, Â.M.; Santos, G.B.; da Silva, D.B.; Boas, B.M.V.; Garcia, J.A.D. Dry Extract of *Passiflora incarnata* L. Leaves as A Cardiac And Hepatic Oxidative Stress Protector In Ldlr-/-Mice Fed High-Fat Diet. *Braz. Arch. Biol. Technol.* **2018**, *61*, e18180147. [CrossRef]
43. Huang, X.-L.; He, Y.; Ji, L.-L.; Wang, K.-Y.; Wang, Y.-L.; Chen, D.-F.; Geng, Y.; Ouyang, P.; Lai, W.-M. Hepatoprotective Potential of Isoquercitrin against Type 2 Diabetes-Induced Hepatic Injury in Rats. *Oncotarget* **2017**, *8*, 101545. [CrossRef] [PubMed]
44. Khlifi, R.; Dhaouefi, Z.; Toumia, I.B.; Lahmar, A.; Sioud, F.; Bouhajeb, R.; Bellalah, A.; Chekir-Ghedira, L. Erica Multiflora Extract Rich in Quercetin-3-O-Glucoside and Kaempferol-3-O-Glucoside Alleviates High Fat and Fructose Diet-Induced Fatty Liver Disease by Modulating Metabolic and Inflammatory Pathways in Wistar Rats. *J. Nutr. Biochem.* **2020**, *86*, 108490. [CrossRef] [PubMed]
45. Tajima, K.; Shirakawa, J.; Okuyama, T.; Kyohara, M.; Yamazaki, S.; Togashi, Y.; Terauchi, Y. Effects of Metformin on Compensatory Pancreatic β-Cell Hyperplasia in Mice Fed a High-Fat Diet. *Am. J. Physiol. Endocrinol. Metab.* **2017**, *313*, E367–E380. [CrossRef] [PubMed]
46. Tiwari, B.K.; Pandey, K.B.; Abidi, A.B.; Rizvi, S.I. Markers of Oxidative Stress during Diabetes Mellitus. *J. Biomark.* **2013**, *2013*, 378790. [CrossRef] [PubMed]
47. Samarghandian, S.; Azimi-Nezhad, M.; Farkhondeh, T. Catechin Treatment Ameliorates Diabetes and Its Complications in Streptozotocin-Induced Diabetic Rats. *Dose-Response* **2017**, *15*, 1559325817691158. [CrossRef] [PubMed]
48. Oldoni, T.L.C.; Merlin, N.; Bicas, T.C.; Prasniewski, A.; Carpes, S.T.; Ascari, J.; de Alencar, S.M.; Massarioli, A.P.; Bagatini, M.D.; Morales, R.; et al. Antihyperglycemic Activity of Crude Extract and Isolation of Phenolic Compounds with Antioxidant Activity from Moringa Oleifera Lam. Leaves Grown in Southern Brazil. *Food Res. Int.* **2021**, *141*, 110082. [CrossRef] [PubMed]
49. Goldberg, I.J. Clinical Review 124: Diabetic Dyslipidemia—Causes and Consequences. *J. Clin. Endocrinol. Metab.* **2001**, *86*, 965–971. [CrossRef] [PubMed]
50. O'Brien, T.; Nguyen, T.T.; Zimmerman, B.R. Hyperlipidemia and Diabetes Mellitus. *Mayo Clin. Proc.* **1998**, *73*, 969–976. [CrossRef]
51. Panchanathan, S.; Rajendran, J. Evidence of Anti-Hyperglycemic and Anti-Oxidant Effect of Passiflora Edulis Flavicarpa (Sims.) in Streptozotocin Induced Diabetic Rats. *Not. Sci. Biol.* **2015**, *7*, 383–389. [CrossRef]

52. Sunny, A.; Perumal, V.; Chandy, V. Leaves of Passiflora Edulis. *World J. Pharm. Res.* **2020**, *9*, 1513–1522.
53. Angel-Isaza, J.; Carmona-Hernandez, J.C.; González-Correa, C.H.; Narváez-Solarte, W.V. Potential Hypoglycemic and Antilipidemic Activity of Polyphenols from Passiflora Ligularis (Granadilla). *Molecules* **2023**, *28*, 3551. [CrossRef] [PubMed]

MDPI AG
Grosspeteranlage 5
4052 Basel
Switzerland
Tel.: +41 61 683 77 34

Nutrients Editorial Office
E-mail: nutrients@mdpi.com
www.mdpi.com/journal/nutrients

www.ingramcontent.com/pod-product-compliance
Lightning Source LLC
Chambersburg PA
CBHW061604210926
51850CB00009B/2207